CONSULTANT WRITERS

ADRIENNE ARDIGO, R.N., B.S.

Instructor, Department of Health Occupations and Nursing
Los Angeles Trade Technical Community College
Los Angeles, California

INICE CHIRCO, R.N., M.A., M.S.

Chairman, Allied Health Department
Rio Hondo College
Whittier, California

JANE M. KAHN, R.N., M.S.

Associate Director of Nursing
Hollywood Presbyterian Hospital
Los Angeles, California

BEVERLY J. RAMBO, R.N., M.A., M.N.

Instructor, Department of Health Sciences, Nursing Division
Grossmont Community College
El Cajon, California

BETTIE RICH, R.N., M.S.

Coordinator, Health Occupations Department
Mt. San Jacinto College
Gilman Hot Springs, California

FRANCES ROGOZEN, R.N., M.A.

Assistant Professor
Department of Health Occupations and Nursing
Los Angeles Trade Technical Community College
Los Angeles, California

Nursing Skills for Allied Health Services

Volume 2

Edited by LUCILE A. WOOD, R.N., M.S.

Formerly Associate Director for the Nursing Occupations
U.C.L.A. Allied Health Professions Project
Santa Monica, California

Presently Director of Nursing
Bay Area Hospital
Coos Bay, Oregon

W. B. SAUNDERS COMPANY
PHILADELPHIA · LONDON · TORONTO

W. B. Saunders Company, Publishers: West Washington Square
Philadelphia, Pa. 19105

12 Dyott Street
London, WC1A 1DB

833 Oxford Street
Toronto, Ontario M8Z 5T9, Canada

The project presented or reported herein was performed pursuant to a grant from the U.S. Office of Education, Department of Health, Education, and Welfare. The opinions expressed herein, however, do not necessarily reflect the position or the policy of the U.S. Office of Education, and no official endorsement by the U.S. Office of Education should be inferred.

Nursing Skills for Allied Health Services

VOLUME ONE — ISBN 0-7216-9600-7

VOLUME TWO — ISBN 0-7216-9601-5

Library of Congress catalog card number 79–186957

Printed by W. B. Saunders Company

Print No.:   9   8   7   6   5

To

Hi

and My Parents

ALLIED HEALTH PROFESSIONS PROJECTS NURSING NATIONAL TECHNICAL ADVISORY COMMITTEE

J. P. Myles Black, M.D.
Clinical Instructor, College of Medicine
University of Southern California
Los Angeles, California

Mary Bruton, R.N., M.S., Assistant Professor
St. Anselm's College
Manchester, New Hampshire

Terry Crowley, Educational Consultant
National Federation of Licensed Practical Nurses
New York, New York

Bernice Dixon, R.N., M.S., Director
School of Nursing, Grady Memorial Hospital
Atlanta, Georgia

Phyllis Drennan, R.N., M.S., Coordinator
Associate Degree Nursing Program
Kirkwood Community College
Cedar Rapids, Iowa
(Official Representative of the National League for Nursing)

Elizabeth J. Haglund
Regional Nursing Consultant for the Division of Nursing
Bureau of Health Professions Manpower Training
Department of Health, Education, and Welfare, Region IX
San Francisco, California

William F. Hartnett, R.N., M.S.
Assistant Administrator, Nursing Services
Riverside Methodist Hospital
Columbus, Ohio

Nannette Turner, L.V.N.
Past Executive Director
California Licensed Vocational Nurses Association
Los Angeles, California
(Official Representative of National Federation of Licensed Practical Nurses)

Captain Ouida Upchurch, Captain, NC, USN
Special Assistant for Education and Training R and D
Department of the Navy
Bureau of Medicine and Surgery
Washington, D.C.

George Wells, Associate Director
Health Insurance Council
Chicago, Illinois

Gerry White, R.N., M.S., Director

Allied Health Careers Institute
El Centro College of Dallas County
Dallas, Texas

Lucie Young, R.N., Ph.D., Chairman

Nursing Department of California State College, Los Angeles
Los Angeles, California
(Official Representative of the American Nurses Association)

NATIONAL ADVISORY COMMITTEE
ALLIED HEALTH
PROFESSIONS PROJECTS

FOREWORD

The Division of Vocational Education, University of California, is an administrative unit of the University concerned with responsibilities for research, teacher education, and public service in the broad area of vocational and technical education. During 1968 the Division entered into an agreement with the U.S. Office of Education to prepare curricula and instructional materials for a variety of allied health areas. For the most part such materials are related to instruction for programs ranging from on-the-job training through the Associate degree level. They also are adapted for use in adult and continuation education.

Because of the crucial staff shortages in the nursing occupations, the Allied Health Professions Projects undertook a national functional analysis of the activities of persons actually employed in health care facilities. This survey was designed to determine what skills were required by personnel employed in the several nursing occupations. The results of this survey have been incorporated into the present text, which covers the activities of entry-level personnel and comprises a comprehensive introduction to nursing. It also presents material which is adaptable to the training of other allied health personnel and seeks to provide a basic introduction to patient care services wherever they may be provided.

MELVIN L. BARLOW,
Director, Division of Vocational Education
University of California

Professor of Education, U.C.L.A.

Principal Investigator
Allied Health Professions Projects

PREFACE

Nursing, like all other health professions, has been undergoing monumental change since 1965, when major health legislation was begun at the federal and state levels of government.

In order to meet the growing health needs of our citizens, the nursing profession is taking some positive steps to make sure that care from competent and concerned health personnel is provided whenever and wherever the need arises.

As a Director of Nursing Service in a large suburban hospital, it was my responsibility and desire to employ nurses whose first concern was for people, and who were also skillful and knowledgeable when administering nursing care to patients. Nursing administrators generally agree that many graduates of recent nursing programs are not able to give such direct bedside care. Hence, when these new nurses are first employed, they face not only the frustrations of evolving from a student to a graduate nurse, but they must also simultaneously develop their clincial competence.

Therefore, when the opportunity presented itself to develop a nursing curriculum based on national occupational statistics for the U.C.L.A. Allied Health Professions Projects, I was eager to accept the challenge.

The Allied Health Professions Projects (AHPP) is a national curriculum research and development program funded in August 1968 as a four-year grant by the U.S. Office of Education. The core curriculum concept and career mobility patterns in allied health were two of its primary considerations.

The instructional materials in this textbook are built around the 184 activities designated in the AHPP national survey as those which are accomplished by all levels of nursing — N.A., L.P.N. (L.V.N.), and R.N. These activities were incorporated into the 36 instructional units which comprise this text.

Because AHPP was attempting something new in media methodology, the process of developing the materials was a difficult one. Initially, the activities defined in the national survey were outlined in a job breakdown (i.e., subdivided into a logical, orderly sequence which was designated as "Important Steps"). Then, each Important Step was supported by practical content under the heading "Key Points," giving related theory which clarified this step. This included factors that make or break the successful attainment of a skill, e.g., safety precautions; suggestions for making the step easier to do (special timing, handling, positioning, or sequencing); related biological concepts or principles of microbiology where applicable; communication and human relations skills required to assure successful completion of the activity; and pertinent ethical or legal concepts.

The sequence of units was established on the premise of progression from the general and simple to the more specific and complex subjects. It should be noted here that all nursing personnel, regardless of their final exit point on the nursing career ladder, should be well-grounded in the theory and practice of these basic nursing skills before moving on to more advanced responsibilities. Successful completion of this text should assure a competent practitioner who can interrupt the nursing educational process to work as a nursing assistant (entry-level practitioner). It should also provide a sound basis for moving on to the complex skills and theoretical knowledge required in the succeeding levels of nursing practice.

These materials represent an example of media methodology which, on the one hand, permits the student to move at his own rate of speed through the background information and procedural skills and, on the other hand, permits the instructor to be released from the need to repeat information to each incoming student. This allows the instructor additional time that can be spent more productively and creatively in the practice and clinical laboratories, assisting the students to polish their performance, expand their interests and comprehension, and to apply the knowledge and skills related to the care of their patients in the clinical assignments.

The materials are adaptable to a variety of teaching settings; they can be used for on-the-job training through the Associate degree in nursing as well as for adult education and staff development programs for nursing personnel and other allied health professionals who require these skills.

LUCILE A. WOOD

ACKNOWLEDGMENTS

I am deeply grateful to the many people who have assisted in the completion of this textbook:

The students and faculty members who have given many valuable suggestions at the following test sites: St. John's Hospital, Santa Monica, California, where the materials were utilized in nurse aide training programs; Santa Monica College, which used the materials in a community nurse aide program as well as in the beginning semester of its LVN program; the Secondary School Pilot and Demonstration Project of the U.C.L.A. Allied Health Professions Projects, which incorporated selected modules into its 10th grade curriculum; West Valley Community College, Saratoga, California, where the materials were utilized to upgrade employed nurse aides in local convalescent hospitals; Grossmont College in El Cajon, which incorporated the units into the beginning semester of its Associate degree RN program; The Center for Allied Health Careers at the Johns Hopkins Medical Institutions, Baltimore, Maryland, which tested the materials in its Family Health Team Curriculum; Charlotte Memorial Hospital, Charlotte, North Carolina, which tested them as a staff development program for nursing assistants; Central Piedmont Community College, Charlotte, North Carolina, which tested the units in its nursing assistant program as well as the beginning semester of its LPN program.

I would also like to thank the writer consultants and the members of the National Advisory Committees for Nursing and the AHPP Project, as well as individual members of the AHPP Staff who assisted in many aspects of the developmental phases. In particular, I would like to thank Melanie Herrick, my secretary, who efficiently fulfilled many demands throughout the numerous revisions. The Project administrators, Dr. Thomas Freeland, Dr. Katherine L. Goldsmith, and Dr. Miles Anderson, worked unstintingly to help me clarify my progress and goals at various critical junctures along the way. My grateful acknowledgment goes to Mrs. Seba Kolb, our staff editor, for her many hours spent deliberating over the drafts.

And finally, my thanks to Mr. Robert E. Wright, Nursing Editor for the W. B. Saunders Company, Publishers, for his enthusiasm, support, and practical suggestions given throughout the prepublishing phases.

L.A.W.

CONTENTS

Volume 1

Volume 2

Unit 21

URINE ELIMINATION

I. DIRECTIONS TO THE STUDENT

You are to proceed through the lesson using this workbook as your guide. You will need to practice the tasks using the different kinds of equipment with the mannequin (Mrs. Chase), with student partners in the skill laboratory, or with other persons. After you have completed the lesson and practiced the tasks, arrange with your instructor to take the post-test.

For this lesson you will need the following items.

1. This workbook.

2. A pen or pencil.

3. A bedpan.

4. A fracture pan.

5. A female urinal.

6. A male urinal.

7. Wash basin.

8. Wash cloth.

9. Towel.

10. Bedside stand.

11. Mannequin (Mrs. Chase).

12. Toilet tissue.

Please read the following paragraphs carefully. They will tell you what you will be expected to know, how you will be expected to assist the patient to use such equipment as a bedpan, female urinal, fracture pan, and male urinal. If you feel that you have the necessary skills and would be wasting your time studying this material, discuss this with your instructor. You would then arrange to take the post-test. All students are expected to demonstrate accurately the skill required in the post-test.

II. GENERAL PERFORMANCE OBJECTIVE

When you have finished this lesson, you will demonstrate your ability to assist the patient (or another person) to use the designated equipment to void in a safe and effective manner; to collect specific urine specimens; and to test urine for sugar and acetone content, using the prescribed procedure.

III. SPECIFIC PERFORMANCE OBJECTIVES

Upon completion of this lesson you will be able to:

1. Assist the patient to safely and modestly use the equipment to void so that the urine can be measured with 100 per cent accuracy.

2. Obtain a specified urine specimen (routine, clean catch, timed), correctly label and provide for immediate transfer of specimen to the laboratory for analysis, and record appropriate information on the patient's chart.

3. Record significant observations about the urinary output: amount, color, odor, time, etc.

4. Enter accurate intake and output measurements on the Intake and Output Record.

5. Remove, clean, dry, and return to storage the designated equipment used in urinary elimination and the testing of diabetic urine.

6. Provide opportunity for the patient to wash and dry his hands following elimination.

7. Obtain and test specimen of diabetic urine for sugar and acetone, and record appropriate information on the patient's record.

IV. VOCABULARY

Some of the words used in this lesson may be new and unfamiliar to you. You should go over the following list several times. When you see the word used in the lesson, refer back to this section unless you are sure of its meaning.

bedpan—the receptacle used by bed patients for urine and bowel elimination.
catamenia—the menses, the periodic menstrual discharge of blood from the uterus.
fracture pan—a specific type of shallow bedpan used by bed patients who have difficulty raising their hips to mount the pan.
frequency—to urinate often.
genital area—the area between the legs where the external excretory and reproductive organs are located.
incontinence—inability to retain feces or urine, lack of voluntary control over the sphincters.
micturition (urination, voiding)—the act by which urine is expelled.
organ—a group of tissues working together to carry on a particular function or work (i.e., the kidney, the bladder, etc.).
preservative—an agent having the power to preserve (to keep from decaying or spoiling).
rectum—distal portion of large intestine located between the sigmoid and the anal canal.
retention—failure to expel the urine from the bladder.
urgency—the immediate need to urinate.
vagina—mucomembranous tube which joins the passageway between the uterus and the external opening (vaginal—related to the vagina).
vulva—the external female genitalia.

V. INTRODUCTION

The urinary system plays a vital role in body excretion; it is one of the most important systems of elimination. Urination is normally accomplished without discomfort and is essential to the well-being of the patient. The amount of urine excreted depends on the amount of liquids ingested into the body, and on the environmental temperature. Burning and pain are symptoms which may be due to concentrated urine or to an infection in the urinary system. Adequate intake of liquids dilutes the toxins (poisons) in the body and aids in their elimination. The tasks and skills carried out by the health workers in this unit are directly related to urinary elimination. Organs in the urinary system will be mentioned only briefly in the enrichment assignment. You will thus acquire the basic information necessary to understand the importance of accurately and safely performing the tasks related to urinary elimination.

ITEM 1.   ASSISTING THE PATIENT TO USE THE BEDPAN

It is necessary for you to know what equipment is needed when the patient has to urinate. The following articles are described so that you will be able to assist the patient to use the appropriate equipment.

Bedpan. Bedpans are made of metal or plastic. Each patient has an individual bedpan stored in the bedside stand during his hospital stay.

Bedpan cover. Bedpan covers are made of cloth or paper, depending upon the agency in which you work. The cover is used to prevent offense from the unpleasant sight and odor of the pan's contents after is has been used.

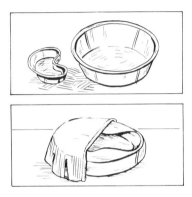

Toilet tissue. Toilet tissue is used either by the patient or you to clean and wipe the vulva and rectal areas.

The washcloth, towel, soap in its dish, and wash basin with warm water, should be available on the patient's bedside stand so that he is able to wash and dry his hands and genital area after using the bedpan.

Now that you know what equipment is needed for this lesson, read the following paragraphs carefully. Remember that perfecting your skills enables you to perform a particular task effectively and confidently and gives you an opportunity to listen thoughtfully to the patient's comments.

When you are assisting the patient to use the bedpan, explain the necessary steps that will be taken to make the task safe and easily accomplished.

Note: The female patient usually uses the bedpan for both urine and bowel elimination, whereas the male patient uses the bedpan for bowel elimination only.

Important Steps	Key Points
1. Wash your hands. 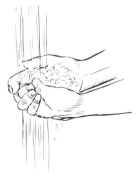	Before starting this task, wash your hands at a sink so that the patient can either see or hear the running water. If this is not possible, tell her that you will assist her as soon as you wash your hands. This will reassure her that you are concerned about her health and are doing everything possible to prevent cross-infection or contamination in your working relationship with the patients.

Important Steps	**Key Points**
2. Approach and identify the patient. Explain what you are going to do, and gain her cooperation and confidence.	Adjust the bed to a comfortable working height. This will prevent unnecessary back and leg strain while you are working. Assess the patient's condition. If she is unable to help, you may need to call for assistance.
3. Raise the siderail.	It should be up on the distal side to assure the patient's safety.
4. Obtain the bedpan, its cover, and toilet tissue.	Remove them from storage either in the bedside stand or the patient's bathroom. Since metal bedpans conduct heat and cold, rinsing the pan with warm water will heat the metal so that it will not be uncomfortably cold when the patient sits on it. Place the bedpan cover between the mattress and springs on the side of the bed nearest you so that you can easily obtain it later. Place the toilet tissue conveniently at the patient's side.

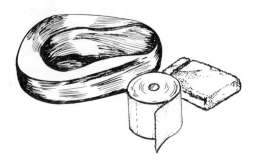

5. Position the patient on the bedpan.	Ask her to roll toward the distal side of the bed, where the siderail is up. While she is lying on her side, place the bedpan under her buttocks with the open, pouring side of the pan toward the foot of the bed. Have the patient return to the supine position and adjust the pan for her comfort and for normal body alignment. Elevate the head of the bed so that the patient is in a sitting position.

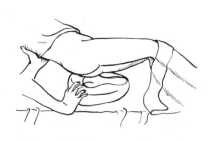

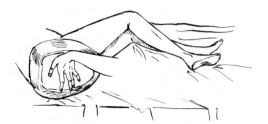

Important Steps	Key Points
6. A. Provide privacy for the patient.	Keep the patient covered with a bath blanket or a sheet to avoid exposure or embarrassment. If she is in a single room, close the door; if it is a room for two or more, pull the curtains around the bed.
B. Take safety precautions.	Pull up the siderail nearest you. Place the call signal within easy reach, and leave the bedside to give her privacy. NOTE: Sometimes patients attempt to get on the bedpan. This method is usually difficult both for the patient and the nursing helper because patients usually overestimate their strength. They are frequently so weak that they are unable to lift themselves high enough off the bed for adequate clearance to slip a bedpan under them easily or without assistance. *Do not attempt to lift the patient by this method.* You will risk hurting yourself and the patient. Encourage her to use the roll method. However, if she needs assistance in being placed on the bedpan, obtain *additional aid* from your co-workers.
7. Remove the bedpan.	Before removing the bedpan, lower the head of the bed.
8. Have patient roll to the distal side of the bed.	Hold the bedpan to avoid spilling its contents while she rolls to her side.
9. Wipe the genital area dry with toilet tissue.	Use a continuous stroke from the vulva across the vaginal opening to the rectum (anterior to posterior). This method of cleansing will help prevent rectal bacteria from contaminating or entering the vaginal opening or urinary tract.
10. Place the bedpan cover on the bedpan.	Empty the urine in the toilet. But before doing so, observe the following characteristics: color, sediment, amount, and any unusual material in the urine.
11. Wash the bedpan thoroughly.	Use a brush with a germicidal solution that is usually kept in the bathroom. Remember to return the cleaned equipment to its proper place.
12. Make the patient comfortable.	Give the wash cloth, towel, soap, and wash basin containing warm water to her so that she can wash, rinse, and dry her hands and genital area.
13. Provide safety and comfort for the patient.	Place the bedside stand and the call signal so that the patient can reach them without strain or discomfort. Adjust the bed to the low position, raise the siderails, and leave the patient in comfort.
14. Obtain the chart.	Record accurately all significant observations made of the urine.

ITEM 2.   ASSISTING THE PATIENT TO USE THE FEMALE URINAL

The female urinal is a plastic bottle with a long, wide, spout-like top; it has a handle, a rectangle base along the side, and a flat round base at the bottom. It is used by the female patient when she is unable to use other equipment to void.

The preliminary and concluding steps in this task are the same as those in the foregoing item, Steps 1 through 4.

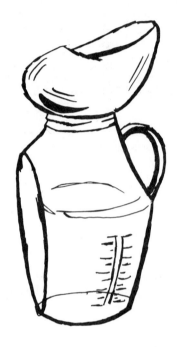

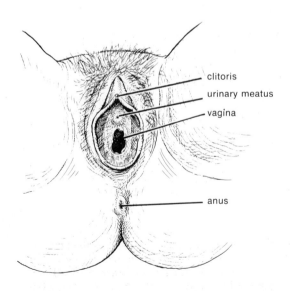

clitoris

urinary meatus

vagina

anus

External Female Genito-urinary Organs

5. *Position the patient to use the female urinal.* The patient's position will depend on the amount of physical movement and activity that she is permitted to make.

A. If she is able to stand at the bedside, ask her to stand with her legs apart and bent slightly at the knees. Either you or the patient should hold the urinal in place between her legs. The spout side should be pointing toward the patient's rectum. The handle should be toward the front of the patient. The opening of the urinal should be in direct contact with the genital area. The extent of body contact with the urinal opening should reach from the rectum to the vagina.

B. If the patient is permitted to be in a sitting position, elevate the head of the bed and place two pillows under her buttocks so that she is sitting on the spout of the urinal edge; this will help prevent spilling the contents of the urinal.

If she is permitted to sit on the edge of the bed (dangle position), she will be able to use the urinal without discomfort or difficulty. If this position is used, remember that you must utilize all known safety skills, particularly locking the wheels of the bed.

C. When the patient must remain flat in bed, yet is permitted to roll from side to side, the urinal can be used. Place it between the patient's legs using the technique described at the beginning of this lesson. Remember that it is necessary to keep the urinal in direct body contact with the patient (skin to urinal) so that the urine does not leak out.

6. *When she is finished, permit her to wipe the genital area dry.* Place wash basin, soap, towel, and washcloth within her reach so that she can wash herself.

7. *Empty, wash and return the equipment to its proper place.*

8. Record all significant observations relating to urine.

Note: Utilize every means available to help the patient maintain her sense of modesty.

ITEM 3.   *ASSISTING THE PATIENT TO USE THE FRACTURE PAN*

The fracture pan is used when female patients are unable to sit on a regular-size bedpan. The fracture pan is made of metal or plastic. It is smaller in surface area and height than the regular bedpan. The back part of the pan is approximately 2½ inches high with a wide strip of metal across the top so that the patient is able to sit comfortably. The front, pouring side is high enough to prevent urine from being splashed or spilled in the bed.

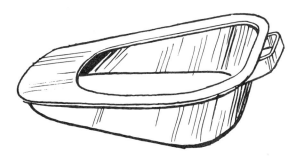

1. Wash your hands.

2. Approach the patient.

3. Obtain the equipment.

4. Position the siderails.

5. Position the patient on the fracture pan.

Expose the patient just enough so that you can see what you are doing. Have her sit with her knees in a flexed, upright squatting position. Separate her legs so that the pan can be placed between them and slipped under her buttocks. This method is to be used if the patient is able to assist you. If she is unable to do so, use the roll-to-the-side method.

6. Place the call signal within easy reach, raise the siderails, and leave the room to insure privacy.

7. Remove the fracture pan.

Use the same technique as for putting the patient on the fracture pan while she was in the sitting position, with one exception: reverse the initial motion. In other words, pull the pan out from under the buttocks.

8. Dry the genital area, cover the fracture pan, and then empty the pan.

If the roll method is used, refer to this step in Item 1. Utilize the concluding steps in Item 1 for completion of this task.

9. Wash the fracture pan.

10. Make the patient comfortable.

ITEM 4. ASSISTING THE PATIENT TO USE THE MALE URINAL

The male urinal is a plastic or metal bottle with a long, round neck, a handle, a rectangular base along one side, and a flat base at the bottom.

The urinal is used by male patients who are limited in physical activity by their illness or injury.

The preliminary and concluding steps used in this task are the same as those learned in Item 1, "Assisting the Patient to Use the Bedpan." There is one exception to be noted: the use of toilet tissue is omitted. It is not customary for the male patient to use toilet tissue when he urinates since the urine is expelled in a straight single stream and the skin surface of the penis does not get wet.

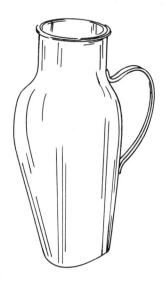

1. Wash your hands.

2. Approach the patient.

3. Obtain the necessary equipment.

4. Position the patient to use the male urinal.

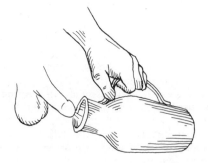

The male patient is able to use the urinal when he is in any one of four positions: lying supine (on back), lying on either the right or left side, in a Fowler's position, or standing at the bedside.

Without Assistance. Give the urinal to the patient so that he can utilize the equipment without assistance. Place the bedpan cover between the mattress and springs of the bed, to be accessible when you carry the bedpan and empty it in the toilet.

With Assistance. If the patient is unable to place the urinal in the proper position to urinate, you will do this for him.

Expose the patient just enough so that you can see what you are doing. Separate the patient's legs so there is enough space to permit the urinal to be placed between them without causing pain or discomfort. Hold the urinal with one hand and with your other hand place his penis into the urinal, far enough that it does not slip out when the patient begins to urinate. Hold the urinal in place if the patient is unable to maintain a supporting position with his legs.

The most important aspect of this task is to remember that this is an embarrassing situation for the patient. The task is to be performed in a skillful, matter-of-fact manner, and every effort made to keep the patient covered with the bath blanket or sheet.

5. If the patient can keep the urinal in place unassisted, put the call signal within easy reach, raise the siderails, and leave the room to insure privacy.

6. Remove the urinal, empty, wash, and store the equipment in its proper place.

Refer to the concluding techniques and steps used in Item 1.

Note: Often the patient will avoid asking the female health worker to assist him with the urinal. He will ask that it be placed on the bedside stand or overbed table and will say that he does not want to bother anyone because "They are always so busy." The true reason is that he is embarrassed to ask for assistance. Therefore, it will be necessary for you to expect and accept this emotional factor and carry out the task in a manner which indicates that you know and understand his feelings and will do everything possible to help him overcome or minimize them.

ITEM 5. ASSISTING THE PATIENT TO THE BATHROOM

The methods to be used for safety in assisting the patient to the bathroom depend on the degree of physical activity ordered by the physician.

1. Wash your hands.

2. Obtain the patient's robe and shoes from closet or bedside stand.

3. Approach and identify the patient.

4. Adjust the bed to low position and lower the siderail nearest you.

5. Position the patient and assist him to the bathroom.

Ask the patient to turn so that he is sitting on the side of the bed nearest you. Help him put on his shoes and robe while he is in this position.

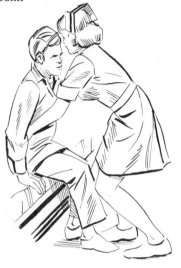

6. Have patient stand and then lean on you for the necessary support while walking to the bathroom.

If the patient is using a walker or a pair of crutches to aid him in ambulation, refer to the unit on Mechanical Aids for Ambulation and Movement.

7. Help the patient to sit down on the toilet.

When he is seated comfortably, remind him *not to flush the toilet.* Explain that you will do so later after you see the results so that accurate observations can be recorded. Close the bathroom door to insure privacy. If there is a lock on the door, remind him not to lock it. In the event anything happens to the patient, you will need to help immediately, and of course a locked door would prevent this.

8. Remain within immediate hearing distance of the bathroom.

Never leave the patient unattended.

9. When the patient is finished, have him wash his hands.

Turn the water on and adjust the temperature so that the patient does not burn himself.

10. Assist the patient to return to bed.

Use the same method to help the patient return to bed as in assisting him to the bathroom.

11. Leave the patient safe and comfortable in bed.

12. Return to the bathroom to clean it up.

ITEM 6. METHODS OF COLLECTING SPECIMENS FOR DIAGNOSTIC TESTS

A. Routine Urines

You have learned how to assist the patient, using designated equipment for urination, and now it is necessary for you to learn about tests of urine that are used by physicians to help in making an accurate diagnosis. This part of the lesson will be concerned with obtaining the urine specimen from the patient so the tests can be accomplished.

The first task to be learned is the collection of a routine specimen:

1. Wash your hands.

2. Obtain the equipment. Bedpan, or urinal, specimen container, specimen label, and laboratory requisition slip.
   Note: Specimen containers may vary. Some are disposable.

3. Approach and identify the patient.

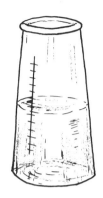

4. Obtain the urine specimen.

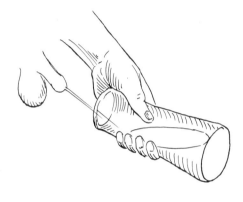

Ask the patient to void into a bedpan or urinal. Refer to the steps in Items 1, 2, 3 and 4. If the patient is ambulatory and has orders that permit him to go to the bathroom, ask him to do so. If possible, the patient may prefer to void directly into the urine specimen container. The male patient will be able to do this without contaminating the container since he usually voids in a standing position, excreting the urine in a straight single stream. He can thus easily hold the specimen container in front of him and, as he voids, "catch" the urine in the container.

The female patient will be able to void directly into the urine specimen container if she is able to stand in a squatting position over the toilet bowl; while she is in the process of voiding, she can hold the urine specimen container underneath the genital area to catch the urine.

5. After voiding is finished, put the lid on the container tightly.

6. Clean and dry the outside of the container.

If any urine has contaminated the outside of the specimen container, take it to the sink in the bathroom and rinse the outside of the container under running water. Dry it with a paper towel and then discard the towel in the wastebasket.

7. The patient will wash her hands at the sink in the bathroom.

8. Measure the urine.

If the patient voids in the bedpan or urinal, pour the urine into a measuring pitcher (commonly called a graduate) and note the amount. Pour at least 4 ounces into the specimen container. If the patient voids directly into the container, you will be able to measure and record only the amount in the container, not the total amount of urine that was voided.

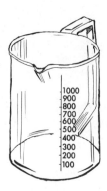

9. Wash the equipment and return it to the proper storage place.

Refer to this step in Item 1.

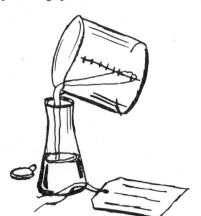

10. Return the patient to bed and provide for his safety and comfort.

11. Remove the container of urine from the patient's room.

12. Label the container with the patient's name and room number.

Use the addressograph plate (similar to a charge plate in a department store) to print the patient's name and hospital number of the laboratory requisition and charge voucher. Enter the type of test that is ordered so that the laboratory technician will know what test to perform.

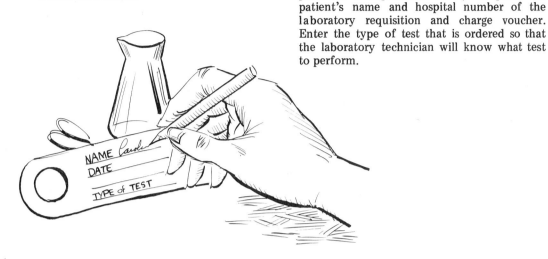

13. Take specimen to laboratory immediately. Urine specimens very quickly deteriorate while standing at room temperature. The chemical composition of the urine changes rapidly if kept at room temperature for more than 15 minutes. Should the urine specimen be left on the nursing unit for a longer period of time, the laboratory would obtain incorrect readings. The laboratory results provide the basis upon which physicians frequently order their treatment and medication. Thus, an incorrect laboratory report, due to delay in delivery of the specimen, could cause an incorrect diagnosis and medication for your patient.

Note: Occasionally all urine specimens are strained to catch stones from the kidney or bladder which may be discharged through the urine.

The most common method to strain the urine is to place a fine gauze 4 × 4 dressing over the spout of the graduate (some agencies may use a special sieve). Pour the urine carefully into the graduate; all stones will be caught in the fine mesh gauze. (Discard gauze after use—take clean gauze for each straining.)

14. Obtain the patient's chart.

Accurately record all pertinent information concerning this task in the nurse's notes.

Record time, amount, color, odor, any unusual characteristic, and disposition of specimen to the laboratory.

Charting example:

6:15 P.M. Urine specimen with requisition and voucher sent to laboratory. Specimen appeared cloudy and slightly pink. No complaints of pain on voiding. Catamenia present.

J. Jones, SN

B. Mid-Stream or Clean-Catch Urine Specimen.

This procedure, occasionally done in place of the routine urine specimen, can be obtained as free from contamination as possible without having to catheterize the patient. It is often used when the urine specimen is to be collected for culture and sensitivity.

Important Steps	Key Points
1. Assemble supplies.	Obtain from Central Supply: sterile urine specimen bottle, cleaning agent, water, and cotton balls.
2. Wash your hands, approach the patient, and explain what you will be doing.	Identify the patient with her identification band. You need the cooperation of the patient. Although this procedure is usually done in private, you may need to provide the patient with some assistance.
3. Drape the patient.	Use the bath blanket to drape over legs.
4. Cleanse vulva.	Expose urinary meatus. (Spread vulva open using the index finger and thumb of left hand.) Moisten cotton ball in cleaning agent (usually a liquid soap). Cleanse area with one wipe from pubis to anus. Discard cotton ball. Repeat cleansing (with approximately 4 cotton balls until area around urinary meatus is free of secretions. Rinse with water. Dry area with remaining cotton balls.
5. Assist patient to bathroom.	Ask patient to void and discard first voiding into toilet.
6. Ask patient to interrupt the stream of urine.	Collect remaining urine specimen in the sterile jar by having patient void directly into the jar.
7. Take specimen bottle from patient.	Have patient dry herself. Wash your hands. Close specimen bottle with cap. Wipe outside of bottle. Clean and dry with paper towel and discard paper towel in waste basket.
8. Assist patient back to bed.	
9. Label specimen with patient's name, room number, and other identifying information used by your agency.	
10. Make arrangements for labeled specimen with requisition and charge vouchers to go immediately to the laboratory.	Remember the change in chemical composition that occurs when urine is left standing.
11. Return to patient's room	Make patient comfortable. Adjust bed and side-rails. Leave signal light and bedside stand close by. Tidy the room. Tell the patient when you expect to return.
12. Clean the bathroom area.	See that soiled supplies have been properly discarded and unused supplies returned to the proper storage place. Leave area clean, neat, and dry. Remember, germs grow in dark, damp, soiled areas.

Important Steps	Key Points

13. Record on patient's chart.

Charting example:
2:30 P.M. Clean catch urine specimen obtained. Sent to laboratory with requisition and charge vouchers for culture and sensitivity.

J. Jones, SN

C. 24-Hour Urine Collection

A number of urine tests require a collection of urine for 24 hours. The most important aspect of this task is that the urine collection must be 100 per cent accurate (i.e., every drop of urine must be kept). The laboratory analysis is done to determine the amount of a specified chemical which is excreted through the urine in 24-hour period. It is the responsibility of all health workers to perform this task skillfully and without error.

1. Obtain the equipment.

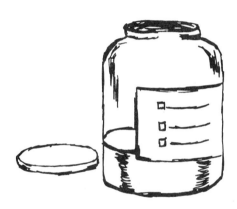

You will need one-gallon jugs obtained either from Central Service or the general laboratory (check your agency procedure). The gallon jug is used because it will usually hold the total amount of urine that is voided by the patient over a 24-hour period. *Note:* If the amount voided over the 24-hour period is more than the gallon jug will hold, add another properly marked jug to the collection. You will put labels on the jug(s) with the patient's name, date and time that the collection was started, and the date and time the collection ended. You will need the designated equipment for the patient to use for voiding, as well as a graduated measuring cup to measure each voided specimen.

Caution: One of the preservatives used in the collection jar, hydrochloric acid, is *very caustic* (capable of burning). If you should accidentally spill some of the solution, wash vigorously with running water and report immediately to your charge nurse.

Most special urine specimens will be collected in containers which have at least one strong preservative; therefore, take great care for yourself and your patient when handling these items.

2. Identify and approach the patient.

Give a detailed explanation to the patient concerning this task. Stress the importance of collecting the urine accurately. The 24-hour urine specimen is collected for a variety of reasons: to check total volume of output in a 24-hour period; to detect certain renal (kidney) diseases; and to detect certain cardiac (heart) conditions. Check with your team leader to find out why your patient is to have a 24-hour urine collection. When you believe the patient understands, proceed with the task.

3. Take the equipment to the patient's room.

Label the jug(s) with the patient's name and room number. Write the time and date the collection is to be started, and the time and date it is to be finished. Place the jug(s) in the patient's bathroom.

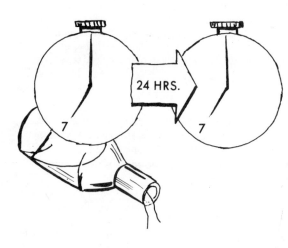

After you have put the equipment in the designated area, make a couple of signs (6 × 8 cards will do) stating that a 24-hour urine collection is in progress. Tape one at the head of the patient's bed and one at the foot of the bed. (Labels may also be inserted in the Hollister Bed Signs. Check with your agency for its procedure.) When the patient voids, ask him to remind the health worker to save the urine and place it in the appropriately marked jug.

Some tests require that the urine be kept cold over the 24-hour collection period. If the urine is to be kept cold, place the labeled jug(s) in the refrigerator used for specimen collections. If there is no refrigerator on the unit for this purpose, place the jug(s) in a pan of ice in the patient's bathroom. You will have to add ice to the pan as it melts over the 24-hour period. Remember to empty the water from the melted ice so there is room in the pan for ice to be added.

4. Begin the urine collection.

Approximately five minutes before the starting time of the collection, ask the patient to void in the designated equipment. Discard this urine specimen into the toilet. Now you begin the collection. *Every voided urine specimen* should be measured and poured into the appropriately marked gallon jug.

5. Have the patient void approximately five minutes before the end of the last hour of the collection.

Add this specimen to the collection.

6. Send the marked gallon jug(s) with the appropriately marked requisition slip and charge vouchers immediately to the laboratory.

Send the specimens to the laboratory immediately by messenger service, dumbwaiter, or staff. Remember the chemical disintegration which can quickly take place when urine specimens are left at room temperature for long periods of time.

7. Tell the patient when the collection is completed and remove all written notations and equipment from the patient's room and bathroom.

8. Obtain the patient's chart.

Record the starting time and date, and ending time and date of the collection in the nurse's notes. Include in the nurses' notes the measured amount of each voiding with a notation that it was part of the collection. The last notation in the nurses' notes will be the time the collected specimen was sent to the laboratory. *Remember, the test is useless if any of the urine specimens are discarded.* If this should occur, notify the charge nurse and she will notify the physician. The physician will have to decide if the collection is to be restarted. An incomplete collection could add another day to the patient's hospital stay. This is costly to the patient, and therefore it is vital that the task be performed accurately and completely during the first collection period.

Charting example:
3/4/71 7:30 A.M. 24-hour urine specimen collection initiated.   J. Jones, SN
3/5/71 7:30 A.M. 24-hour urine specimen collection completed. Sent immediately to
lab. with requisition and charge vouchers.
J. Jones, SN

D. Timed Urine Collection

In this lesson you will learn to obtain a timed urine collection. This procedure is determined by the kind of test to be done and the reason the physician is asking that it be done. The physician will determine the fluid intake, the time, and number of specimens that are required to complete the test. (Some laboratory procedure manuals give the specific procedures for collection of timed urine specimens. Check your agency's Laboratory Procedure Manual.)

1. Obtain the equipment.

Obtain the number of urine specimen bottles that will be required from Central Service or the general laboratory. Label each bottle with patient's name and room number and the date and time of each voiding. Wash your hands.

Note: If some of the specimen collection bottles contain preservatives, remember to use *extreme caution* to avoid spilling any on you or your patients. If the solution does spill, rinse area vigorously with running water and report at once to your charge nurse.

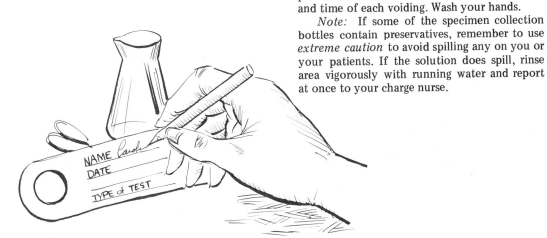

2. Identify and approach the patient.

Check the patient's identification. Call him by name. Give a detailed explanation to the patient concerning this task. Stress the importance of collecting the urine accurately. Timed urine specimens may be collected to aid in the diagnoses of a variety of diseases. Although the doctor has probably told his patient the reason for the test, you should ask your team leader why the test is being ordered. Timed urine tests are done to determine or confirm some renal and cardiac diseases. When you think the patient understands, proceed with the task.

3. Begin the collection.

Place the labeled bottles in the patient's bathroom. Ask the patient to void. Pour this specimen in the bottle labeled for the appropriate time. The labels may also be numbered in sequence, e.g., 1st specimen, 2nd specimen, 3rd specimen.

4. Liquid intake required.

Ask the patient to drink the kind and amount of liquid the physician has requested for the specimen: water is taken at stated intervals to determine the volume and concentration of the urine; glucose solution is taken to determine if the patient is a diabetic.

5. Instruct the patient to void at the specified times designated by the physician or laboratory procedures.

6. Measure every voided specimen and pour each specimen into the properly marked bottle.

7. Place 6 X 8 cards in easily observed places in the patient's room stating that the collection is in progress.

8. Tell the patient when the collection is completed, and remove all written notations and equipment from the patient's room and bathroom.

9. Take the specimens with requisition and charge vouchers to the laboratory for testing and evaluation.

Refer to this step in Item 6-C.

10. Obtain the patient's chart.

Record the time, amount, and each voided specimen in the nurse's notes. State that it was a timed urine collection. The last notation will tell where the specimens were sent.

Note: Remember, the collection will be useless if the time of each voiding is not accurate. If an error is made, notify the charge nurse. She will notify the physician, who will decide the proper course to take, i.e., whether to start the specimen collection over. This could mean an added day of hospitalization for the patient, which is costly. Remember, specimen collections are extremely important in determining the medical plan of care. *Extreme accuracy and attention to detail are mandatory.*

ITEM 7.   COMMON TESTS FOR SUGAR AND ACETONE CONTENT IN THE URINE

Patients with diabetes mellitus (commonly called diabetes or sugar diabetes) have difficulties burning (or using) the sugars in food. Sugar is used by the body for energy. Insulin is a normal hormone produced by endocrine cells called the islets of Langerhans, located in the pancreas. This hormone assists in the oxidizing (burning) of sugars in the blood and thereby maintains the normal limits of blood sugar. However, in the diabetic patient there is less insulin, or none at all, manufactured by the body to aid in the process of burning sugars. A medication (insulin administered by hypodermic or an oral synthetic insulin) is therefore given to the patient to assist him in using the sugars from foods.

To determine how much medication is needed, the doctor will order certain doses dependent on the amount of sugar which is excreted in the urine. The simple urine test for sugar content is called Clinitest. It is done four times a day (q.i.d.), usually before meals and before bedtime. The testing may be done more frequently if the patient's condition warrants it. Depending on the accurate reading of the urine test, a prescribed amount of insulin will be given.

A. *Clinitest Test*

A Clinitest set which includes Clinitest tablets, test tube, eyedropper, and color chart will be ordered for each diabetic patient. These items usually are kept in the patient's bathroom.

Important Steps	Key Points
1. Wash your hands. Approach and identify the patient.	Explain what you are going to do. Part of the Diabetic Teaching Program may be to teach him how to perform this simple test. Therefore, it is extremely important that you understand the procedure completely.
2. Obtain a urine specimen from the patient.	Have the patient void into a clean urinal or bedpan. *Note:* A urine specimen can be obtained for testing diabetic urine from the Foley catheter by disconnecting the catheter at the drainage tube site and allowing some urine to run into a graduate. Care must be taken to keep the specimen clean. Reconnect catheter to drainage tube.
3. Take the specimen to the utility area (or patient's bathroom).	Assemble the test tube, Clinitest tablet, and eyedropper on the table surface near running water.
4. Hold the test tube in your left hand and add 5 drops of urine to the test tube. 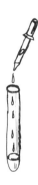	Hold the test tube between the thumb and forefinger of your left hand about one-fourth inch from the top of the tube. With your right hand, use the eyedropper to draw up 5 drops of urine from the bedpan or urinal. Extreme accuracy is necessary. Drop the urine into the center of the test tube; do not let it drop along the sides of the tube. You are working with a very small amount of solution.
5. Turn on the water faucet and rinse the eyedropper in running water.	Then draw up 10 drops of water and add to the urine in the test tube. Again, drop freely into the center of the test tube. All 15 drops (urine and water) must combine for this test. *Extreme accuracy* is essential.
6. Gently rotate the test tube.	Rotate it between your left forefinger and thumb to mix the urine and water thoroughly. (Reverse hands if you are left-handed.)
7. Remove one Clinitest tablet from the bottle and drop it into the test tube.	Be careful not to use tablets which are moist or have changed color. If so, they will not react correctly with the solution to give you an

Important Steps	Key Points

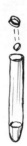

accurate reading. Good tablets are lightly spotted and bluish-white in color. If a tablet differs from this, do not use it; order a new supply. Handle the tablets cautiously because they contain a caustic soda and may irritate your skin.

Continue to hold the test tube *near the top.* The dissolving tablet causes a boiling reaction and the test tube becomes hot. If you hold the bottom of the test tube, you might drop it when it becomes hot. *Do not rotate* the test tube during this step.

WARNING: If Clinitest tablets are mistakenly swallowed, they may cause severe burns of the esophageal tissues. Call a doctor at once. *Do not* have the patient vomit.

8. Compare the color of the specimen in the test tube with the color chart.

After 15 seconds (or after boiling stops), shake tube gently and compare with Clinitest Color Chart.

9. Wash, rinse, and dry equipment.

Return the bedpan or urinal to storage space. Close Clinitest bottle tightly, wipe up spills, and tidy work area.

10. Record readings on patient's chart.

Record color reaction. Usual color designations are:

Negative—the fluid will be blue, indicating no sugar present.

Positive— the fluid changes in color from dark green to orange; check the color change in the test tube with the block on the color chart indicating the degree of sugar content: trace, 1+, 2+, 3+, and 4+.

The dosage of insulin is based on the amount of sugar in the urine. The higher the sugar content, the more insulin will be given. Therefore, report the results of the test immediately to your team leader so she can give the insulin. Diabetic patients are usually taught to carry out this procedure themselves.

B. Tes-Tape Test

Another method for testing the content of sugar in the urine is with the use of Tes-Tape. As in the preceeding item, you will be testing the urine at least q.i.d. (or oftener if the condition so indicates).

Important Steps	Key Points

1. Wash your hands. Approach and identify the patient.

Explain what you are going to do. It may be part of a Diabetic Patient Teaching Program.

2. Obtain a urine specimen from the patient.

Have him void into a clean bedpan or urinal.

3. Take the specimen to the patient's bathroom or utility room.

Assemble the Tes-Tape and specimen on a counter top for convenient working.

Important Steps	Key Points
4. Withdraw 1½ inches of Tes-Tape from its dispenser.	This is similar to a Scotch tape dispenser. (Do not use if the tape has turned brown.) On the outside of the dispenser there is printed a color code with percentages indicated for each color.

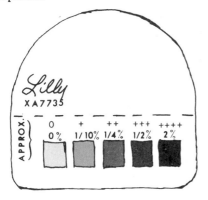

5. Tear off the piece of tape.	Holding it between your forefinger and thumb, pull the tape up against the cutting edge on the dispenser and cut it free.

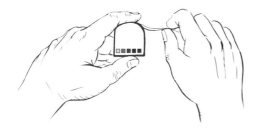

6. Dip the distal end of the tape into the urine specimen.	Then remove the tape immediately from the urine. However, be sure it has been moistened uniformly throughout the tape. (Keep your fingers dry.)

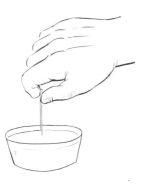

7. Wait one minute.

8. Compare the tape with the color chart on the exterior of the dispenser.	Match the tape with the darkest square of color shown on the dispenser. If the tape indicates ½ per cent or higher, wait one additional minute for final comparison.

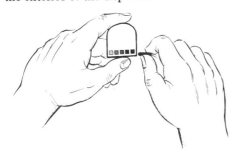

Important Steps	Key Points
9. Wash, rinse, and dry equipment.	
10. Record the readings on patient's chart.	Record the color reaction, coded as follows: Yellow — zero per cent (or sugar-free). Varying shades of green range from light to dark green — they indicate: 1+ (1/10 per cent); 2+ (1/4 per cent); 3+ (1/2 per cent); and 4+ (2 per cent or more). Again the dosage of insulin given is dependent on the amount of sugar in the urine. Report the results immediately to your team leader so that she can give the prescribed dose of insulin.

C. Test for Ketone Bodies (Acetone) in the Urine

Another commonly performed urine test is the one for ketone bodies (acetone) in the urine. The test can also be used on blood to determine the amount of acetone in the blood. This test is used as an indicator for specific treatment of patients with diabetes, and for unconscious patients to determine whether the coma is due to ketosis, hypoglycemia (low blood-sugar), stroke, or other disorders. The *Acetest tablet* is used for this test.

Important Steps	Key Points
1. Wash your hands. Approach and identify the patient.	You may be teaching the patient how to do this test himself as a part of the Diabetic Teaching Program. Follow your agency procedure for this.
2. Obtain a urine specimen from the patient.	Ask him to void into a clean bedpan or urinal.
3. Take the specimen to the work area.	This may be in the patient's bathroom or in the utility room. Assemble the bottle of Acetest tablets and an eyedropper on a flat work surface near the bedpan or urinal.
4. Place a clean paper towel on the work surface.	
5. Place one Acetest tablet on the paper.	Draw urine up in the eyedropper. Drop *one* drop of urine on the tablet.
6. Wait 30 seconds.	Compare the color of the tablet with the color chart on the bottle. Reactions can be negative or positive. If the color of the tablet remains unchanged or becomes a cream color, it is considered to be a *negative reaction*. If the tablet turns from a lavender to a deep purple, it is considered a *positive reaction*. It is recorded as slightly, moderately, or strongly positive.
7. Record and report.	Report the results to your team leader and record this information on the patient's chart.
8. Wash, rinse, and dry equipment.	Return it to the storage area. Check to be sure the cap is secured tightly on the Acetest bottle. Be sure to wipe up spills in the work area. Leave the work area neat and tidy.

Important Steps	Key Points

9. Record the readings on the patient's chart.	Record color reaction and report them to your team leader so that she can take the appropriate action.
	    The color reaction is as follows:
	Negative: buff color
	Positive: slightly — lavender
	        moderately — dark lavender
	        strongly — purple

D. Ketostix Test

Another frequently used method to determine the amount of acetone (or keytones) in the urine is the Ketostix. It can also be used to determine the amount of ketones in blood. The specially treated strips react when moistened with urine or blood. The variations in color determine the amount of acetone in the urine or blood and the reaction is similar to that of the acetest tablets.

Important Steps	Key Points
1. Wash your hands. Approach and identify the patient.	Explain what you are going to do. You may be teaching the patient this procedure as a part of his Diabetic Teaching Program. If so, follow your agency procedure.
2. Obtain a urine specimen.	Ask the patient to void in a clean bedpan or urinal.
3. Take the specimen to the work area.	Assemble the equipment on a convenient table top.
4. Remove one Ketostix strip from the bottle.	Close the jar tightly.
5. Dip the designated tip into the urine and then remove it immediately.	The tip is indicated with an arrow-type point. Remember, this must be freshly obtained urine so that you will obtain an accurate recording.
6. Tap the edge of the strip against the bedpan.	This will remove excess urine.
7. After 15 seconds, compare the Ketostix with the color chart.	The color chart is printed on the container which holds the Ketostix.

8. Record your readings on patient's chart.	Indicate the color reaction.
	    Usual color designations are:
	Negative: buff color
	Positive: slightly — lavender
	        moderately — dark lavender
	        strongly — purple
	
	Report the results to your team leader.

E. *Keto-Diastix Test*

A newer method that is in use is the reagent strip which combines in one strip the test for sugar and acetone. The strip changes the urine color by a reaction similar to that in the Ketostix Test. The color variation determines the amount of sugar and acetone in the urine. A bottle of the Keto-Diastix is ordered for the patient and kept in his bathroom or bedside stand.

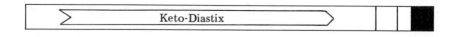

Important Steps	Key Points
1. Wash your hands. Approach and identify the patient.	Explain what you are going to do.
2. Obtain a urine specimen.	Ask the patient to void in a clean bedpan or urinal.
3. Take the specimen to a work area.	Assemble the equipment on a convenient table top.
4. Remove one Keto-Diastix from its bottle.	Close the jar tightly.
5. Dip the designated tip into the urine for *two seconds* and then remove it.	Tap the strip gently against the urine container to remove excess urine.
6. Compare Ketone Reagent area on strip to the chart.	Be sure to match it with the Ketone Chart on the Keto-Diastix package.
7. Compare Glucose Reagent area on the strip after *30 seconds.*	Check the results with the Glucose Chart on the package for the closest matching color.
8. Record your readings on the patient's chart.	Indicate the color reaction; report the results to your team leader immediately.

ITEM 8. METHOD OF COLLECTING URINE FROM FOLEY CATHETER

In this procedure you will learn how to care for the Foley catheter, or the indwelling catheter, as it is often called. Inserted into the bladder to maintain a continuous free flow of urine, it is used for a variety of reasons: (a) emptying of the bladder to allow healing of an infected area, free of contaminated urine; (b) keeping an incontinent patient dry; (c) retraining or restoring normal bladder function; and (d) keeping an accurate intake and output record.

Foley catheters come in various sizes; the size to be used depends on the physical structure of the patient. (The physician may designate the size when he writes the order for the catheter to be inserted.) The Foley catheter has two rubber tubes; the main line is identified by the openings at the tip and at the wide base on the opposite end. The second tube is connected and sealed along the side of the main tube; the end of the tube is fixed in a manner that allows it to be inflated with air or sterile liquid, causing the formation of an inflated balloon around the main tube. The balloon prevents the catheter from slipping out of the urinary tract.

After the catheter has been inserted well into the bladder, the balloon is inflated. You can test to see if the catheter is in place by gently pulling the catheter toward you.

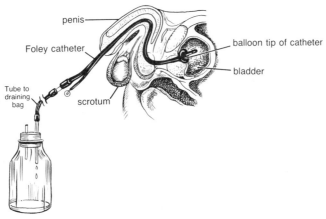

Foley catheter drainage

The plastic drain tube with the attached plastic drain bottle or pouch is inserted onto the main drain tube of the catheter. The complete catheter drainage setup is known as a *closed drainage system.* The cap which has been removed from the end of the drainage tube is placed in a germicidal solution and kept at the patient's bedside. When the patient wants to walk, you may (on doctor's order) disconnect the catheter from the drainage tube and place the clean cap on the end of the drainage tube to prevent germs from entering the tubing while the patient is unattached. The distal end of the Foley catheter is covered with a sterile 4 X 4 protective dressing or bandage and secured with a clamp to prevent the urine from draining out while the patient is ambulatory. This also prevents germs from entering the open catheter. *(Many agencies avoid disconnecting the tubing to decrease possibility of contamination.)*

Important Steps	Key Points
1. Wash your hands.	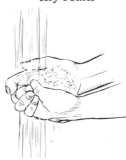
2. Approach and identify the patient.	
3. Position the patient.	
4. Observe his skin at the place of insertion and surrounding area.	Be certain there is no redness, skin eruption, or swelling at the insertion site or surrounding area. If there are any of these signs, report immediately to your team leader so that she can begin recommended treatment at once.
5. Cleanse area gently with warm water and soap, rinse and gently pat dry.	Usually this is done as part of the daily bath. However, if the patient has a Foley catheter in for several days, the proximal end of the catheter should be inspected frequently throughout the day and night and kept free of dried crusts and blood.
6. Keep the tubing close to the patient's body.	Put tape around the drain tube about 12 to 18 inches from the entry site and secure it to the skin on the patient's thigh. Place the tube so that it is comfortable for the patient and there

Important Steps	Key Points

is no tension or unnecessary pull on the skin. Use non-allergenic tape so that it can be changed when necessary without causing skin irritation.

Some agencies recommend placing a piece of tape around the drainage tube about 18 to 24 inches from the entry side into the urethra, making a side loop through which a safety pin can be placed and in turn be pinned to the bottom sheet. Provide enough length on the drainage tube to allow the patient to move freely in bed.

7. Maintain tubing alignment.

The drainage tube should lie on top of the bed in a straight alignment. It must be kept free of "kinking or twisting" and added weight pressure. This prevents the tubing from being clamped together and allows urine to flow freely into the bottle at all times.

8. Keep the gravity flow drainage even.

Pin or tape the longest part of the tube to the bed linen. This prevents the tubing from falling over the side of the bed and keeps it above the drainage bottle to maintain an even free gravity flow. Attach the drainage container to the side of the bed frame. Some agencies use a glass drainage bottle which can be set on the floor beside the patient's bed or placed in the special metal rack which is attached to the bed. It should be placed frontally when the patient is turned to his side. The bed should be slightly elevated, if necessary, so that the container is off the floor. If the container rests on the floor, it can be kicked over easily by a worker and the contents spilled. If this occurs, wipe up immediately with a mop. Stale urine odor quickly becomes offensive. If the urine was being collected as a specimen, report immediately to your team leader so she can take the appropriate action.

9. Empty the drainage container.

Most disposable drain containers have a short tube extending from a bottom corner so that the urine can be easily emptied without disconnecting the whole system. Remove the cap from the drain tube and let the urine flow into the graduate pitcher.

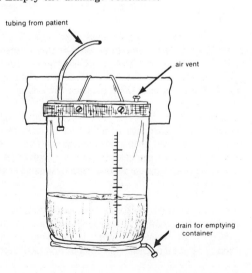

tubing from patient

air vent

drain for emptying container

Important Steps	Key Points
10. Measure and discard or save the urine as indicated by the order.	Utilizing this method of urine drainage helps to prevent the risk of reinfection of the urinary tract and contamination from the environment. Wash your hands.
11. Position the siderails.	Leave the patient safe and comfortable. Refer to this step in Item I.
12. Obtain the chart.	Record all pertinent information in the nurse's notes.

Note 1: Some disposable catheter sets have a sterile solid plastic plug included with the set. If the drain tube has to be disconnected from the catheter, insert the plug into the catheter end. This will prevent urine from spilling on the patient or the surrounding area. The open end of the drain tube should be covered with the cap that was placed in the small container of germicidal solution and kept at the patient's bedside. Before the drain tube is reinserted into the catheter, wipe the outside of the tube clean with a germicidal sponge (alcohol sponges are frequently used).

Note 2: At times the patient will state that he has the urge to urinate. You are to check the catheter and drainage through the tubing. The catheter openings in the bladder may be clogged with solid matter, and the catheter may need to be irrigated with sterile saline to remove it. This, of course, will depend on the doctor's order and your agency procedure. Another source of discomfort may be the position of the catheter in the bladder. The opening may be lying against the bladder wall, or the opening may be above the urine level so that it is impossible to remove the urine. Gently rotate or move the catheter so the flow will be continuous. The size of the catheter may affect the urine flow, particularly if the catheter tube is too small for adequate drainage. This can cause the bladder to be distended, and internal pressure will be exerted on the sphincter so the patient feels the urge to void.

Note 3:   Remember, the reproductive organs are in the genitourinary area of the body. Do not be surprised if the male patient expresses concern about a sexual stimulus reaction that may occur while he has the Foley catheter in place. Reassure him that it is a natural phenomenon because these organs are extremely sensitive to external and internal stimulation. You should maintain a matter-of-fact, gentle, and comforting manner while you care for the patient.

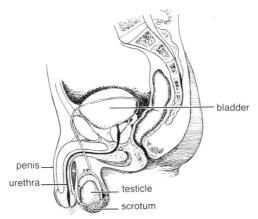

Male urinary system

V. ADDITIONAL INFORMATION FOR ENRICHMENT

You are now beginning with the basic knowledge of the urinary system. The identification and purpose of the organs are as follows:

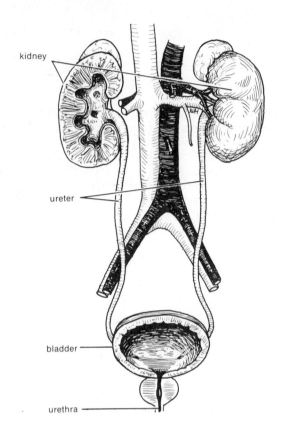

kidney

ureter

bladder

urethra

Urinary system

A. *Organs of the Urinary Tract*

There are *two kidneys*, which are glandular organs that secrete urine. Urine is composed of the waste products which are filtered through an elaborate system of coiled tubes (nephrons) within the kidney. As the blood flows through these tiny tubules, the liquid waste products are filtered (sifted) out of the blood and diluted with water—this then becomes urine.

The *two ureters* are ducts (tubes) which carry the urine from the kidneys down to the urinary bladder.

The *urinary* (cystic) *bladder* is a hollow, muscular organ which serves as a temporary reservoir for urine. By contraction of the muscular wall of the bladder, urine is expelled from the body through a tube called the urethra. When the amount of urine in the bladder reaches a certain level, it exerts pressure on certain nerve endings in the bladder wall and causes the individual to have the urge to empty his bladder. Expelling the urine from the bladder is called *urination* or *micturition.*

Urination is a natural function that is not usually discussed openly and frankly in public. It is for this reason that you can expect the patient to be ill at ease, or to indicate verbally (by speaking) or non-verbally (e.g., facial expressions, body posture) his embarrassment when asking for assistance with the bedpan. Your behavior, verbal and nonverbal, should convey an attitude that is helpful and nonjudgmental. You should utilize your skills confidently, efficiently, and effectively to give the patient a feeling of modesty, security, and dignity at all times.

The *urethra* is a small tube approximately ¼ inch in diameter, 1½ inches long in the female, and 8 to 9 inches long in the male. The urethra extends from the bottom end of the bladder to the exterior (outside of the body). The external opening of the urethra is concealed between the folds of the labia in the female and at the distal end of the penis in the male.

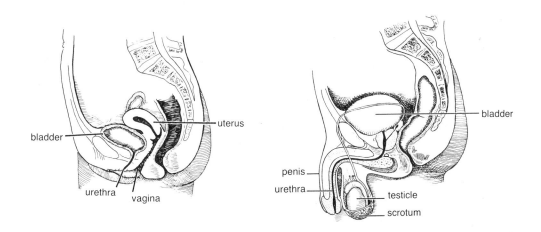

Female urinary system   Male urinary system

B. Components of the Urinary Bladder

The mucous membrane is the continuous lining inside the urethra, the ureter, and the kidney pelvis. You will remember that a mucous membrane secretes a lubricating fluid; in other words, it keeps the tissue moist.

The *musculature* of the bladder wall enables it to expand and hold the accumulating urine. Excessive expansion of the bladder wall causes a condition known as *bladder distention.* The capacity for urine accumulation varies in relation to the patient's health, disease, fluid intake, the action of food and drugs on the kidneys and the weather. The normal adult urine secretion is 1300 to 1500 cc (2 to 3 pints) within 24 hours. The desire to empty the bladder occurs when approximately 300 cc of urine has accumulated. Thus, most adults void (urinate) 5 to 9 times daily. Most healthy adults do not urinate during their sleeping hours, although healthy people do so occasionally. In certain diseased conditions, the bladder may hold as much as 3,000 to 4,000 cc of urine (3 to 4 quarts). When the bladder is severely distended, extreme caution must be taken to prevent any blow or heavy weight on the bladder region which could rupture (break) the bladder wall. In case of *bladder rupture* the patient can die within 8 hours if surgical intervention (a special operation to sew up the bladder wall) is unavailable. Death is due to generalized uremia (waste products of the urine accumulating or backing up into the general blood circulation). Therefore, it is wise to remember to empty your bladder before traveling in your car. Should you have a car accident when driving with a full bladder, you may be thrown against the seat belt or the steering wheel and rupture your bladder.

C. Common Urinary Infections and Pathogens

Because the urinary tract is dark, moist, and warm, it is therefore an excellent breeding place for germs or pathogenic bacteria.

Cystitis (inflammation of the urinary bladder) is a very common bladder infection caused by any of the following: highly concentrated urine, pathogenic bacteria, injury, irritation, or instillation of an irritating substance.

There are a number of pathogenic bacteria which cause urinary infections. The most common are coliform bacilli (i.e., *E. Coli*), streptococci, staphylococci, typhoid bacilli, gonococci, and tubercle bacilli.

D.   Characteristics and Components of Urine

The *normal components* are: 95 per cent water, 3.7 per cent organic wastes, and 1.3 per cent inorganic wastes, mineral salts, toxins, pigments, and sex hormones.

The *color* of normal urine is described in terms of varying shades of yellow. The color is due to the presence of pigments in the urine. Normal urine is a straw yellow or amber color (a darker yellow, due to more concentration of pigments and a smaller amount of water to dilute it). The lighter the shade of yellow, the more it is diluted with water.

Abnormal pigments are often found in the urine and they, too, are designated or indicated by color of the urine. Smoky red or dark brown urine denotes presence of hemoglobin or many red blood cells (erythrocytes) from bleeding in some part of the urinary tract. Blue or blue-green urine may be due to a dye or medication the doctor has ordered for his patient.

The *odor* of freshly voided urine is faintly aromatic but not unpleasant. Variations occur from certain foods, drugs, or a decomposition of bacteria which changes the urea to ammonium carbonate and then to ammonia. An unpleasant (putrid) odor may indicate pathology.

Note: Since sediments alter the composition of urine when it stands at room temperatures for short periods of time (as little as 20 to 30 minutes), it is urgent that urine specimens be sent to the laboratory immediately upon collection. Otherwise laboratory personnel may give an erroneous (wrong) urine report and the doctor may in turn prescribe a wrong treatment, based on the laboratory report. Therefore, although this is a small task, it is vitally important to the patient's recovery.

The *specific gravity* is the weight of a given volume of urine as compared with the weight of an equal volume of pure water. In simple terms, it is the thinness or thickness of the liquid urine. The specific gravity is measured by an instrument called the *urinometer* or a refractometer. The normal numerical range is 1.010 to 1.030. Variations of the numerical values are due to the amounts of solids dissolved in the urine. The specific gravity of a healthy individual changes during a 24-hour period within the above normal limits.

The acidity or alkalinity of the urine is measured in units called *pH*. A neutral urine would have a pH of 7.0. The pH of normal urine is slightly acid, ranging from 5.5 to 7.0. A persistent (continuing) acid condition of the urine may indicate a metabolic disease. An alkaline reaction of the urine is due to the production of ammonia, bacteria, food, and drugs. The alkaline reaction is recorded at a pH greater than 7.0. If there is a consistent alkaline reaction reported, the patient may have a urinary infection, a metabolic disorder, or be on some special medication.

The following *chemicals are inorganic salts*, which constitute 20 per cent of the solid matter of urine. They compose 1.3 per cent of the urine: nitrogen, sulphate, chloride, phosphate, calcium, magnesium, potassium, ammonium, bicarbonate of sodium, and sodium chloride.

Other *chemicals* which are called *organic matter* include urea (which forms 50 per cent of the urine solids), creatinine, and uric acid. A few white (pus) cells and epithelial cells are normal.

The abnormal matter in the urine is composed of many pus cells, red blood cells, hemoglobin, occasional kidney stones (calculi), casts (rectangular cells), acetone bodies, albumin, sugar, bacteria, and some parasites. Other chemicals and drugs may be present.

The urine output can be affected by two kinds of drugs: *diuretics*, which increase the flow of urine, and *antidiuretics*, which decrease the flow of urine.

POST TEST

A. Following are 10 statements. If the statements are true, put a + (plus) sign before the number. If the statements are false, put a 0 (zero) sign before the number.

_0_ 1. When the patient is in the hospital, bedpans are generally used as mop buckets.

_0_ 2. Bedpan covers are placed under the patient's buttocks to protect the linen when the patient is urinating.

_+_ 3. The wash cloth, towel, soap in dish, and wash basin with warm water should be available on the bedside stand so the patient can wash her hands and genital area after she uses the bedpan.

_+_ 4. It is a good idea to tell the patient you are going to wash your hands before you give the bedpan to her.

_0_ 5. When you are working with the patient, you will always leave the bed in the low position and with both siderails down.

_+0_ 6. The easiest method for the patient to be positioned on the bedpan is to have her roll from side to side while she is in the supine position.

_+_ 7. Remember, both the health worker and the patient should be in good body alignment while the patient is being positioned on the bedpan.

_0_ 8. Remove the bedpan by lifting the patient's hips approximately two feet from the bed.

_+_ 9. The genital area should be wiped dry and cleaned, using downward strokes, from the vulva across the vaginal opening to the rectum.

_+_ 10. The bedpan should be rinsed and then stored in the bedside stand.

B. Fill in the blank spaces with the word or words that will correctly complete the statements.

1. There are two kinds of ___Urinals___, male and female.

2. The use of the female urinal depends on the amount of activity and physical ___movement___ the patient is permitted to make.

3. The opening of the female urinal should be in direct contact with the ___genital___ area.

4. When the patient uses the urinal while she is in the "dangle position," utilize all known safety skills, particularly ___locking___ the wheels of the bed.

5. The unique characteristic about the ___fracture___ pan is that part of the pan is lower than the front pouring side.

6. The preliminary and concluding steps used in the task "assisting the male patient to use the urinal" are the same as for the female with one noted exception, and this is using ___toilet tissue___.

7. The male patient is able to use the urinal when he is in one of four positions: lying in the ___supine___ position; lying flat rolled to either the right or left side; in a ___Fowlers___ position; and ___standing___ at the bedside.

8. The male patient usually prefers to use the ___urinal___ without assistance.

9. If the male patient is unable to place the urinal in the proper position to ___urinate___, you will have to do it for him.

10. The most important aspect for you to remember is that this is an ___embarassing___ situation for the patient.

C. The following questions are to be answered in brief descriptive statements.

1. When you are assisting the patient to the bathroom, what are three specific areas of safety to be considered?

Bed in low position

siderails down

Keep bathroom door unlocked

2. What is the primary purpose for obtaining a "routine urine specimen"?

provide for lab information for which the doctor may order treatment & meds.

3. After a urine specimen is obtained, what is the most vital step to take before it is sent to the laboratory?

label the container c̄ pt name room #

4. Name at least three reasons for obtaining urine by catheterization.

Keeps accurate I & O.

Emptying the bladder allows healing infected areas

Keeps incontinent pt. dry

5. What are four important steps to constantly remember when the patient has an indwelling catheter in place?

Keep distal end clean when tubing is disconnected.

Observe skin around meatus for redness + drainage

Maintain gravity flow

Empty + record as ordered

6. Why does the patient with a urinary catheter feel the urge to urinate?

tubing may be clogged & urine not draining

7. The "clean voided" urine collection is ordered for what reason?

So it will be free of contamination

8. What is to be done if a urine specimen is discarded during the process of obtaining a 24-hour specimen?

Report to doc. & start over again

9. State at least 6 steps that the individual tasks (within this lesson) have in common.

wash hand

identify pt.

position pt.

explain procedure

assemble equipment

assist pt. as needed

10. Name the 2 most important aspects considered in the timed urine collection.

(1) *provide safety measures for pt.*

(2) *convey a helping nonjudgmental attitude*

Now that you have completed this lesson, briefly state what you think are important aspects for you to be constantly aware of while you are performing these tasks for the patient:

POST-TEST ANNOTATED ANSWER SHEET

A.
1. F (p. 397
2. F (p. 397)
3. T (p. 397)
4. T (p. 397)
5. F (p. 398)
6. T (p. 398)
7. T (p. 399)
8. F (p. 399)
9. T (p. 399)
10. T (p. 399)

B.
1. urinals   (pp. 399 and 402)
2. movement   (p. 400)
3. genital   (p. 400)
4. locking   (p. 400)
5. fracture   (p. 401)
6. toilet tissue   (p. 402)
7. supine, Fowler's, standing   (p. 402)
8. urinal   (p. 403)
9. urinate   (p. 402)
10. embarrassing   (p. 403)

C.
1. Adjust the bed to the low position; lower the siderail; have patient lean on you for support (if necessary); stay nearby when patient is in bathroom; keep bathroom door unlocked; adjust water temperature to prevent burning when patient washes his hands. (pp. 403-404 — any order)

2. Provide a basis of laboratory information upon which the physician may order treatments and medication. (p. 404)

3. Label the container with the patient's room number and other identification. (p. 407)

4. Emptying the bladder allows the healing of an infected area; keeps the incontinent patient dry; retraining or restoring normal bladder function; keeping an accurate intake and output record. (p. 418)

5. Keep the distal end of catheter clean when tubing is disconnected from catheter when patient is ambulatory; observe skin around meatus for redness or discharge; secure catheter tubing to leg area to prevent undue pulling on catheter as patient moves about; maintain gravity flow for urine; empty and record urinary drainage as ordered. (pp. 419 and 420)

6. Tubing is clogged and urine is not draining, catheter is too small to promote adequate drainage; internal pressure on the sphincter. (p. 421)

7. To obtain a urine specimen which is as free of contamination as possible without having to catheterize the patient. (p. 408)

8. Report to the physician and start the 24 hour collection over again. (p. 410)

9. Wash your hands; identify the patient; position the patient; explain the procedure; assemble equipment; assist patient as needed; obtain specimen; observe; discard or save specimen as ordered. Clean equipment, return to storage; label specimen and send to laboratory as indicated; record observations on chart. (pp. 404-421)

10. To provide safety measures for patient (infection, pain, prevent falls, burns, etc.), convey a helping nonjudgmental attitude. (pp. 396, 421)

NOTES

PERFORMANCE TEST

In the skill laboratory, you will be asked to perform the following activities for your instructor without reference to any source material. You will need another person to take the part of the patient.

1. Given a patient who is unable to move her legs and assist herself on the bedpan, you will explain to the patient how she is to roll and how you are going to place her on the bedpan. In this movement you will assist her to roll safely to the far side of the bed, place the bedpan under the buttocks, position her for comfort, and keep her modestly covered with the bath blanket.

2. Given a patient who is to have a 24-hour urine collection, you will explain the task to the patient, stressing the importance of obtaining all the urine voided in the 24-hour period, and explaining that if one specimen is lost, the test is useless. You will obtain the equipment from the laboratory, mark the labels correctly on the bottle, and then indicate by signs placed on the bed and in the bathroom that the 24-hour urine collection is in progress.

3. Given a patient who is to have a clean voided urine specimen obtained, you will explain the task to the patient. You will obtain and set up the necessary equipment, position the patient standing over the toilet bowl, and go through the motions of cleaning the patient for the task.

4. Given a diabetic patient who has voided a urine specimen, you will test the urine for sugar and acetone (using your agency procedure) and practice recording the results on the chart forms.

INTAKE – OUTPUT RECORD
BEDSIDE RECORD

PATIENT'S NAME   ROOM NO.

INTAKE		INTRAVENOUS SOLUTIONS	OUTPUT		
7-3:30 LIQUIDS	C. C.	C. C.	VOIDED	EMESIS	DRAINAGE ETC.
3-11					
11-7					

EQUIVALENTS

CUP	180 CC	SOUP BOWL	CHILDS	110 CC
PAPER CUP LG	210 CC	SOUP BOWL	ADULTS	190 CC
PAPER CUP MED	150 CC	SOUP BOWL	LARGE	210 CC
WATER GLASS	210 CC	WATER PITCHER		950 CC
FR JU GLASS	150 CC			
TEA POT	250 CC			
JELLO	100 CC	EMESIS BASIN	STD	500 CC
ICE CREAM	120 CC	EMESIS BASIN	SM	300 CC

Saint John's Hospital — Santa Monica, California

PERFORMANCE CHECKLIST

URINE ELIMINATION

24-HOUR URINE COLLECTION

Student to demonstrate procedure for 24-hour urine collection.

1. Identify patient.

2. Obtain equipment with preservative and transport to patient's room.

3. Post warning signs.

4. Store collection jugs in refrigerator or buckets if indicated.

5. Request patient to void approximately 5 minutes *before* collection begins.

6. Transfer urine to appropriate jug after each voiding; make sure to measure quantity and record.

7. Have patient void approximately 5 minutes prior to end of 24-hour collection.

8. Mark jugs appropriately.

9. Mark laboratory slip appropriately.

10. Mark charge vouchers appropriately.

11. Arrange for immediate transfer of specimen to laboratory.

12. Inform patient that the collection period is completed.

13. Remove written warnings and equipment from room.

14. Obtain patient's chart and record pertinent information pertaining to collection.

COLLECTION OF A CLEAN-CATCH SPECIMEN

Student to demonstrate procedure for collection of clean-catch specimen.

1. Identify patient.

2. Obtain supplies and equipment.

3. Wash hands.

4. Explain procedure to patient.

5. Provide for patient's privacy.

6. Cleanse genital area.

7. Assist patient to bathroom.

8. Request patient to void.

9. Ask patient to interrupt voiding.

10. Collect specimen after interruption.

11. Transfer specimen to specimen jar.

12. Assist patient to bed; provide opportunity for patient to cleanse self.

13. Label specimen with all appropriate information.

14. Arrange to have specimen transported to laboratory with all pertinent information.

15. Return to patient's room and provide for patient's comfort and safety.

16. Restore bathroom to clean condition.

17. Record activity on patient's chart.

DIABETIC TESTING

Student to demonstrate procedure for diabetic testing of urine specimen.

1. Wash hands.

2. Identify patient.

3. Explain procedure.

4. Obtain urine specimen.

5. Transport urine specimen to work area.

6. Perform indicated diabetic test.

7. Compare reading of test to color chart.

8. Record reading on patient's chart.

POSITIONING THE BEDPAN

Student to demonstrate procedure for positioning bedpan.

1. Wash hands.

2. Identify patient.

3. Explain procedure to patient.

4. Obtain necessary materials.

5. Raise distal siderail.

6. Assist patient to lateral position.

7. Place bedpan appropriately.

8. Return patient to supine position.

9. Elevate patient to sitting position.

10. Provide patient with privacy and safety.

11. Lower head of bed.

12. Help patient return to lateral position.

13. Hold bedpan during move to avoid spilling contents.

14. Remove bedpan.

15. Assist patient with personal cleansing if necessary.

16. Provide for patient's comfort and safety.

17. Empty contents of bedpan.

18. Wash bedpan thoroughly.

19. Record significant observations of urine.

Unit 22

BOWEL ELIMINATION

I. DIRECTIONS TO THE STUDENT

You are to proceed through this lesson using the workbook as your guide. In the skill laboratory you will need to practice the enema and irrigation procedures on the Chase doll. After you practice the procedures and complete the lesson, arrange with your instructor to take the post-test for this lesson.

You will need the following items for your study and practice.

1. This workbook.

2. A pen or pencil.

3. Disposable or reusable enema unit.

4. Lubricant.

5. Solution as ordered by doctor.

6. Bedpan and cover.

7. Irrigating graduated pitcher, 1000 ml.

8. Roll of toilet tissue.

9. Chux, or pad for buttocks.

10. Irrigating bag, plastic apron, and tubing.

11. Stool specimen container.

12. Rectal tube.

13. Examining or rectal gloves.

Please read the following paragraphs carefully. They will tell you exactly what you will be expected to know and how to assist the patient to establish and maintain regularity in the elimination of waste products from the large intestine. If you feel that you have sufficient knowledge and skills to do the performance test accurately without further study of the lesson, please discuss this with your instructor. All students are expected to perform accurately the skills required in the test without use of reference materials.

II. GENERAL PERFORMANCE OBJECTIVE

You will be able to demonstrate your ability to assist the patient to establish and maintain regular elimination of waste products from the large intestine using methods appropriate to the patient's age, physical condition, and disease.

III. SPECIFIC PERFORMANCE OBJECTIVES

Upon completion of this lesson, you will be able to:

1. Identify some of the abnormal conditions manifested in the appearance of the patient's stool, such as the presence of blood, mucus, iron, worms or other parasites.

2. Collect a stool specimen and prepare it correctly for examination in the laboratory.

3. Promote the patient's regular elimination of waste products from the large bowel through nursing measures related to the patient's prescribed diet, fluid intake, exercise, and rest.

4. Reduce incontinence of feces in patients of any age through methods of habit training and retraining.

5. Assist evacuation of feces and flatus in the hypoactive bowel through the use of the enema, rectal tube, or Harris flush.

6. Examine for the presence of constipated stool in the rectum and promote its evacuation by the use of suppositories, cleansing or retention enemas.

7. Assist and teach the patient with a colostomy or ileostomy to irrigate his bowel to cleanse it of fecal material, to prevent obstruction, and to establish a habit of regular evacuation.

IV. VOCABULARY

Many new words are introduced in this lesson. These words are frequently used by doctors and nurses, and you will need to learn their meanings. Because there are so many new words, some related words will be grouped together.

1. The small bowel (total length 22 to 23 feet in the adult):
duodenum—an 8- to 10-inch portion of the small intestine connected to the lower end of the stomach and to the jejunum.
jejunum—the section of the intestine between the duodenum and the ileum; about 9 feet long in the adult.
ileum—the twisting intestine between the jejunem and the large intestine; about 13 feet long in the adult.
ilium—part of the pelvic bone.
2. The large bowel (total length 4 to 6 feet in the adult):
colon—the large intestine from the cecum to the rectum which is divided into the ascending colon, the transverse colon, the descending colon, and the sigmoid.
anus (anal)—the outer opening of the rectum between the buttocks and beyond the lower tip of the sacrum.
appendix—a small wormlike pouch about 7.5 cm long at the end of the cecum.
cecum—the pouch at the junction of the small intestine and the ascending colon with the appendix at the lower end.
rectum—the lower part of the large intestine between the sigmoid and the anus; about 5 inches long.
sigmoid—the lower part of the descending colon which is shaped like the letter "S."
3. Some diseases and surgical conditions:
appendicitis—inflammation of the appendix.
colitis—inflammation of the colon.
diverticulitis—inflammation and distention of little pouches throughout the colon.
colostomy—an incision into the colon to form an artificial anus (stoma).
hemorrhoids—dilated blood vessels in the anal area.
ileostomy—an incision into the ileum of the small intestine to form an artificial anus (stoma).
polyps—growths attached to mucous membranes of the nose, bladder, colon, or uterus.
ulcerative colitis—a severe inflammation of the colon with open sores of the membrane lining.
4. Contents of the bowels:
bile—an important digestive juice secreted by the liver, stored in the gall bladder; substances in bile give the brown color to feces.

chyme—the partially digested food and digestive juices; the liquid mass found in the
    intestines.
electrolytes—substances of a solution capable of conducting an electrical impulse or charge.
    Important electrolytes in the body are sodium, chlorides, calcium, potassium, iron, and
    others.
feces—the waste material following digestion; the stool.
flatus—gas in the digestive tract. (Flatulence is the distention of the abdomen due to gas in
    the intestines.)
mucus—a slippery, slimy fluid secreted by mucous membranes and glands.
parasites—organisms that live upon or in another organism or body called the host. Common
    parasites in the intestinal tract are amoeba, flukes, pinworms, roundworms, hookworms,
    and tapeworms.
stool—feces; the waste matter discharged from the bowel.
5. Words pertaining to movement of the intestines:
constipation—sluggish action of the bowels; compacting of the feces into a hard, dense mass.
defecation—the evacuation of the bowel.
diarrhea—frequent movement of the bowels, increased number of stools per day, often liquid
    or semiliquid.
hyperactive—excessive movement; irritable.
hypoactive—decreased movement; less than normal.
incontinence—inability to retain feces or urine; lack of voluntary control over sphincters.
peristalsis—contraction of successive portions of the intestines followed by relaxation which
    propels food content, fluids, and flatus onward.
sphincter—a circular muscle that opens and closes an opening, such as the sphincter of the
    anus.
6. Other words used in the lesson:
hemorrhage—excessive flow of blood out of the blood vessels; an abnormal amount of
    bleeding.
suppository—a semisolid, medicated substance that is inserted in the rectum, vagina, or
    urethra where it dissolves and is absorbed.
proctoscopy—examination of the rectum by instrument.
sigmoidoscopy—examination of the sigmoid colon by instrument.
stoma—mouth or opening, or an artifically created opening.

A. That makes quite a vocabulary list. Now let's see what progress you have made in
    learning what the words mean. In the following list, all but one of the words on each line
    are related to the others. Place a checkmark before the word that does not belong.

(1) ____sigmoid   ____rectum   ✓ mucus   ____ anus

(2) ✓ cecum   ____ ileum   ____duodenum   ____ jejunum

(3) ____ intestine   ✓ tract   ____bowel   ____colon

(4) ____appendicitis   ____diverticulitis   ____ colitis   ✓ flatus

(5) ____chyme   ____ electrolytes   ✓ suppository   ____ bile

(6) ✓ polyp   ____ feces   ____waste products   ____ stool

B. Three of the words in your vocabulary are spelled in an unusual way with the letters
    "r-r-h" in sequence. Match the word with its meaning and spell the word correctly.

(1) _hemorrhage_____ an excessive amount of bleeding.

(2) _diarrhea_____ increased number of bowel movements.

(3) _hemorrhoids____ dilated blood vessels around the anus.

ITEM 1. THE IMPORTANCE OF BOWEL ELIMINATION

Why do you need to learn about the elimination of wastes from the bowel? Emptying a bedpan filled with stool, or feces, seems to be one of the more unpleasant tasks that nursing workers do. The sight and odor are often very unpleasant. To some of you, it might seem that we should rush through this part and get on to some more important lesson. Unfortunately, bowel elimination happens to be one of the most important things we study.

What are the functions of the bowel that make it so important to health? They can be stated simply as those related to the absorption of nutrients and those related to the elimination of waste products.

Absorption of vital nutrients, electrolytes, and water takes place in the small intestine and a portion of the large intestine as the liquefied food mass moves out of the stomach and down the bowel. Elimination of the waste products at regular intervals indicates free passage of the food mass through the bowel in the time allowed for the absorption process. Absorption is reduced when the bowel moves the food mass along too quickly, when the bowel moves so slowly that waste products collect in the absorbing parts, and when the bowel becomes obstructed or blocked. The causes of these conditions in the bowel *may be* serious enough to endanger the life of the patient.

The body must get rid of the waste materials that are produced in the process of converting food into usable substances delivered to the cells with oxygen. These waste products of the body are eliminated through the skin, lungs, kidneys, and the bowel. The bowel is the most important excretor of the more solid wastes of the body. The solid wastes consist of by-products of the digestive process, indigestible stuffs, water, and matter from the intestinal tract itself, such as secretions, dead bacteria, and sloughed cells.

The appearance and the composition of the stool are important indicators of conditions in other parts of the digestive system. Obstruction or disease of the bowel may be detected by observing the stool for changes in color, the absence of color, and the presence of unusual matter such as blood. Changes in bowel habits may indicate a growth, obstruction, or disease.

In this lesson, you will learn more about the functions of the intestinal tract; conditions which change the normal composition and appearance of the stool; such problems related to elimination as distention, constipation, diarrhea, and incontinence; and ways to assist the patient to achieve and maintain regular elimination of waste matter from his bowel.

C. The two main functions of the intestines are: _absorption_ and _elimination of waste products_

D. Select the best answer(s) to complete the following statement. The patient's life may be endangered when absorption in the bowel is reduced by:

___√_(1) blockage of the bowel by twisting itself closed.

___(2) change in the color of the stool.

___√_(3) slow movement with no stool passed in five days.

___√_(4) quick movement with ten stools in one day.

___(5) all of the above.

E. Four of the problems related to elimination are:

distention , _diarrhea_ ,

constipation ; _incontinence_ .

ITEM 2. BRIEF DESCRIPTION OF THE INTESTINAL TRACT

The intestinal tract is a muscular tube that extends from the stomach to the anus opening at the skin surface. The intestines are approximately six times the length of the body. In the adult, this would average about 8.5 meters, or 33½ feet.

The inner surface of the intestine is not smooth, but has innumerable circular folds that greatly increase the area for absorption. It is through this surface that nutrients, water, vitamins, and electrolytes are absorbed into the blood stream. A rich supply of blood vessels around the intestines transports the absorbed materials to all cells of the body.

In addition, the walls of the intestines have circular muscle fibers which contract or enlarge the size of the tube, and longitudinal and oblique muscle fibers which allow stretching and turning of the tube.

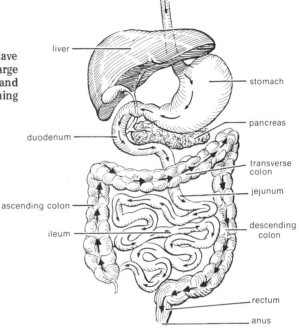

The intestinal tract.

The *small intestine* is composed of the *duodenum*, the *jejunum*, and the *ileum*. The duodenum is connected to the lower end of the stomach. The jejunum is the middle section of the small intestine, and the ileum, or twisted intestine, is the lower section that is joined to the cecum of the large bowel. As the liquefied food mass *(chyme)* enters and passes through the small intestine, it is mixed with intestinal digestive juices. The greatest absorption of nutrients takes place in the small intestine. Electrolytes are also absorbed in the upper portion of the small intestine, and some water is absorbed in the ileum.

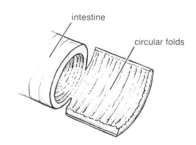

Cut-away section of intestinal folds.

The *large intestine* provides a frame for the small intestines in the abdominal cavity. The *cecum with the appendix* is at the lower right corner of the frame and is attached to the *ascending colon*. The *transverse colon* crosses the abdomen at about the level of the navel, and the *descending colon* goes down the left side where it joins the *sigmoid*. The sigmoid colon, which gets its name from its "S" shape, crosses the abdominal cavity toward the back.

The lower segment of the large intestine is the *rectum*, and the *anus* is the outer opening of the bowel to the skin.

The main functions of the large intestines are: (1) to absorb water and electrolytes, and (2) to temporarily store the residual waste products as feces. As an example of the water absorbing capacity of the large intestine, about 500 ml. of chyme enters the bowel daily and all but 50 to 100 ml. of water is absorbed.

Numerous bacteria are present in the normal bowel. They are found in the absorbing portion of the large intestines where they digest small amounts of food roughage, form some of the vitamins, and produce gas, or *flatus*, as a result of this bacterial activity.

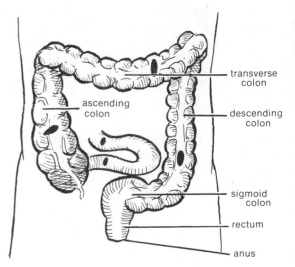

The large intestine.

F. A child's intestinal tract is approximately _____6_____ times as long as his body.

G. The long length of the intestinal tract and the circular folds provide greater surface for _absorption_ to take place.

H. The various parts of the intestinal tract have been described. For the following, indicate the parts of the small intestine with an "S" and those of the large intestine with an "L".

S (1) ileum   L (2) rectum   L (3) colon

S (4) jejunum   L (5) cecum   S (6) duodenum

L (7) Anus

I. The two functions of the large intestines are (1) _absorption of water + electrolytes_ and (2) _storage of waste products_

ITEM 3. CHARACTERISTICS OF FECES

The digestion of food is similar to the refining of oil. Food enters the body as raw fuel and is changed by the digestive juices. The usable parts are converted to nutrients, and these are absorbed into the small and large intestines. The unusable part, or the waste product, is passed into the colon where most of the water and electrolytes are absorbed. It is then passed into the sigmoid and rectum for storage as feces until it is evacuated from the body.

Normally, the feces are three quarters water by weight and one quarter solid material. The solid material consists of about 30 per cent dead bacteria and 70 per cent undigested roughage from food, fat, protein, and inorganic material. The brown color of the normal stool is caused by *bile* (one of the digestive juices), and the odor is the result of bacterial action on the foods which are eaten.

In the newborn infant, the stool is characteristically dark greenish black (meconium) for the first two to three days of life. The breast-fed baby will have an orange-yellow colored stool which has a strong smell, and the bottle-fed baby will have a brownish-yellow stool if the formula contains malt sugars.

The color of the feces may be changed by certain drugs the person may be taking. Vitamins and other drug preparations containing iron give the stool a black color throughout. Chlorophyll may cause a green color in the stool.

J. Feces are made up of one-fourth _solid material_ and three-fourths _water_ .

K. The color of the normal stool in an adult is _brownish_ , and in the bottle-fed baby the color is _brownish-yellow_

ITEM 4. BLOOD IN THE STOOL

Before you empty feces from any patient's bedpan or flush the toilet, you should know whether a specimen of the stool is required for laboratory examination *and* you should observe the stool for any noticeable changes from the normal-appearing stool. The most serious change is the presence of blood in the stool.

Blood in the stool should always be regarded as a serious matter until it has been determined otherwise. A small amount of bleeding from hemorrhoids or an irritation caused by straining at stool may clear up without any treatment. Most serious causes of blood in the stool include hemorrhage from ulcer in the stomach or duodenum, severe inflammation or irritation as in ulcerative colitis or diverticulitis, cancer, or diseases which cause hemorrhage. When you *observe blood in the stool,* you should *report it promptly, record* it on the patient's chart, and *save* the stool so it can be inspected by the doctor for amount of blood and clues as to when the bleeding occurred.

Bleeding which occurs in the upper gastrointestinal tract (usually the stomach or the small intestine) will show up in the feces as dark, almost black in color and tarlike in consistency. During the hours that it takes the blood to move through the intestines, it undergoes partial digestion which changes blood to the dark tarry substance. Therefore, a dark tarry stool usually indicates that the hemorrhage occurred hours earlier, probably from the area of the stomach or the small intestine, and the partially digested blood is found thoroughly mixed in all of the stool.

Bright red blood in the stool is a sign of a recent hemorrhage, or one that occurred in the large bowel. The bright red blood will be found on the surfaces of the stool and in pools, but is not mixed throughout the stool. The color indicates that the blood has not undergone digestion in the upper part of the bowel, and that it has not been in the intestinal tract for hours.

L. One of your patients, Mr. Long, has just had a bowel movement which is black in appearance and tarry in consistency. This means that the stool contains _blood_ which probably came from the (duodenum) (cecum) (sigmoid colon). (Circle one.)

M. Mr. Long's hemorrhage probably occurred (10 minutes) (10 hours) (10 days) ago.

N. Hemorrhage in the large intestine produces a _bright red blood_ appearance of the stool.

ITEM 5. OTHER ABNORMALITIES OF THE FECES

One of the most easily observed changes in the stool is the change in color. Color changes according to the foods eaten, but the normal stool is brown, except in infants or patients receiving formula in tube feedings, and in these cases the stool is a dark yellow color. The color of the stool is important in the care of patients with disease of the digestive system because it may indicate need to change the diet. This is important for the patient with an ileostomy since his stool is evacuated through an opening in the ileum of the small bowel before maximum absorption of nutrients, electrolytes, and water has occurred.

Some of the abnormalities in the color of stools are listed along with the condition that this color indicates. *Clay color*, or pale white, indicates the absence of bile or an obstruction that prevents its passage into the intestines. *Chalky white color* is due to chalky substance swallowed by the patient or instilled into the lower intestinal tract for X-ray purposes. *Light tan color* indicates undigested fat in the stool. *Green, watery* indicates too much sugar in stool, most often seen in infants.

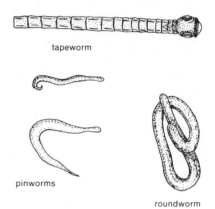

tapeworm

pinworms

roundworm

Types of parasites.

Other abnormal characteristics of feces are the presence of large amounts of mucus, pus, or the presence of parasites, such as worms. Unusual amounts of mucus in the stool indicate an irritation or inflammation of the inner surface of the intestines. The mucus coats the stool and gives it a slimy appearance. The presence of pus results from drainage of an ulcer that is inflamed or infected. The most *common parasitic worms* found in the intestines are the *tapeworm*, the *pinworm*, and the *roundworm*.

O. Too much sugar in a baby's diet irritates the bowel to cause stools that are
   green and _watery_ .

P. Pale, clay-colored stools are due to the absence of _bile_ .

Q. _mucus_ causes a slick slimy look to the stool.

ITEM 6.   MOVEMENT IN THE INTESTINES

The *chyme* (liquefied food mass) is passed along the intestines by means of movement of the muscular tube. This movement is called *peristalsis*. In peristalsis the circular muscle layer of the intestine contracts to squeeze the portion of chyme and gas ahead of it. The circular, longitudinal, and oblique muscle layers in the segment ahead of the contracted part will expand and lengthen to accommodate the mass entering it. When you hear the rumbling noise in your abdomen, it is caused by peristaltic movement of liquid mass and gas along the intestinal tract.

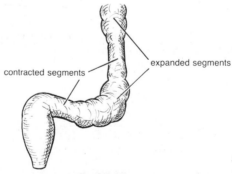

contracted segments

expanded segments

Peristalsis.

The feces are moved along the lower intestines by peristalsis until they reach the storage portion in the lower sigmoid colon and the rectum. As more feces collect here, the rectum is filled, and the pressure on the sphincter of the anus causes the urge to open and defecate. The abdominal muscles contract to help force the evacuation of the rectum and pass the feces through the anus.

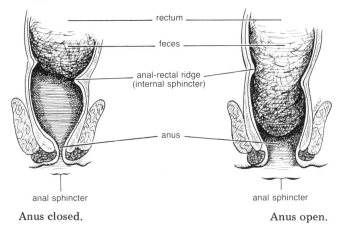

rectum

feces

anal-rectal ridge
(internal sphincter)

anus

anal sphincter   anal sphincter

Anus closed.   Anus open.

R. Movement in the intestines is caused by contraction and expansion of the __circular__ , __longitudinal__ , and __oblique__ muscle layers.

S. The movement is called __peristalsis__ .

T. The urge to defecate results from __pressure__ of feces filling the rectum.

ITEM 7. PROBLEMS CAUSED BY THE HYPOACTIVE BOWEL

A reduction or absence of peristaltic movement of the bowel results in the hypoactive bowel. The more common conditions which cause the hypoactive bowel are surgery, injury, disease, and bed rest. In the normal person, lack of sufficient roughage in the diet and decreased exercise may produce sluggish or hypoactive bowel. Certain drugs, such as narcotics and tranquilizers, also reduce the activity of the bowel.

Constipation is one of the more common problems of the hypoactive bowel. It is the irregular evacuation of feces from the bowel so that the feces become more compacted and hard while in the rectum. As more feces are formed, they will fill more and more of the colon as well as the rectum. People tend to have constipation when they lack muscle tone due to little exercise, lack regularity of bowel movements, lead a sedentary life, or have worry, anxiety, or fear. The treatment includes plenty of exercise, lots of liquids, a good diet with sufficient roughage, setting a regular time for defecation, and avoiding emotional stress. When ordered by the doctor, enemas are used to empty the rectum, laxatives are used to stimulate bowel activity, and suppositories are used to stimulate the urge to defecate.

ITEM 8. FECAL IMPACTION

Fecal impaction means that the rectum and sigmoid colon become filled with fecal material. As the fecal material remains in the bowel for several days, it becomes more compacted, contains less water, and consequently becomes quite hard and difficult or painful to pass through the anus.

The most obvious sign of fecal impaction is the absence of (or only a small amount of) bowel movement for more than three days. Another important sign of a possible fecal impaction is the passage of small amounts of semi-soft or liquid fecal stool so that there is staining and soiling of the bed linens. This occurs as bacterial action of the fecal material continues to work on the outer surfaces of the hardened impacted mass, liquefying small portions of it, and results from the body's effort to remove the obstructing mass.

Fecal impaction should be suspected when a patient has a hypoactive bowel with constipation, or lack of bowel movement for three days or more. As in the case of bowel incontinence, this condition usually occurs in patients who may not be fully aware of their surroundings due to their physical condition, illness, or mental state of confusion. The very young and the very old patients are especially prone to develop fecal impaction.

The nursing treatment of a fecal impaction is to *examine* for the presence of an impaction, *manually break it up*, and *remove* portions of the fecal mass. This should be followed by the use of suppositories, enemas, or laxatives as ordered by the physician. Again, emphasis should be on the *prevention of fecal impactions* through the promotion of measures to insure regular evacuation of the waste products from the bowel in each patient.

ITEM 9. PROCEDURE FOR REMOVAL OF FECAL IMPACTION

In the skill laboratory, you should run through the steps of the procedure several times until you are familiar with it. If a lifelike model of the anus and rectum is available, it can be used to help you get the feel of examining the rectum for impacted stool before you perform the procedure in the clinical area.

In this procedure, you are to examine the rectum for the presence of hardened stool, manually break it up, and remove such portions as you can in an older patient who is able to turn on his side.

Important Steps	Key Points
1. Collect the items you will need: a pair of rubber or plastic gloves, toilet paper, bedpan with cover, paper towel, lubricant, and a Chux pad.	Check with the team leader or the nurse in charge to find out if there are any reasons for not carrying out the procedure. Gloves need not be sterile unless specified by the RN. The Chux is used to protect the sheets from possible soiling during the procedure.
2. Approach the patient, check his identification band, explain what you plan to do, and enlist his cooperation.	This procedure is often *uncomfortable for the patient*, so when possible you should have someone assist you who can reassure and comfort the child, aged patient, or one who may be mentally disturbed. Wash your hands.
3. Prepare the patient.	Provide for privacy by closing door, screening, or pulling cubicle curtain. Raise bed to working height; place it in flat position and lower the siderail. Place the patient in the Sims position, and slip the Chux under his hips. Fold the top bedding back obliquely over his hips to expose the buttocks. Fold the hospital gown out of the way or lower the pajama pants. Place the bedpan and toilet tissue on a chair which is close to the bed and within your convenient reach, to avoid strain or injury to yourself.
4. Examine him rectally for fecal impaction.	The person assisting you should reassure the patient, hold his hand or support his shoulder in the Sims position, and help explain what is being done. Put on the gloves, use lubricant on index finger, and *gently* insert in the anus. The index finger should follow the wall of the rectum in a slightly curving motion. As the finger comes in contact with feces in the rectum, note consistency. Then move the finger into the lower portion of the fecal mass, again noting the consistency.

Important Steps	Key Points
5. Break up and remove the fecal impaction.	With the examining index finger, dislodge or break off small amount of fecal material and gently remove it, placing it in the bedpan. Continue removing as much fecal material as you can reach with your finger, or until the patient's discomfort warrants discontinuing the procedure. Remove soiled gloves and place them in paper towel.
6. Remove remaining fecal material.	Often, the stimulation of removing the impaction manually will create the urge in the patient to defecate. Place the patient on a clean bedpan and provide toilet paper. If he is unable to defecate, follow up by carrying out the doctor's order for a suppository, enema, or laxative.
7. Provide for the patient's comfort.	Wash and dry the patient's anal area. Remove the Chux from under his hips. Position him comfortably in good alignment and adjust his bed to the desired position. Leave his call light within reach, raise the siderail if used, and ventilate the room or use deodorizer if necessary to get rid of odors.
8. Remove used items.	Observe the characteristics of the fecal material in the bedpan; then remove it from the room, empty the pan, clean it, and return it to its proper place, along with the roll of toilet paper. Remove the soiled Chux and the gloves in the paper towel. Rinse the gloves in soap and water if they are reusable rubber ones and return them to the Central Processing Department or discard them if they are the disposable type.
9. Report and record as appropriate.	Record the presence of the fecal impaction, the time, and characteristics of the feces, such as color and consistency. Record any additional procedures, such as giving an enema or a suppository. Report the results of these procedures to the team leader or the nurse in charge.

ITEM 10. ADDITIONAL PROBLEMS CAUSED BY THE HYPOACTIVE BOWEL

A second problem related to the hypoactive bowel is that of distention. Abdominal distention is caused by flatus (gas) stretching and inflating segments of the intestines when peristalsis is reduced or absent. Distention and "gas pains" occur frequently following abdominal surgery. The discomfort and pain are due to the stretching of the intestines, and the spasms of the muscle layers. The goal of treatment is to reduce the amount of flatus in the bowel. Procedures that you will use include the enema, irrigations such as the Harris flush, and use of the rectal tube.

U. In the hypoactive bowel, peristaltic action is (increased) (decreased).

V. Two common conditions which result from a hypoactive bowel are,
(1)___distention___ and (2)___constipation___.

W. Name five possible causes of a sluggish or hypoactive bowel.
(1)___surgery___ (2)___illness___ (3)___worry___
(4)___bed rest___ (5)___certain drugs___.

ITEM 11.   THE IRRITABLE OR HYPERACTIVE BOWEL

Hyperactivity of the bowel is excessive movement. Any condition that causes irritation of the intestines can cause hyperactivity of the bowel. The hyperactive, irritable bowel is seen in diarrheas of all kinds, in ulcerative colitis, diverticulitis, and certain other diseases.

Excessive strong and frequent peristaltic action moves the chyme rapidly through the intestines because the food mass may also serve as an irritant to an already irritated bowel. This rapid movement of the chyme in the bowel reduces the amount of time available for the intestines to *absorb* the nutrients, electrolytes, and water. It results in numerous bowel movements per day which generally are liquid or semiliquid in consistency.

The problems related to the hyperactive bowel are: lack of enough food to nourish and repair the cells of the body; loss of electrolytes, which disturbs the chemical composition of the body fluids; and dehydration, which reduces the amount of water available for the body fluids. These conditions pose a serious threat to the patient's life. For example, infants and small children may die in a matter of 24 hours or less as a result of severe diarrhea.

The goal of treatment of the hyperactive bowel is to reduce the irritability *and* to maintain adequate levels of nutrition, electrolytes, and water in the body. This requires vigorous treatment by the doctors and nurses. It is very important for the nurse worker to record the number and character of the stools per day and the amount of food and fluid intake of the patient, and to provide an emotionally calm atmosphere for the patient.

X. In the hyperactive bowel, _absorption_ of nutrients, water, and electrolytes is reduced.

Y. An increase in the number of bowel movements per day is called _diarrhea_ .

Z. Disturbance of the chemical composition of body fluids is caused by loss of _electrolytes_

ITEM 12.   BOWEL CONTROL TRAINING

In almost every culture, the child is expected to learn early in life to control the elimination of stool from his bowels. Control is usually accomplished between the ages of two and three. The child can then curb the urge to defecate for a period of time to allow him to get to the bathroom or toilet. The child's success in controlling his bowels becomes a sign of progress toward personal independence, a step toward growing up; and it gives him the feeling of being more socially acceptable to his family and others.

To establish bowel control in the child, attention must be given to the child's diet, fluid intake, exercise, and rest inasmuch as these will influence the child's ability to regulate his bowels.

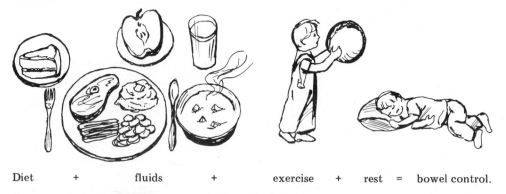

Diet   +   fluids   +   exercise   +   rest   =   bowel control.

The diet should contain roughage adequate to give bulk to the stool. The young child should take 800 to 1000 ml. of fluids per day, which include water, milk, juices, soups, jello, and others. Adequate sleep and exercise are necessary for health and the proper functioning of the intestinal tract.

The frequency of bowel movements depends on many factors and will vary among individuals. It is normal for some people to have a movement every day, for others to have one every other day, and for a few to have a movement every three days. The important thing is that the bowel movements occur on a regular basis. The time of the bowel movement also varies. Many adults have elimination following breakfast, but it can occur at other times of the day. Infants will usually have two or three movements per day following feeding, and the young child will often have his bowel movement shortly after breakfast or lunch.

Habit training for bowel control depends on recognizing the urge to defecate, establishing a regular time for elimination, providing a comfortable position, and allowing sufficient time.

Signs of the urge to defecate are a rumbling noise in the abdomen, expelling of flatus, and restlessness due to the feeling of fullness in the rectum. The child should be toiletted at a regular time each day, usually after breakfast or after lunch. He should be placed in a comfortable position on a potty chair, a small commode, or toilet with a child-sized seat on it. No more than 20 minutes should be allowed. The child should be reminded frequently and encouraged to move his bowels. Playing with toys distracts the child from the task to be done.

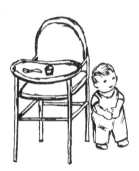  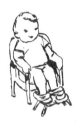

Bowel training.

AA. Bowel control in children is usually accomplished by age___3___ .

BB. To help establish bowel control, attention should be given to the child's
(1)___diet___ , (2)___fluids___ , (3)___rest___ and
(4)___exercise___ .

CC. It is essential for your good health to have a bowel movement every day.
True_____ False___√___

ITEM 13.   INCONTINENCE OF FECES

Some patients lose the ability to control their bowels during a serious illness or hospitalization. This condition is called *incontinence*. The patient may become incontinent of feces whether his bowel is hypoactive, hyperactive, or normal. Incontinence generally occurs in patients who are not fully aware of where they are or what is going on. This lack of awareness may be due to the physical disease or illness, or to the mental condition. However, whenever possible you should attempt to retrain and assist the incontinent patient to control the regularity of his bowel movements.

Even patients who are not fully aware of what is going on about them often realize that they have had a bowel movement and have soiled themselves or the bedding. The patient often has feelings of being less of a person, loses some of his self-respect, becomes embarrassed or humiliated, or suffers from anxiety and fears that he has lost all control over what is happening to him. When caring for the incontinent patient, it is important not to judge, scold, or fuss at him.

The treatment for incontinence is *retraining* in *bowel control habits.* In the beginning, it will take more time to try to establish bowel control habits than to clean up the soiled patient and change his bed. In the long run, however, you will help the patient to regain his self-respect as well as control of his bowels. Special effort should be taken to help the very elderly patient overcome incontinence. Incontinence of urine or feces is one of the major reasons for admitting the elderly patient to the extended care facility or nursing home.

The method of retraining the incontinent patient is the same as that used for training a child to control his bowels. You must see that the patient eats an adequate diet, that his fluid intake is at least 2500 ml., that he gets the proper amount of sleep and rest, and that he gets exercise within the limits imposed by his illness. You need to set a regular time for evacuation based on his prior bowel habits and your observation of when the incontinent movements tend to occur. The patient should use the bedpan or commode, or be taken to the toilet. He should be given privacy and allowed at least 20 minutes for his bowels to move. Many doctors order rectal suppositories to stimulate defecation on a regular schedule in the retraining period. One way of using suppositories in habit training is to give a suppository every day for the first week, then every other day for the second and third week, and thereafter only as needed to maintain regularity of every two to three days.

DD. Incontinence of feces means _unable to control feces elimination_

EE. The treatment for incontinence is _Retraining bowel control_ .

FF. Two benefits to the patient that result from retraining bowel control habits are
(1) _control of BM_ , and (2) _regain self-respect_ .

ITEM 14. THE USE OF RECTAL SUPPOSITORIES

In some settings the beginning worker in nursing may not be allowed to insert rectal suppositories. *Check with your instructor; she may omit the next two items.*

Rectal suppositories consist of a semisolid material that melts readily; they are somewhat cone-shaped and are approximately 1½ inches long. They are made for many different purposes: some relieve pain or irritation, some contain drugs which the patient cannot take by mouth, and others promote bowel movements. The latter may do so (1) by stimulating the inner surface of the rectum and increasing the urge to defecate, (2) by forming gas that expands the rectum, or (3) by melting into a lubricating material to coat the stool for easier passage through the anal sphincter.

Rubber or plastic gloves should be worn when inserting the suppository into the rectum. After it has been inserted through the anal sphincter, the suppository should be guided by the index finger along the wall of the rectum to a point beyond the anal rectal ridge which is about 2 to 3 inches from the outer sphincter. The suppository will be ineffective if it is pushed into the fecal mass. Correct and incorrect placement of the suppository are shown in the following sketches. Correct placement aids melting and action of the suppository.

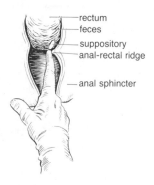

Correct placement.

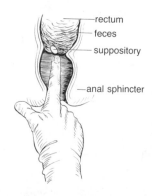

Incorrect placement.

GG. Rectal suppositories are used to (1) *relieve pain*, (2) *give meds*, or (3) *promote B.M.* .

HH. When placed correctly, the rectal suppository:
Check correct answer(s)

_____(1) stimulates the outer surface of the rectum.

__X__(2) is in contact with the inner surface of the rectum.

_____(3) melts inside the fecal mass in the rectum.

_____(4) lies between the anal sphincter and the anal rectal ridge.

ITEM 15. PROCEDURE FOR INSERTING RECTAL SUPPOSITORIES

You should run through the steps of this procedure several times in the skill laboratory in order to become familiar with it. Most schools do not have life-like models of the anus and rectum, and you will not be able to insert the suppository and get the "feel" of it in the rectum until you reach the clinical area.

For your practice situation, you are to insert a rectal suppository to stimulate a bowel movement in a bed patient who can be turned on his side.

Important Steps	Key Points
1. Collect the items needed: the correct suppository, a rubber or plastic examining glove, lubricant and a paper towel.	Check the doctor's orders for the type of suppository to be used and obtain it from the team leader or nurse in charge. The glove used to protect your hand need not be sterile unless specified because of surgery or chance of infection in the anal region.
2. Approach the patient, check his identity, explain what you plan to do, and enlist his cooperation.	The crucial point is to identify the patient correctly. The name on the patient's wrist-band should be identical to the name on the doctor's order. Unless it matches, do not proceed further. Most adult patients will be cooperative and eager for relief from their constipation. Children cooperate better if they have become used to having rectal temperatures taken, and if it is explained that the suppository will not cause pain.
3. Prepare the patient. 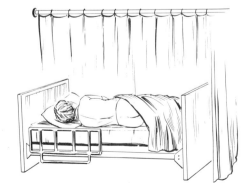	Provide for privacy by closing door, screening, or pulling cubicle curtain. Wash hands. Place suppository, glove, and towel on the bedside table. Place the bed in a nearly flat position, and lower the side if it is used. Place the patient in a Sims position with his uppermost leg flexed and his back to the proximal side of the bed. Fold the top bedding obliquely back over the hips to expose the buttocks. Lower the pajama pants or fold the hospital gown out of the way.

Important Steps	Key Points
4. Insert the suppository rectally.	Unwrap the foil or plastic covering of the suppository, leaving it on the wrapper. Put the glove on your dominant, or working hand and take the suppository between thumb and index finger and lubricate. With other hand, draw the top gluteal fold upward and toward the head to expose the anus. Slip the suppository into the anus and with gloved index finger guide it along the wall of the anus and rectum for 3 inches or the length of your finger. Ask the patient to take a deep breath at the time you insert the suppository, because this helps to relax the anal sphincter. Withdraw your finger, and hold both buttocks tightly together for a few seconds while the patient breathes deeply until the urge to expel it has passed.

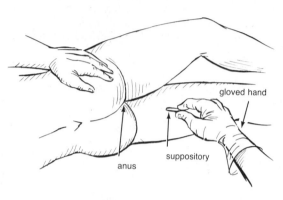

gloved hand

suppository

anus

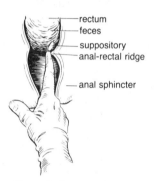

rectum
feces
suppository
anal-rectal ridge

anal sphincter

Correct placement.

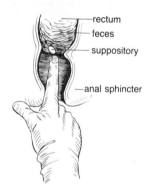

rectum
feces
suppository

anal sphincter

Incorrect placement.

5. Remove the glove	Take the cuff of the glove and pull it down over the hand so that the glove turns inside out. Place the soiled glove on the paper towel and fold it closed.
6. Provide for the patient's comfort.	Turn the patient to his back. Inform him that he should retain the suppository for 15 to 20 minutes if possible. Leave his call light so that he can signal you to assist him to the toilet, onto a commode, or onto the bedpan. Adjust the top bedding neatly; adjust the bed for the patient's comfort; and raise the siderail. If the patient can get onto the bedpan himself, he may feel more secure if the bedpan is placed under the covers at his side and a roll of toilet paper placed within his reach.
7. Remove used items.	Take the suppository wrapper and the towel containing the soiled glove from the room. Discard the wrapper and towel, and rinse the glove in soap and water and return it to the Central Processing Department or discard it if it is a disposable one.

Important Steps	Key Points
8. Report and record as appropriate.	Record the type of suppository given, the time given, the time it acted, and the results. Note the color, amount, and other characteristics of the feces. Charting example: 9:30 A.M. Glycerine suppository inserted. <div align="right">J. Jones, NA</div>10:05 A.M. Large amount of soft brown formed stool expelled with large amount of flatus. Patient states he is much relieved. <div align="right">J. Jones, NA</div>

ITEM 16. COLLECTION OF A STOOL SPECIMEN

You should review the following procedure several times to become familiar with it before you collect a stool specimen from a patient in the clinical area.

Given a doctor's order to obtain a stool specimen for specific laboratory tests, you are to inform the patient, and after he has had a bowel movement, collect a portion of the stool, place it in a specimen container, complete the laboratory request for examination, and then assure prompt delivery of the specimen and request slip to the laboratory.

Important Steps	Key Points
1. Gather the items needed: two tongue blades, a plastic or cardboard container with lid, and a paper towel.	Take them to the patient's unit and store near the bedpan or the bathroom. This will serve to alert whoever cares for the patient that a stool specimen is needed. When the nurse answers the patient's light to remove the bedpan, supplies will be convenient for use in collecting the specimen.
2. Approach the patient, check his identification band, explain that a stool specimen is needed, and enlist his cooperation.	It is necessary to inform and get the cooperation of all patients, but especially the patient who has bathroom privileges so that he won't flush the stool away and delay the collection of the specimen for a day or more.
3. Tell the patient how to assist in the collection of the specimen. 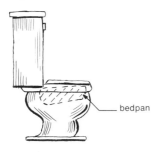 bedpan	The patient should be asked to: (a) use the bedpan or bedside commode when he has the next bowel movement, (b) save the stool, and (c) notify the nurse that he has had a stool for the specimen. The bedpan may be placed on a chair for use by the patient who has bathroom privileges, or the bedside commode may be used. In some cases, a bedpan will fit in the toilet bowl under the toilet seat as shown, but not always.

Important Steps	Key Points
4. Collect a specimen of the stool after the patient has defecated.	Take the bedpan and your supplies to the bathroom where you will empty the pan after obtaining the specimen. Write the *patient's name, room number* or *ward*, and the *date* on the lid of the container. Often the label is on the container. You may need to put the information in both places. Use one or both of the tongue blades to transfer approximately one tablespoon of stool to the container. Put the lid on the container, wrap the soiled tongue blades in the paper towel, and drop into the wastebasket. Empty and clean the bedpan or commode pan, and return it to its proper place.

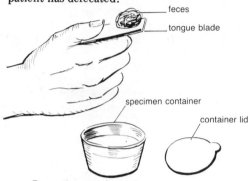

feces

tongue blade

specimen container

container lid

Preparing stool specimen.

5. Complete the laboratory request (requisition) slip.	Check the name of the patient and the name on the lab slip to see that they are identical. This is *vitally important.* An incorrect label will cause the laboratory to give the wrong information on a patient. The doctor could therefore order incorrect medicines or treatments for his patient because of an error in labeling a specimen.
6. Assure prompt delivery of the specimen and the request slip to the laboratory.	Stool specimens should be examined while still warm (at or near body temperature) and while still fresh. Time and changes in temperature alter the stool. As an example: bright red blood begins to clot, dry out, and turn dark, and certain disease-causing organisms may die and thus fail to be detected. *Make sure the specimen is taken to the lab immediately.* (Some laboratories accept stool specimens only during specified hours. Check your agency procedure.)
7. Record and report as appropriate.	Report to the team leader or nurse in charge that the specimen has been obtained and sent to the laboratory. Record on the patient's chart that specimen has been sent to lab, the date and time, and anything unusual about the stool. Charting example: 11.10 A.M. Stool specimen with requisition to lab. No unusual characteristics noted. J. Jones, NA

ITEM 17. THE ENEMA

An enema is the introduction of fluid into the rectum and colon. The most common reason for giving rectal enemas is to stimulate peristalsis and the urge to defecate. The cleansing enema is used to wash out the waste products or feces from the bowel when these have not been properly eliminated, when the bowel is to be examined by X-ray or proctoscopy, and when the bowel is distended by flatus.

The *kind* and the *amount of fluid* used in the enema will often be prescribed by the doctor and will vary depending on the age and condition of the patient, the preference of the doctor, and the purpose of the enema. The most common solutions are the tap water enema (TWE) using water obtained from the faucet, the saline enema using a saline (salt) solution usually made up in Central Supply, and the soap suds enema (or SSE) using a small amount of liquefied soap in water. Commercially prepared enema units, such as Fleet's enema, contain a solution of various salts. When other types of enemas are ordered, you may need to consult the nursing procedure book of the hospital for the ingredients and the proportions to use in the enema.

The amount of solution to be used is usually between 500 ml. (cc.) to 1000 ml. (cc.) for adults, with a lesser amount for children. The solution should run in slowly to avoid discomfort and pain to the patient as the rectum is distended by the fluid. The solution container should be between 12 to 18 inches above the anus. Any height more than 18 inches causes too much pressure so that the fluid runs in too rapidly and causes painful distention of the rectum and colon. It will also stimulate the urge to defecate immediately so that the patient cannot retain the fluid.

The temperature of the solution should be about 40.5°C. (105°F.). If a bath thermometer is not available, you can test the temperature of the fluid by pouring a small amount over your inner wrist. It should be warm to touch, but not hot. Solution which is too cool usually can't be retained, while hot solutions may damage the tissues of the rectum.

The position of the patient receiving an enema may be supine or lateral. The lateral position is most widely used, and better results are achieved by elevating the hips slightly. Enemas should not be given to a patient seated on the toilet unless it is given just to stimulate the urge to defecate. In a sitting position, the fluid cannot flow to other parts of the colon, but dilates the rectum and is rapidly expelled.

II. For a cleansing enema given to an adult, indicate the specific information for the following:

(1) Kind of solution used _SSE or TWE_.

(2) Amount of solution _500 – 1000 cc._.

(3) Temperature of the solution _105 F_.

(4) Height of solution container above the anus _12-18 in._.

JJ. The patient will not be able to retain the solution when:

(1) ~~if height is more than 18 in.~~ Rectum overdistended.

(2) ~~if fluid runs to fast~~ solution is too cool.

ITEM 18. PROCEDURE FOR GIVING A CLEANSING ENEMA

In the skill laboratory, you should practice assembling the supplies needed for giving an enema, and the procedure using the Chase doll or other model with an anal opening. Go over the procedure several times until you are familiar with it before you give an enema to a patient in the actual clinical setting.

Given a patient in bed who can turn to his side, you are to assemble the supplies, prepare the enema, and give it to the patient so that it will produce an emptying of the rectum without undue discomfort to the patient.

Important Steps	Key Points

1. Collect the materials needed: the enema tray or disposable enema unit with cover, lubricant, solution, paper towel, Chux or pad for placing under the buttocks.

The enema tray or the disposable unit should contain the same items: a container to hold the solution, tubing with a clamp to regulate the flow, and a rectal tube with rounded tip to insert into the rectum. In the commercial enema, such as Fleet's, these are in one unit.

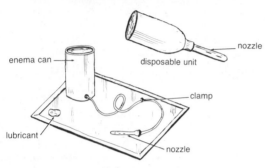

Enema tray.

2. Prepare the solution as ordered by the doctor.

For tap water enema (abbreviated to TWE) fill container with warm water from the faucet (approximately 1000 ml.). For soap solution enema (abbreviated to SSE) add 1 ounce of liquefied mild soap, like Ivory, to 1000 ml. of warm water.

For saline enema, use prepared solution which has been warmed to 105° by setting the flask in a pan of hot water. The temperature of all solutions should be about 105°F (40.5°C). Carry the enema unit to the patient's room.

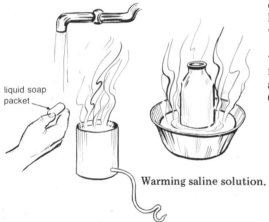

Warming saline solution.

Preparing soap suds enema.

3. Approach and identify the patient, explain what is to be done and why, and enlist his cooperation.

Wash your hands. Check the patient's wristband to assure that the name is the same as the one for whom the enema is ordered. While few patients like the idea of an enema, the vast majority do cooperate.

4. Prepare the patient.

Provide for privacy by closing the door, screening the bed, or pulling the cubicle curtains. (Avoid giving enemas at mealtimes, when other patients are eating in the same room, or during visiting hours unless visitors are asked to leave the room.) It is embarrassing to the patient and others.

Important Steps   **Key Points**

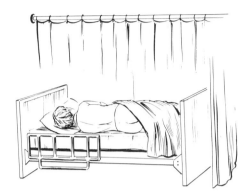

5. Prepare to give the enema.

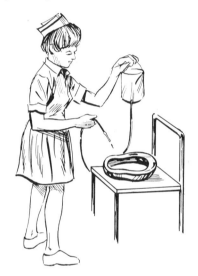

6. Insert the rectal tube.

7. Instill the solution into the bowel.

8. Remove the rectal tube.

If at all possible, work from the right side of the bed so that the patient can turn on his left side. (The enema solution flows through the rectum and sigmoid colon to the descending colon more easily in this position.) Raise the bed to a comfortable working height. Lower the siderail, if one is used, and adjust the bed in a flat position. Place the Chux or pad under the buttocks. Fold back the upper bedding and replace it with a bath blanket. Avoid exposing the patient's body. Turn patient on his left side.

Place enema unit on chair near area where you are working and place bedpan near it. Put small amount of lubricant on paper towel and lubricate the end of the rectal tube for about 1 inch. Open the clamp and allow the solution to run through the tubing to expel the air. Use the bedpan to collect this solution. Close the clamp on the tubing.

Tell the patient about each step as you go along. Ask him to take deep breaths through his mouth to relax the anus and rectum. Insert the lubricated rectal tube *slowly* and *gently* about *4 inches*.

Open the clamp on the tube and *allow the solution to flow slowly into the bowel.* Hold the solution *container 12 to 18 inches above the anus.* Regulate the flow according to the patient's ability to retain it. When the patient has discomfort, stop the flow by kinking the tubing or clamping it and instruct the patient to take deep breaths through his mouth until the cramping and urge pass. Then continue until the patient can retain no more, or the can is empty except for the fluid in the tubing.

Do not allow all of the fluid in the tube to flow in, but clamp the tubing. If all the solution runs in, air may get into the rectum and cause more discomfort to the patient. Withdraw the rectal tube gently and quickly. Place the soiled end in the paper towel.

Important Steps	Key Points
9. Assist the patient onto the bedpan.	Roll up the bed so that the patient is in a sitting position, unless contraindicated by his condition. Place the toilet tissue and his call light within his reach.
10. Remove the bedpan when enema and stool have been completely expelled.	Slip the bedpan out from under the patient, have him turn to his side, then finish cleaning his buttocks and anal area with toilet tissue or wash cloth. Observe the results of the enema—the color, amount, and consistency of the stool. Take the bedpan, empty the contents, clean, and return it to the patient's unit.
11. Provide for the patient's comfort.	Remove the Chux or pad from under the patient. Replace the top covers. Provide water and towel so that patient can wash his hands. Place the patient in the desired position, adjust the position of the bed for comfort, and raise the siderail. Ventilate the room when possible to get rid of the odor, or use a room spray deodorizer if needed.
12. Remove all enema equipment.	Wash the enema container, tubing, and rectal tube in soapy water; rinse, and dry. If it is a disposable unit, discard it. Return reusable equipment to proper place for sterilizing, put soiled linen in laundry hamper. Wash your hands.
13. Report and record as appropriate.	Report to the team leader or the nurse in charge that the enema has been given, and describe the results. Record this information on the patient's chart and the time the enema was given. Charting example: 8:30 P.M. Fleet's enema given. Solution returned clear with a large amount of hard dark brown stool. J. Jones, NA

ITEM 19. THE RETENTION ENEMA

Often an oil retention enema is ordered for the patient with constipation. The oil is to be retained in the rectum and serves to soften and coat the hardened feces. Between 120 ml. to 180 ml. of warm oil is instilled rectally in the same manner as with the cleansing enema, except that it should be retained at least 30 minutes. An Asepto syringe, rectal tube or small catheter, and a small pitcher or funnel to hold the oil may be used instead of the usual equipment. Mineral oil or olive oil is most commonly used. Follow same procedure as when giving a cleansing enema.

Note: There are several prepackaged retention enemas on the market. Check your agency for their procedure.

ITEM 20. THE HARRIS FLUSH

One of the most effective methods of stimulating the hypoactive bowel to reduce the abdominal distention due to flatus is through the use of the Harris flush. This is a method of irrigating the rectum and colon with fluid, then, with the rectal tube still in place, lowering the solution container (or irrigating can) 12 to 18 inches below the anus so that the fluid flows back into the container. The *alternate filling and draining of the colon* continues for about 15 minutes, or until there is no further release of gas. Since the fecal material, as well as flatus and the solution, may drain into the container, the contents may become thick and offensive. It must be emptied into the bedpan, and clear solution added to the irrigating container.

KK. The primary use of the Harris flush is to reduce _flatus_ _abd. distention_.

LL. The Harris flush uses the principles of alternately _filling_ and _draining_ the colon and rectum with fluid.

Note: In some parts of the country this procedure may be called colonic irrigation. It is an alternate system to introducing the solution into the colon and draining off the solution.

ITEM 21. PROCEDURE FOR GIVING A HARRIS FLUSH

In the skill laboratory, you will need to practice collecting the equipment and carrying out the steps of the procedure of giving a Harris flush. The Chase doll, or similar model, can be used to demonstrate the procedure, except that you will not be able to let the solution actually run in and out. However, you should be thoroughly familiar with the procedure before performing it in the clinical area.

Given a patient with moderate abdominal distention following surgery of the abdomen three days ago, you are to give a Harris flush to reduce the flatus.

Important Steps	Key Points
1. Collect the equipment needed: an enema unit, a 1000 ml. graduated pitcher with solution, rectal tubing and clamp, lubricant, paper towel, bedpan cover, and Chux or pad for buttocks.	In addition to the regular items used in giving an enema, the pitcher is used to hold the solution. Only 300 ml. of solution is used at one time in the enema container to flow in and out of the bowel.
2. Prepare the solution.	Unless ordered otherwise, tap water is used, 1000 ml. amount, and at 105°F (40.5°C).
3. Prepare the patient.	Same as for the cleansing enema, Step 4, Item 18.
4. Prepare to give the Harris flush.	Same as Step 5, Item 18.
5. Insert the rectal tube.	Same as Step 6, Item 18.
6. Instill the solution into the bowel.	Open the clamp on the tube and allow approximately 250 to 300 ml. of the solution to flow slowly into the bowel. Hold the irrigating can 12 to 18 inches above the anus. Regulate the flow according to the patient's ability to retain it. When the patient has discomfort, stop the flow by kinking the tubing or clamping it, and instruct him to take deep breaths through his mouth until the cramping and urge pass.
7. Drain the solution from the bowel.	Lower the irrigating can to a point 12 to 18 inches below the anus and allow the solution and flatus to flow back into the can. Fecal material may also flow back into the can. If the solution becomes thick with fecal particles, it may be emptied into the bedpan, and more clear solution should be poured from the pitcher into the can.

Important Steps	Key Points
8. Repeat Steps 6 and 7 until there is no further evidence of flatus.	You should continue the flushing of the bowel for at least 10 to 15 minutes to insure release of flatus.
9. Remove the rectal tube.	The key points for the remaining steps are the same as those given for the cleansing enema (Step 8, Item 18).
10. Provide for the patient's comfort.	(See Step 11, Item 18.)
11. Remove all Harris flush equipment.	(See Step 12, Item 18.)
12. Report and record as appropriate.	(See Step 13, Item 18.) Charting example: 8:45 P.M. Harris flush given. Solution returned clear with a large amount of flatus expelled. Patient comfortable. J. Jones, NA

ITEM 22. USE OF RECTAL TUBE FOR RELEASE OF FLATUS

When a patient is uncomfortable due to flatus in the lower bowel, a rectal tube can be inserted in the anus. This allows the gas to be expelled without straining to open the anal sphincter. The procedure is simple and effective. Obtain a rectal tube, lubricate the end, and take it to the patient's bedside in a hand towel or paper towel. Turn the patient to his side and gently insert the rectal tube about 4 inches. The free end of the rectal tube should be placed in the folded hand towel in case there is some expulsion of fecal liquid. The *rectal tube should not remain in the anus more than one-half hour*. It should be removed and reinserted after several hours if the patient again has discomfort. Severe irritation of the lining of the rectum can occur from prolonged insertion. When treatment is completed, rinse the rectal tube and return it to Central Processing Department. If your agency uses disposable rectal tubes, discard it in the designated waste container.
Charting example:
11:15 A.M. Rectal tube inserted. Much flatus expelled.   J. Jones, NA
11:45 A.M. Rectal tube removed. Patient states he is greatly relieved.   J. Jones, NA

ITEM 23. ILEOSTOMIES AND COLOSTOMIES

The patient with an ileostomy or a colostomy has an artificial opening on his abdomen through which the fecal material is eliminated. An "ostomy" is performed to correct an obstruction, to provide a period of rest for a severely inflamed or irritated bowel, or because of cancer when the rectum and anus are removed.

As you might imagine, the patient with an "ostomy" has many problems. First, he wonders whether he will live, and then he has to adjust to a new pattern of living. He has many fears and great anxiety. He often feels that a monstrous thing has happened to him and that he will not be accepted by other people because he is now so different.

Your attitude and reactions to him while giving him care are very important. In order to help the patient, you need to know about the function of the bowel in the "ostomy," avoid showing feelings of disgust, assist the patient to gain control of the "ostomy," and help him to resume his usual pattern of living. The patient often needs reassurance that many people in all walks of life live with an "ostomy" and carry out normal daily activities. The entire colon can be removed without interfering with the life process. When the colon is absent, the small intestines absorb more water, and the storage of waste products is minimized via discharge through the "ostomy."

The common sites of "ostomy" are shown on the facing page, and the characteristics of the fecal material are described.

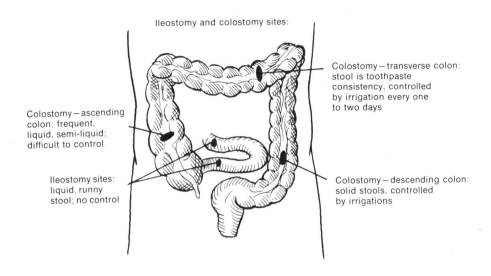

Ileostomy and colostomy sites:

Colostomy—transverse colon: stool is toothpaste consistency, controlled by irrigation every one to two days

Colostomy—ascending colon: frequent, liquid, semi-liquid; difficult to control

Ileostomy sites: liquid, runny stool; no control

Colostomy—descending colon: solid stools, controlled by irrigations

Ileostomy and colostomy sites.

Control of the fecal discharge is most easily achieved in the colostomy of the descending or sigmoid colon, and is the most difficult in the colostomy of the ascending colon, although it can be done.

MM. Your _attitude_ is most important to the "ostomy" patient to help *reduce* his fears, anxiety, and his feeling of rejection by others.

NN. An artificial anus is created on the abdomen for the following conditions:

(1) _correct obstruction_ (2) _rest an inflam. bowel_, and (3) _cancer_.

OO. The control of fecal discharges from the "ostomy" are more easily achieved in a _colostomy_ of a _descending colon_

ITEM 24. CONTROL OF FECAL DISCHARGE FROM "OSTOMIES"

The first discharge of fecal material from an "ostomy" (or stoma) usually occurs two to four days after surgery. The doctor irrigates the bowel at this time to insure that it is working. Thereafter the nurse carries out the irrigations until the patient has learned to carry out his own irrigations.

The colostomy irrigation is done (1) to cleanse the intestinal tract of wastes, (2) to prevent obstruction of the bowel, and (3) to establish control or regular evacuation from the colostomy. The irrigations should be done at the same time each day. This time ordinarily is planned with the patient so that he can continue at the same time when he is discharged. It should be about one hour after his largest meal and when he will be able to use the bathroom undisturbed for about an hour. When the colostomy is irrigated at the same hour every day, control can be established in 3 to 10 days. Irrigations should be continued until there is no spillage from the colostomy during a 24-hour period. Many patients will then be able to maintain control with irrigations every other day or as needed.

The fecal material is very irritating to the skin so that the area around the stoma (artificial opening) must be protected. The skin should be cleaned gently with tissue, washed with mild soap and water, and patted completely dry. (Procedures for skin care of colostomy and ileostomy will be given in the unit Special Skin Care.)

As soon as the colostomy is working, the patient should begin to use an appliance instead of a bulky surgical dressing over the stoma to collect the fecal material. The patient should have his own personal appliance purchased for him as soon as possible. There are many types of appliances available and some are shown to give you an idea of how they look.

cleaned. It is usually of rubber or plastic. The Type B appliance has a disposable plastic bag attached to a ring which is around the stoma. The Type C appliance can be cemented directly to the skin, and is usually disposable.

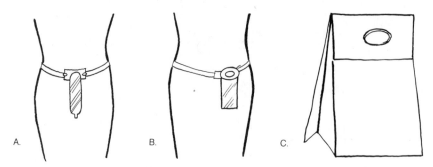

Types of ostomy appliances.

The patient should first be instructed and encouraged to keep the skin around the stoma clean and dry. Next, he should learn to change the bag on his appliance when it has become soiled with fecal drainage. When he has become accustomed to doing these tasks, he should be encouraged to learn to do his own irrigations. He will be able to resume his normal daily living activities sooner if he can irrigate his own colostomy and not depend on someone else to do it.

Note: In some agencies this procedure is not done by the nurse aide, only the LPN (LVN) or RN. Check your agency for their policy on this procedure.

ITEM 25. PROCEDURE FOR IRRIGATING A COLOSTOMY

In the skill laboratory, you should assemble the equipment needed to do an irrigation, prepare to give the irrigation, and practice each step using a Chase doll or similar model. Again, you will not be able to let the solution flow or observe the actual function of the colostomy in your practice, but you should be familiar with the procedure before performing an actual irrigation in the clinical area.

Given a patient who had a colostomy of the descending colon five days ago and is making a good recovery, you are to irrigate the colostomy with the patient sitting on a commode or toilet. Your actions should be skillful and your manner should be accepting of the patient as a person.

Important Steps	Key Points
1. Assemble the equipment needed to give the irrigation: an irrigation can or enema can, a 16 to 18 French catheter, lubricant, 2000 ml. pitcher or graduate for the solution, paper towel, and an irrigating bag or plastic apron. An IV stand may be used.	The equipment should be arranged on a tray to be carried to the room. You may want to have an IV stand in the bathroom from which to hang the irrigating can during the irrigation because the procedure will take almost an hour. The plastic apron or the irrigating bag is attached to the patient's appliance to direct the drainage into the commode or toilet. Wash your hands.

2. Prepare the solution, as ordered by the doctor.

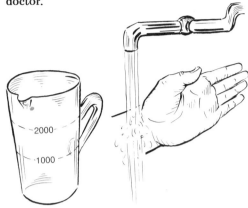

Tap water is most commonly used, but saline or soap solution may be ordered. The temperature of the solution should be 105°F. (40.5°C). The amount needed will be between 1000 ml. and 2000 ml. If tap water is to be used, you can get it in the bathroom where you will do the irrigation. Test the temperature of the water by running it over the inner surface of your wrist. It should be warm, but not hot to touch. Other solution should be put in the pitcher and kept warm by placing it in a basin of hot water. Take the tray of equipment to room and place on chair or the bathroom sink.

3. Approach the patient, explain what is to be done and why, and enlist his cooperation.

Wash your hands. Check the patient's wristband to make sure that you have correctly identified the person to receive the irrigation. Be sure that you will be doing the irrigation at the same time as on the previous day in order to establish control and regularity. The patient may be very depressed and shocked by the colostomy, so you will need to be skillful and sincere in reminding the patient of what he has left in life, not what he has lost.

4. Prepare the patient.

Provide for his privacy so that he will not be intruded upon during the procedure. Assist the patient to the commode or toilet and into a comfortable sitting position. Assist the patient to remove the colostomy bag, and clean or dispose of it if it is soiled. (Patients who are permitted to have the irrigation on the toilet are usually fairly well controlled.)

5. Prepare to give the irrigation.

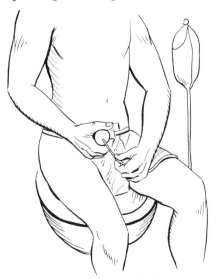

Colostomy irrigation
sitting on a toilet.

Attach the plastic irrigating bag to the appliance ring and arrange just below the stoma of the colostomy, or fasten the plastic apron snugly below the colostomy, and place the end into the toilet or commode to direct the flow of the fecal material. The gown or pajama pants should be placed out of the way to avoid soiling them. Make sure the catheter is attached to the tubing. Clamp the tubing of the irrigating can, pour in about 1000 ml. of solution, and then expel air from the tubing by opening the clamp; run some solution through into the sink or a bedpan, and reclamp. Hang the irrigating can from the IV stand. If saline or soap solution is used, keep remaining amount of solution warm by placing pitcher in warm water in the sink.

Important Steps	Key Points

6. Insert the catheter into the colostomy stoma.

Place small amount of lubricant on a paper towel or tissue and lubricate about 2 inches of the tip of the catheter. Insert the catheter into the colostomy stoma about 6 to 8 inches. It will go in easier if you unclamp the tubing and allow the solution to start flowing.

An alternate position for giving a colostomy irrigation: patient lying in bed. The irrigation is usually given to the new "ostomy" patient and will probably be done by the RN.

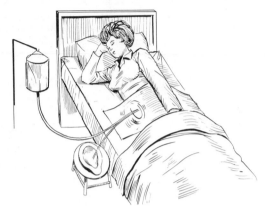

Colostomy irrigation,
in bed.

7. Instill the solution into the bowel.

Run in between 250 ml. to 500 ml. depending on the patient's ability to retain it. If he becomes uncomfortable, stop the flow and ask the patient to breathe through his mouth until he is more relaxed.

Note: The solution may be expelled in a forceful spray. Shield yourself by holding an emesis basin in front of the stoma.

8. Allow the solution to drain out of the bowel.

Remove the catheter after the tubing is clamped. Place the irrigating bag over the colostomy opening so that fecal material and solution will drain into the toilet or commode. Repeat Steps 6, 7, and 8 until the return flow is clear of feces and flatus. More solution may need to be added to the irrigating can to complete the irrigation, but test the temperature before you do to make sure it is the proper temperature.

9. Prepare for the patient's comfort.

Remove the irrigating bag from the colostomy appliance, or remove the plastic apron. (After the toilet has been flushed, these can remain over the side of it to be cleaned and rinsed later.) Assist the patient to clean the skin around the colostomy and dry it completely. Assist the patient to attach a clean bag to the colostomy appliance, and let him wash his hands before you help him return to bed. Adjust the bed to a comfortable position as the patient may desire, with good body alignment. Leave signal light and bedside stand within easy reach of the patient. Ask if there is anything else you can do for him. Tell him when you will return.

10. Clean the equipment and return to its proper place.

Use the pitcher to rinse material from inside the irrigating bag, then wash it in soap and water at the sink. Rinse and fold to store with patient's personal appliance materials. Take the

Important Steps	Key Points
	remaining equipment from the room, wash, rinse, and dry. Return equipment to proper place.
11. Report and record as appropriate.	Report to the team leader or the nurse in charge that the colostomy irrigation has been given, the time it was given, and the results. Also note the patient's reaction to the procedure and any change in his condition, such as extreme weakness, dizziness, or pain.

Charting example:

2:10 P.M. Colostomy irrigation given. Moderate amount of soft brown stool with solution returned. Skin care given. Clean appliance applied.   J. Jones, NA

ITEM 26. CONCLUSION OF THE LESSON

You have now completed the lesson on bowel elimination. When you feel sure that you know the vocabulary, the abnormal characteristics of the feces, problems related to the hypoactive and hyperactive bowel, methods of control of the bowel, and have practiced the procedures used, arrange with your instructor to take the post-test.

V. ADDITIONAL INFORMATION FOR ENRICHMENT

The bowel is part of one of the major systems of the body. In this lesson on bowel elimination it has been possible to include only a small part of what is known about the bowel and its function. Those of you who have a special interest or a desire to learn more about nursing problems related to the bowel may wish to study further.

Some areas that might be of interest to you are listed:

1. Information related to the anatomy and physiology of the intestinal tract.

   A. Absorption of nutrients through the mechanisms of active transport and diffusion.

   B. Electrolytes, their function in body fluids, and imbalance of the body's acid-base balance.

   C. Types of bacteria present in the bowel, the function of the "good guys" and the identity of the "bad guys."

   D. The role of the liver and bile in the digestive process.

2. Causes, treatment, and nursing care of patients with diseases related to the bowel.

   A. Diarrheas and dysentery.

   B. Ulcers of the stomach or duodenum.

   C. Ulcerative colitis.

   D. Diverticulitis.

   E. Cancers of the bowel.

   F. Sprue and other nutritional diseases.

   G. Obstructions and intussusception of the bowel.

   H. Parasite and worm infestations of the bowel. Common in children in underdeveloped countries. Some cases are so severe that worms are regurgitated from the stomach and infest the lungs as well.

3. Other areas suggested by material in the lesson.

   A. Effects of various drugs on the bowel, especially the hypoactive and the hyperactive bowel.

   B. Incontinence problems of elderly patients.

   C. Indications, preparation, and procedure for proctoscopy and sigmoidoscopy.

   D. Preoperative and postoperative care of the colostomy patient.

   E. The altered body image and the psychological impact of the artificial anus.

   F. The special challenges to nursing care presented by the patient with an ileostomy.

   G. Procedure for irrigating a double-barrel, or two-loop, colostomy.

4. It is highly recommended that you contact the local chapter of the Colostomy Club which is part of a national organization, United Ostomy Association, Inc., found in many cities. A member of the club could be invited to speak to a group about his operation, his feelings about it, the problems he has encountered, and how he controls his colostomy.

When you have found a topic of interest to you, you will need to look up reading material on the subject in your library. If you have some difficulty finding material, contact your instructor, who may be able to help you find it.

WORKBOOK ANSWER SHEET

Vocabulary	P. 434	A.	(1)	mucus
			(2)	cecum
			(3)	tract
			(4)	flatus
			(5)	suppository
			(6)	polyp
	P. 435	B.	(1)	hemorrhage
			(2)	diarrhea
			(3)	hemorrhoids
Item 1	P. 436	C.		absorption, elimination of waste products
		D.		Answers (1), (3), and (4)
	P. 436	E.		distention
				diarrhea
				constipation
				incontinence
Item 2	P. 436	F.		6
	P. 437	G.		absorption
	P. 437	H.		1-S, 4-S, and 6-S
				2-L, 3-L, 5-L, and 7-L
	P. 438	I.	(1)	absorption of water and electrolytes
			(2)	storage of waste products
Item 3	P. 438	J.		solid material; water
		K.		brown; brownish-yellow
Item 4	P. 439	L.		blood; duodenum
		M.		10 hours
		N.		bright red blood
Item 5	P. 440	O.		green; watery
		P.		bile
		Q.		mucus
Item 6	P. 440	R.		circular, longitudinal, and oblique
		S.		peristalsis
		T.		pressure (or weight)
Item 10	PP. 441 and 443	U.		decreased
		V.		constipation; distention
		W.		Any five answers of the following: surgery, illness, disease, bed-rest, lack of roughage in diet, lack of exercise, certain drugs, fear, worry, anxiety

Item 11   P. 444   X.   absorption

                                 Y.   diarrhea

                                 Z.   Electrolytes

Item 12   P. 444   AA. three

                                 BB. (1) diet
                                      (2) fluids
                                      (3) exercise
                                      (4) rest

                                 CC. False

Item 13   P. 445   DD. inability to control feces elimination

                                 EE. retraining bowel control

                                 FF. (1) continence or control of bowels
                                      (2) regain self-respect

Item 14   P. 446   GG. (1) relieve pain
                                      (2) give medications
                                      (3) promote bowel movement

                                 HH. two

Item 17   P. 450-451   II. (1) tap water, saline, or soap solution or as
                                           ordered by the physician
                                      (2) 1000 ml.
                                      (3) 105° F. (40.5°C.)
                                      (4) 12 to 18 inches

                                 JJ. (1) rectum is over-distended
                                      (2) solution is too cool

Item 20   P. 454   KK. flatus, or abdominal distention

                                 LL. filling; draining

Item 23   P. 456   MM. attitude, or reaction

                                 NN. (1) to correct an obstruction
                                      (2) to rest an inflamed bowel
                                      (3) cancer

                                 OO. colostomy; descending colon

WORKSHEET

Directions: Read through each situation, then record the appropriate information on the nurse's notes for each situation.

Situation #1

At 2:30 P.M. the postoperative patient in 244 complained of severe cramping pain in his lower abdomen. The abdomen was definitely distended. Dr. Reed was notified by phone, and he ordered that a rectal tube be inserted. This was done at 2:40, and 15 minutes later the patient was comfortable after having expelled much flatus. Forty minutes after insertion, the tube was removed from the rectum, cleaned thoroughly, and returned to the Central Service room.

Situation #2

The patient in room 224 was given an S.S. enema at 2:15 P.M. He expelled the enema as given except for a few hard-formed particles of feces. Half an hour later Dr. Smith called and ordered that within the next 30 minutes a retention enema of 4 ounces of olive oil be given. The oil enema was retained the desired length of time and then expelled without any apparent result. Dr. Reed was notified and he ordered another S.S. enema to be given. This enema was expelled with a copious, soft-formed stool. Fifteen minutes after the second S.S. enema was given, the patient was sleeping.

SAINT JOHN'S HOSPITAL
SANTA MONICA, CALIFORNIA

NURSES' RECORD

DATE	HOSPITAL DAY	POST-OP.DAY	DATE	HOSPITAL DAY	POST-OP.DAY

	NIGHT	DAY	EVENING		NIGHT	DAY	EVENING
CHARGE NURSE				CHARGE NURSE			
MEDICINE NURSE				MEDICINE NURSE			

VISITS DOCTOR		TIME		VISITS DOCTOR		TIME	
DOCTOR				DOCTOR			

WEIGHT	TIME				WEIGHT	TIME			
	BLOOD PRESSURE					BLOOD PRESSURE			

DIET	APPETITE AM	NOON	PM	DIET	APPETITE AM	NOON	PM

O₂ LITERS   □ NASAL   □ TENT   □ CONTINUOUS   O₂ LITERS   □ NASAL   □ TENT   □ CONTINUOUS
_____   □ MASK   □ PRN   _____   □ MASK   □ PRN

□ BED REST □ BED BATH □ ORAL CARE	□ BED REST □ BED BATH □ ORAL CARE
□ CHAIR □ TUB BATH □ EVENING CARE	□ CHAIR □ TUB BATH □ EVENING CARE
□ BRP □ SHOWER □ SIDE RAILS UP	□ BRP □ SHOWER □ SIDE RAILS UP
□ UP AD LIB □ AM □ HS	□ UP AD LIB □ AM □ HS
□ VOIDING □ ENEMA □ HARRIS FLUSH	□ VOIDING □ ENEMA □ HARRIS FLUSH
□ STOOL □ SITZ BATH ____ ____ ____	□ STOOL □ SITZ BATH ____ ____ ____

TIME		TIME	

SAINT JOHN'S HOSPITAL
SANTA MONICA, CALIFORNIA

NURSES' RECORD

DATE	HOSPITAL DAY		POST-OP.DAY	DATE	HOSPITAL DAY		POST-OP.DAY
	NIGHT	DAY	EVENING		NIGHT	DAY	EVENING
CHARGE NURSE				CHARGE NURSE			
MEDICINE NURSE				MEDICINE NURSE			

VISITS DOCTOR			TIME			VISITS DOCTOR			TIME		
DOCTOR						DOCTOR					

WEIGHT	TIME					WEIGHT	TIME				
	BLOOD PRESSURE						BLOOD PRESSURE				

DIET		APPETITE AM	NOON	PM	DIET		APPETITE AM	NOON	PM

O₂ LITERS ____ □ NASAL □ TENT □ CONTINUOUS □ MASK □ PRN

O₂ LITERS ____ □ NASAL □ TENT □ CONTINUOUS □ MASK □ PRN

□ BED REST   □ BED BATH   □ ORAL CARE
□ CHAIR   □ TUB BATH   □ EVENING CARE
□ BRP   □ SHOWER   □ SIDE RAILS UP
□ UP AD LIB   □ AM   □ HS

□ BED REST   □ BED BATH   □ ORAL CARE
□ CHAIR   □ TUB BATH   □ EVENING CARE
□ BRP   □ SHOWER   □ SIDE RAILS UP
□ UP AD LIB   □ AM   □ HS

□ VOIDING   □ ENEMA   □ HARRIS FLUSH
□ STOOL   □ SITZ BATH ____ ____ ____

□ VOIDING   □ ENEMA   □ HARRIS FLUSH
□ STOOL   □ SITZ BATH ____ ____ ____

TIME		TIME	

PERFORMANCE TEST

In the skill laboratory, your instructor will ask you to determine your knowledge and skill in performing four of the following six activities without use of reference material:

1. Describe five unusual or abnormal conditions of the stool that you could observe visually.

2. Given a patient who has called you to empty feces from his bedpan, describe the steps you would take to collect a specimen of the stool and prepare it for the laboratory.

3. Given a patient who is incontinent of feces, you are to describe the factors that you would use in retraining the patient to control his bowels.

4. Given a recent postoperative patient with constipation due to a hypoactive bowel, you are to demonstrate the preparation and the procedure for giving a cleansing enema.

5. Given a recent postoperative patient with abdominal distention, you are to demonstrate the preparation and the procedure for giving a Harris flush.

6. Given a patient with a recent colostomy of the sigmoid colon, you are to demonstrate the preparation and the procedure for irrigating the colostomy as the patient sits on the toilet. (This is an optional performance test—will be used at the discretion of your instructor.)

PERFORMANCE CHECKLIST

BOWEL ELIMINATION

IDENTIFICATION OF ABNORMAL FECES

Identify at least five of the following abnormal conditions of the feces.

1. Brown — normal.

   Green — too much sugar in infant's diet.

   Greenish-black — (meconium) newborn infant.

   Orange-yellow — breast fed infant.

   Green — from chlorophyll.

   Some drugs may color stool.

   Clay — lack of bile secretion.

   Chalky-white — ingestion of X-ray preparation solutions.

   Light tan — undigested fat.

2. Blood: bright red indicates hemorrhage in lower bowel or from hemorrhoids.

   A. Dark brown to black indicates bleeding high in G.I. tract.

3. Mucus indicates irritation or inflammation of lining of intestine.

4. Parasitic worms: tapeworms, roundworms, pinworms.

5. Pus indicates drainage from infected portion of intestinal tract.

6. Constipation.

7. Diarrhea.

COLLECTION OF STOOL SPECIMENS

Student is to demonstrate correct method of stool specimen collection.

1. Gather equipment: two tongue blades; specimen container and lid; paper towel.

2. Wash hands.

3. Collect specimen.

4. Remove bedpan and take to appropriate work area.

5. Write patient's name, room number, and date in proper place on container.

6. Transfer, with tongue blade, at least one tablespoon of stool from bedpan to specimen container.

7. Put lid on container; wrap and discard tongue blade.

8. Empty, clean and return bedpan to storage.

9. Complete laboratory requisition. Check patient's name on requisition and specimen container to be sure they are the same. Be sure to use correct lab slip, indicating type of test ordered, date and time stool was passed.

10. Take to lab stat. Explain why delay in taking specimen to lab would alter the stool and give a false reading.

11. Record on patient's chart.

BOWEL TRAINING

Student is to describe factors in retraining the incontinent patient:

1. Adequate diet.

2. Adequate liquids, at least 2500 cc. liquid daily.

3. Sleep and exercise within patient's physical limits.

4. Regular time for bowel evacuation based on his prior habits.

5. At least 20 minutes allowed for bowels to move.

6. Suppository may be used on doctor's order. Given daily at same time for first week, then every other day the second and third weeks, and then PRN.

ENEMA

Student is to demonstrate steps in giving enemas.

1. Collect materials needed and wash hands.

2. Prepare solution as ordered (temperature at 105° F.).

3. Take to patient's room and place on chair near bed.

4. Identify patient.

5. Explain procedure and enlist patient's cooperation.

6. Wash hands.

7. Correctly prepare patient: screen for privacy, drapes, position patient, adjust bed height, and lower siderails.

8. Prepare to give enema:

   A. Lubricate tube about one inch.

   B. Expel air from tube.

   C. Allow solution to run into bedpan.

   D. Clamp tube.

9. Insert rectal tube, slowly and gently, four inches.

10. Open clamp.

   A. Run solution slowly.

   B. Hold can 12 to 18 inches above anus.

   C. Clamp tubing and wait if patient complains of cramps. Instruct patient to breathe deeply through mouth.

11. Remove rectal tube and place in paper towel.

12. Remove bedpan.

   A. Empty (observe contents).

   B. Clean bedpan.

   C. Store bedpan.

13. Leave patient comfortable.

    A. Permit patient to wash and dry hands.

    B. Use deodorizer if available and needed.

14. Record activity on chart.

HARRIS FLUSH

Student is to demonstrate method for performing Harris flush.

1. Collect equipment.

2. Identify and inform patient of procedure.

3. Prepare patient.

4. Wash hands.

5. Prepare rectal tube:

    A. Lubricate tube.

    B. Expel air from tube.

6. Insert tube, four inches.

7. Raise can 12 to 18 inches above anus.

8. Unclamp tube and insert 250 to 300 cc. solution.

9. Regulate flow with patient's ability to retain.

10. Drain solution from colon by lowering can to 12 to 18 inches below anus.

11. Repeat steps 4, 5 and 6 until no more flatus. (Procedure will take at least 15 minutes.)

12. Remove rectal tube and place in paper towel.

13. Provide for patient's comfort.

14. Remove equipment; clean; return to storage.

15. Record treatment on patient's chart.

COLOSTOMY IRRIGATION

Student will demonstrate procedure for colostomy irrigation.

1. Assemble equipment.

2. Wash hands.

3. Prepare solution (temperature 105°F. or 40.5° C) 1000 to 2000 cc.

4. Identify patient and inform him of procedure.

5. Prepare patient for procedure and provide for his privacy.

6. Attach plastic irrigating bag to appliance, or place plastic apron over patient.

7. Place distal end in commode (toilet) to direct flow.

8. Clamp tubing.

   A. Pour 1000 cc. solution into irrigating can.

   B. Expel air.

   C. Hang can on IV stand.

9. Lubricate tip of catheter.

   A. Place in stoma about 6 to 8 inches.

   B. Unclamp tubing as inserted for easier insertion.

10. Insert 250 cc. solution.

11. Remove catheter.

12. Place irrigating bag over stoma and allow solution to drain out.

13. Repeat step 8 until solution returns clear, no flatus.

14. Remove irrigating bag (or apron).

15. Cleanse skin and dry.

16. Attach clean colostomy bag (patient may do this himself). Let patient wash hands.

17. Leave patient comfortable.

18. Clean, dry, and return equipment to storage.

19. Record treatment on patient's chart.

Unit 23

COLLECTION OF SPUTUM AND GASTRIC SPECIMENS, AND CARE OF THE VOMITING PATIENT

I. DIRECTIONS TO THE STUDENT

Please read the following paragraphs carefully. They will tell you what you will be expected to do and know with respect to the collection of sputum and gastric content specimens, and how to care for the vomiting patient.

Proceed through the lesson. Practice the steps of the procedures on the laboratory mannequin (Mrs. Chase). It will not be necessary at this point to obtain an actual specimen of sputum or emesis.

After you have practiced and are well-acquainted with the steps of the procedures, you should arrange with your instructor to take the post-test. You will be expected to perform the activities accurately.

II. GENERAL PERFORMANCE OBJECTIVE

After completing this unit, you will be able to assist the patient to provide a sample of sputum and to collect and label sputum and gastric content specimens for the laboratory.

You will also be able to take care of the vomiting patient in a skillful and effective manner while giving him emotional reassurance and physical support.

III. SPECIFIC PERFORMANCE OBJECTIVES

When you have finished this lesson, you will be able to:

1. Instruct and assist the patient to produce sputum without undue discomfort and distress, and collect the sputum specimen correctly for delivery to the laboratory.

2. Collect a gastric content specimen and prepare it correctly for delivery to the laboratory.

3. Provide care for the patient who is or has been vomiting in such a manner that he will feel more comfortable, and so reduce the stimulation of the "gagging" or vomiting reflex.

IV. VOCABULARY

aspiration—to draw in or out of a cavity of the body by suction; withdrawal of fluid from a body cavity by suction with an instrument called an aspirator.

bronchitis—inflammation of the mucous membrane of the bronchi (airway) into the lung.

diagnosis—the process of identifying a disease from its signs or symptoms: reflexes, general appearance, laboratory and X-ray examinations, etc.

emesis—vomiting.

expectorate—spitting out or expulsion of mucus or phlegm from the throat or lungs.

projectile vomiting—forceful and sudden ejection of stomach contents, usually without preceding nausea.

pneumonia—inflammation of the lungs caused by various organisms which produce a high fever, a collection of mucus in the lungs, and pain when breathing.

saliva—a liquid secreted by the salivary glands in the mouth which moistens food and assists in the digestive process, acting mainly on starches.

sputum—substance from the lungs which is coughed up and spit out of the mouth; it contains saliva, mucus, and sometimes pus.

tuberculosis (TBC)—an infectious disease caused by the tubercle bacillus, commonly affecting the lung or other organs.

vomitus—gastric contents ejected through the mouth during the act of vomiting.

V. INTRODUCTION

In this unit, we will be considering primarily the patient with a possible respiratory problem and cough, and the patient who is vomiting. It may be necessary to obtain specimens of sputum from the coughing patient to aid in the diagnosis and determination of his disease. It is important to know that the patient may be encouraged to cough (in certain medical and postoperative situations) in order to clear mucus from the respiratory tract and from the lungs. This promotes adequate expansion and ventilation of the lungs. However, in other postoperative conditions, such as eye surgery or hernia repair, it is advisable to inhibit (prevent) coughing. Sputum specimens are requested most often from patients who are suspected of having a respiratory disease such as pneumonia, tuberculosis, or bronchitis. Obtaining the specimen may be difficult, painful, or unpleasant for the patient, and so you must know how you can best assist the patient.

A specimen of gastric contents obtained from the patient vomitus is seldom required for laboratory examination in the hospital. Often a visual inspection of the vomitus by the doctor or the nurse is sufficient to provide the necessary information. Most specimens of gastric content are obtained by inserting a tube down the patient's nose into his stomach in order to aspirate some of the gastric contents for the specimen. This is the procedure used by the doctor when he wants to determine the presence or absence of normal stomach acids, the presence of poisons or drugs, etc. You will learn more about this in the unit on gastro-intestinal tubes. You may be called upon to prepare such a specimen for the laboratory so that this unpleasant procedure need not be repeated by the patient.

One of the most common discomforts of the patient in the hospital is vomiting. Various medications are now used that help control vomiting and the accompanying nausea. However, some patients may vomit because of their disease, or before the medication is ordered for them. You should know how to care for the patient who is or has been vomiting. Various nursing measures can be used to make the patient more comfortable and to reduce the possible recurrence of nausea and vomiting.

ITEM 1. COLLECTION OF THE SPUTUM SPECIMEN

In the classroom or the skill laboratory, you should practice the steps of the procedure until you are familiar with them and can carry them out skillfully.

Important Steps	Key Points
1. Wash your hands.	

Important Steps	Key Points

2. Obtain the materials needed for the specimen.

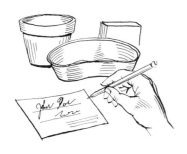

Container and cover for the specimen, a small paper bag, tissues, a label for the container, and the laboratory requisition slip.

The label should have the patient's full name, room number, hospital unit or floor number, date, and time of collection. The laboratory slip should be properly marked with the patient's identifying information, the tests to be done, and signature. Most hospitals now have mechanical recorders (Addressograph) that imprint identifying patient information from a metal or plastic card.

Take all items except the laboratory slip to the patient's room.

3. Approach and identify the patient.

Check the patient's identification band, read his name aloud, and have him confirm it.

4. Give instructions to the patient on how to collect the sputum specimen.

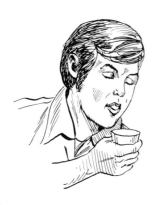

Explain that sputum is the mucus coughed up from his lungs, and *not* the saliva in his mouth. Ask him to cover his mouth with tissues when coughing. (This will prevent him from coughing germs into the air you and others breathe.) Have him hold the sputum container close to his mouth and spit the coughed up sputum into the container.

5. Assist the patient to provide an immediate specimen, if possible.

Provide for the patient's privacy. If he is able, he may go to the bathroom while trying to produce the sputum. If he is not able to get up and if other patients are in the room, pull the curtain to provide visual privacy. The curtain will not shut out the sound of coughing, but it keeps others from seeing the effort involved.

Ask the patient to breathe deeply and cough to bring up the sputum from the lungs, and not merely from the back of the throat.

Collect at least one to two tablespoons of sputum, unless directed otherwise. Observe the patient carefully and assist him when necessary; offer encouragement.

Avoid contamination with his sputum. Keep the outside of the container and your hands free of sputum when you are collecting and transporting it to the laboratory.

After getting the sputum in the container, seal it with the lid. Wash and dry the outside of the container (paper towels from the patient's bathroom may be used). Put the labeled con-

Important Steps	Key Points
	tainer in the paper bag for delivery to the laboratory with the lab requisition slip. (Some agencies do not require that the specimen be enclosed in a paper bag. Follow your agency procedure for transporting sputum specimens to the laboratory.)
6. Give the patient instructions again if he is unable to produce an immediate specimen and ask him to notify the nurse when he is able to get the specimen.	It may be easier for the patient to produce the specimen early in the morning. Mucous that collected in the lungs during the night is more apt to be coughed up at this time. Have the patient notify the nurse who will pick up the specimen.
7. Provide for the patient's safety and comfort.	
8. Arrange for delivery of the specimen to the laboratory.	Use the appropriate method designated by the hospital. If there is any delay in delivering the specimen, put it in the refrigerator used for specimens.
9. Record all pertinent information concerning this task in the nurse's notes of the patient's chart.	The following descriptive terms used in charting include statements on the color, amount, odor, consistency, date, and time: hemoptysis — blood in sputum. color variations — clear, gray, yellow, red, brown, green, and black. consistency — liquid; thick and sticky (tenacious); mucous-like (mucoid). profuse — large amount. scanty — small amount.

ITEM 2. ASSISTING THE PATIENT TO COUGH

There are times when it is very painful for the patient to cough. If the patient has pain in the abdominal or chest area when he coughs, obtain a drawsheet or folded large sheet and wrap it around the painful area of his body. Hold the sheet securely with minimal pressure so that the body walls of the affected area are supported. This gives the patient the external pressure necessary to equalize the internal pressure occurring during the coughing period, and minimizes the pain and discomfort. *Do not hold the sheet too tightly* so that you defeat your purpose by causing pain and increased difficulty in breathing.

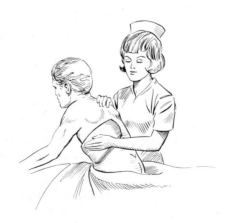

ITEM 3. CARE OF THE VOMITING PATIENT

This part of the lesson is concerned with the physical cleanliness and the emotional support you can provide the patient who has been vomiting or who is now vomiting. Often the patient is fearful and apologetic during an episode of vomiting. He is distressed by his illness, his discomfort, and often by the fact that he is dependent upon someone else to clean up after he has vomited. You must reassure the patient that you will help him and provide for his comfort. It is important that you perform this task skillfully and effectively in a matter-of-fact, pleasant, and gentle manner.

Important Steps	Key Points
1. Closely observe patients who complain of nausea or who may vomit (e.g., those recovering from anesthesia, those who have taken certain medications or therapy, those who are acutely ill).	Place emesis basin and tissues within reach of the patient. Ask him to put on his call signal if you can be of help, or when he vomits.
2. Assist the patient by telling him how to reduce the nausea and vomiting.	Resting quietly and avoiding sudden movements, or resting on one side with his knees flexed may be helpful. It is important to remove or reduce odors which may stimulate nausea and the "gagging" reflex (e.g., strong, sweet perfume of flowers, smell of food or smoke, disagreeable odors of feces or drainage). Remember, it is particularly important for you to be scrupulously clean and free from heavy perfumes, lotions, cigarette smoke, and other odors because sick people are often hypersensitive. Have the patient take short, panting breaths through the mouth when he feels acutely nauseated.
3. Provide assistance to the patient who is vomiting or has vomited. 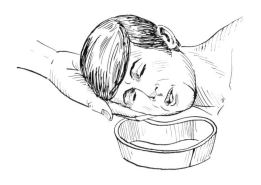	Wash your hands. Position the patient's head on one side and place the emesis basin under his cheek to catch the emesis. Use tissues to wipe vomitus from nose or mouth, to avoid possible *inspiration* of the vomitus material into the patient's lungs. This may cause "aspiration pneumonia," which could be fatal. *Note:* Provide for the patient's privacy as soon as you can by closing the door if he is in a single room; if not, pull the curtains around the bed, or ask others in the room to step outside the room if they are able. After the patient has vomited, take the emesis basin to the bathroom or utility room. Note the color, odor, consistency, and other characteristics of the vomitus. Measure the amount of emesis before discarding. Record amount as output if the patient has an Intake and Output record. Wash and dry the basin, and return it for future use by the patient.
4. Leave the patient safe and as comfortable as possible.	Prepare mouth wash or toothbrush and dentifrice so the patient can use them to refresh his mouth. Vomiting leaves a foul taste in the mouth. Some patients may simply wish to rinse out the mouth with tap water to avoid further nausea or vomiting. Provide wash basin with warm water, washcloth, towel, and soap and assist or wash the patient's face and hands.

Important Steps	Key Points
5. Remove soiled linen and tidy up the room.	Change all soiled linen. Remember, the odor of vomitus lingers if the immediate area is not cleaned thoroughly. This odor will often induce further nausea and vomiting. If it is possible, open the window to air the room for a few minutes, or use an unscented room deodorizer.
6. Record all pertinent information on the nurses' notes of the patient's chart.	The following descriptive terms are used in charting: hematemesis — blood in the vomitus. tarry — looks black, usually from old blood. partially digested food — this is from a recent meal and should be described. odor — any unusual smell: sweet, fruity, sour, fecal, etc. amount — scanty, moderate, or large. projectile vomiting — sudden, forceful emesis.

ITEM 4. COLLECTION OF A GASTRIC CONTENT SPECIMEN

There are two ways of obtaining a sample of the gastric contents for a specimen to be sent to the laboratory: (1) from the emesis produced by a vomiting patient, and (2) by passing a tube into the stomach and aspirating the amount of contents needed for the specimen. Regardless of the method used to obtain the gastric contents, you should know how to prepare the specimen for the laboratory.

Important Steps	Key Points
1. Wash your hands and obtain the necessary items to prepare a gastric specimen for the laboratory.	You will need a specimen container with a lid, labels and laboratory requisition slip marked with the patient's name, room number, hospital unit or floor number, and the tests to be done. Some specimens obtained from passing a tube and aspirating are put into test tubes instead of a container, but *all tubes should be labeled and numbered in the sequence* that they were obtained or at the time they were collected.
2. Identify the patient and ascertain that he is the one who produced the specimen.	Be sure the name on the identification band of the patient and the name on the lab slip are the same. A common and costly error is the mislabeling of specimens. *Extreme caution must be taken* to correctly label every specimen.
3. Obtain the sample of gastric contents either from the emesis basin of the vomiting patient, or from the aspirated material.	Pour it into the specimen container and apply the lid. If it is put in test tubes, apply a stopper type of lid. Avoid contaminating the specimen container or tube while pouring the specimen in it. Wash and dry the outer surface if it has been soiled. Use paper towels. Attach the labels to the specimen container or test tubes. Check labels again to be sure they correspond to the patient's identification band.
4. Prepare for delivery to the laboratory.	Be *sure* to include the laboratory requisition slip. Some hospitals require that the specimen and the lab slip be put in a paper bag for delivery to the laboratory. Some agencies use some other methods, so you should check with

Important Steps	Key Points
	your nurse. Arrange for the specimen to be taken to the laboratory by messenger service or place it in the refrigerator used for storing specimens.
5. Wash and dry all of the equipment you have used and store it in the proper place.	Paper towels are very convenient for drying equipment; they are clean and disposable; use them, but don't waste them. Return the patient's emesis basis to his bedside if this was used to obtain the specimen.
6. Indicate on the nurses' notes of the patient's chart that the specimen was obtained, sent to the laboratory, and note the time.	Charting example: 10:30 A.M. Gastric specimen sent with requisition to laboratory. J. Jones, LVN

ITEM 5. CONCLUSION OF THE LESSON

You have now completed the unit on the collection of sputum and gastric contents and the care of the vomiting patient. When you have practiced the steps of the procedure so that you are very familiar with them, you should arrange with your instructor to take the post-test and demonstrate your skills in performing these procedures accurately.

POST-TEST

Multiple Choice: Select the best answer and check it.

1. A specimen of sputum is often required from the coughing patient in order to:

____A. Provide for adequate ventilation of the lungs.

____B. Determine the presence of a respiratory problem.

____C. Determine the nature of a respiratory disease.

2. Visual inspection of a specimen by the doctor or the nurse is often adequate to provide the needed information in the case of:

____A. Aspirated gastric contents.

____B. Vomitus.

____C. Mucous.

____D. Sputum.

3. The fluid which is secreted by a gland in the mouth is called:

____A. Sputum.

____B. Saliva.

____C. Phlegm.

____D. Emesis.

4. All but one of the following may be ways to reduce the recurrence of nausea and vomiting in the patient. The item that does not apply is:

____A. Rest quietly and not move around much.

____B. Take short, panting breaths through the mouth.

____C. Rest on one side with knees flexed in Sims' position.

____D. Provide close observation of the patient.

5. The presence of blood in the sputum is called:

____A. Tenacious.

____B. Hematemesis.

____C. Hemotysis.

____D. Tarry

6. The process of drawing in or out by suction is called:

____A. Aspiration.

____B. Expectoration.

____C. Irrigation.

____D. Elimination.

7. Before emptying the emesis basin after the patient has vomited, you should:

____A. Air the room to reduce the odor.

____B. Encourage the patient to drink a glass of water.

____C. Remove flowers and meal trays from the room.

____D. Measure the amount of emesis.

8. Many patients may be unable to produce an immediate specimen of sputum when it is requested. It is often easier for the patient to produce the specimen:

____A. During the night.

____B. When he is alone.

____C. Early in the morning.

____D. After a meal.

9. After a patient has vomited, you can provide for his comfort by:

____A. Assisting him to brush his teeth.

____B. Having him rinse his mouth out.

____C. Changing any soiled bed linen.

____D. All of the above.

____E. A. and C only.

10. In preparing an aspirated gastric specimen for the laboratory, the laboratory requisition slip should contain the following information:

____A. Name, date, age, and tests to be done.

____B. Room number, sequence of specimen, and name.

____C. Tests to be done, name, and room number.

____D. Hospital unit number, birthdate, and tests to be done.

POST-TEST ANNOTATED ANSWER SHEET

1. C — p. 474
2. B — p. 474
3. B — p. 475
4. D — p. 477
5. C — p. 476
6. A — p. 474
7. D — p. 477
8. C — p. 476
9. D — p. 477
10. B or C — p. 479

PERFORMANCE POST-TEST

In the classroom or the skill laboratory, your instructor will ask you to demonstrate the following procedures. You should be able to do so accurately without reference to your study guide, notes, or other source material.

1. Given a patient with a suspected respiratory disease who is allowed bathroom privileges, you are to instruct and assist the patient to produce a specimen of sputum, and prepare the specimen for delivery to the laboratory.

2. Given a patient who has just vomited the lunch he had eaten a half hour ago, you are to provide for the patient's comfort and assist him by suggesting ways to reduce the recurrence of the nausea and vomiting. The pillow case and spread have been soiled by the emesis.

3. Given the patient who has had some gastric contents aspirated by the physician, you are to prepare the specimen correctly for delivery to the laboratory.

PERFORMANCE CHECKLIST

COLLECTION OF SPUTUM AND GASTRIC SPECIMENS, AND CARE OF THE VOMITING PATIENT

COLLECTION AND PREPARATION OF GASTRIC SPECIMEN

Student will demonstrate correct method for collecting and preparing a gastric specimen.

1. Obtain necessary items and prepare labels after washing hands.
2. Identify patient as the one who produced the specimen.
3. Pour basin of aspirated gastric contents into specimen container or test tube.
4. Put lid or stopper on container, clean outer surfaces, and attach label.
5. Arrange for delivery of specimen and laboratory slip to laboratory.
6. Wash, dry, and return all equipment to proper place.
7. Record pertinent information on patient's chart.

CARE OF VOMITING PATIENT

Student will demonstrate steps in the care of a vomiting patient.

1. Approach patient and provide for his privacy after washing hands.
2. Position patient's head to the side, with emesis basin under cheek.
3. Use tissues to wipe vomitus from mouth, nose, and face.
4. Measure emesis, note characteristics, and discard it.
5. Wash, dry, and return emesis basin to bedside.
6. Provide oral hygiene for patient, or solution to rinse out his mouth.
7. Wash patient's face and hands.
8. Change any soiled linen on bed.
9. Air room, if possible.
10. Instruct patient on ways to reduce feelings of nausea and vomiting.
11. Provide for patient's safety and comfort.
12. Remove soiled linen from room.
13. Record pertinent information on patient's chart.

COLLECTION OF SPUTUM SPECIMEN

Student will demonstrate necessary steps in the collection of a sputum specimen.

1. Wash hands.
2. Obtain necessary items and prepare labels correctly.
3. Identify the patient.
4. Instruct patient on how to collect specimen.

5. Provide for patient's privacy.

6. Assist patient as needed.

7. Avoid contamination of hands, uniform, and container with patient's sputum.

8. Seal container, wash and dry outside of container.

9. Apply label to container.

10. Put labeled container and laboratory slip in paper bag for delivery to laboratory.

11. Provide for patient's safety and comfort.

12. Arrange for delivery of specimen to laboratory.

13. Record pertinent information on patient's chart.

U
N
I
T
23

NOTES

Unit 24

PERINEAL CARE

I. DIRECTIONS TO THE STUDENT

Please read the following paragraphs carefully. They will tell you what you are expected to know about perineal care. You are to practice the procedure in your classroom or laboratory until you feel confident of your ability and skills. You will need the following items for the procedure:

1. A perineal care tray containing:

   a. A graduate or pitcher

   b. Cotton balls or gauze squares

   c. Dressing — sanitary pad, ABD, or 4 x 4's

   d. T-binder for male or female

   e. Chux pads

   f. Dressing forceps — optional

   g. Paper (newspaper, paper bag, wax paper, etc.)

2. Bedpan

3. Mrs. Chase, or similar type mannequin, for practice purposes

4. Bath blanket

When you have had sufficient practice in the procedure, you should arrange with your instructor to take the performance test. You will be expected to perform the procedure to demonstrate your knowledge and skill.

II. GENERAL PERFORMANCE OBJECTIVE

As a health worker, you will be able to assist the patient with the care and cleanliness of his perineal area, and to give perineal care as required. You will perform this task skillfully, effectively, and in a reassuring manner to reduce or avoid embarassment to the patient.

III. SPECIFIC PERFORMANCE OBJECTIVES

Upon completion of this lesson, you will be able to:

1. Provide perineal care for the female patient by pouring warm solution over the perineal area, cleansing and drying the area properly, applying a dressing or pad, if required, and securing it in place.

2. Provide perineal care for the male patient by pouring warm solution over the perineal area, cleansing and drying the area properly, applying a pad or dressing, if required, and securing the dressing in place.

3. Approach the patient, explain the procedure in an objective or matter-of-fact way, and give reassurance in a nonjudgmental way in order to avoid embarrassing the patient.

IV. VOCABULARY

A-P repair—corrective surgery of the female perineum which includes repair of anterior and posterior muscle defects, tears or weakness usually occurring after the birth of a baby.

genitalia—the reproductive organs of the male and the female.

hysterectomy—surgical removal of the uterus (womb).

perineal—refers to the perineum.

perineum—the area between the vulva and the anus in the female; and between the scrotum and the anus in the male.

lochia—the discharge from the uterus of blood, mucus, and tissue in the period immediately following the delivery of a baby.

scrotum—the double pouch containing the testicles and part of the spermatic cord in the male.

uterus—the muscular, hollow, pear-shaped organ of the female, located within the abdomen; the womb.

vulva—the external female genitalia.

vaginal hysterectomy—surgical removal of the uterus (womb) through the vaginal opening.

V. INTRODUCTION

Perineal care (usually referred to in the hospital as "peri care") is necessary for the health and well-being of the patient. It is the term usually applied to the external irrigation or cleansing of the vulva and perineum following voiding or defecation. The procedure is performed to prevent contamination or infection in the genital area, and to remove drainage or odors through cleansing. The procedure is used following the birth of a child, or following an operation involving surgery on the perineum, the vagina, the lower urinary tract, or the anus. Although the procedure is more commonly performed for the woman patient, it may be required for the male patient following surgery on the perineum or the anus.

You will find that some health workers use the term "peri care" to refer to the portion of the patient's bath when the genital area is washed and dried. Usually the patient is able to perform this part of his bath, but you may need to complete this portion for certain patients who are helpless. The use of the term "peri care" is correct in this situation, but this lesson will be concerned with cleaning the perineal area by external irrigation, or pouring of solution.

ITEM 1. DEALING WITH PATIENT EMBARRASSMENT

The procedure of giving perineal care to the patient may cause embarrassment to the patient as a result of the nurse's close contact with the patient's genitals. Most patients will accept the nurse's assistance and make very little fuss about having the procedure done. A few, however, may find it very difficult to overcome their feelings of embarrassment and will try to avoid the perineal care even when they know it might be necessary.

Why do patients become embarrassed and reluctant about using the bedpan or having perineal care? We all know some of the reasons. In this country, until very recent changes of attitude, our cultural and social customs were such that certain parts of the body and its functions were not seen, discussed, or even acknowledged in public. The genital part of the body was considered very private, and the person raised in this kind of culture and according to these customs regards it as so. When this person becomes a patient, his attitude about the privacy of his body does not change much.

As a nursing worker, how can you deal with this problem? First, you need to understand that *you* may have some embarrassment initially if you have been raised in a similar culture with similar customs. Your own embarrassment will be reduced if you remember that your purpose is to *assist the patient.* By regarding the patient as a whole person, you can develop a calm and matter-of-fact attitude and a nonjudgmental manner while accepting his right to have and express his feelings. Explaining the need for perineal care and the reasons for it can reassure the patient so that he will willingly cooperate in the procedure without undue embarrassment. When performing the procedure, you should be matter-of-fact and objective, and avoid any suggestive conversation or actions.

ITEM 2. PROCEDURE FOR PERINEAL CARE FOR THE FEMALE PATIENT

Important Steps

Key Points

1. Wash your hands. Refer to the unit on handwashing for instructions.

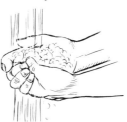

2. Obtain necessary supplies and equipment. Use the perineal tray if one is provided and take it to the patient's bedside table.

You will need the following: a pitcher or graduate, 500 cc. of water or other solution at approximately 105°F., cotton balls or gauze squares for cleaning, dressing, T-binder, Chux pad, and dressing forceps if used. If the dressing to be used is a sanitary pad, most women will prefer to use an elastic sanitary belt to secure the pad, rather than a T-binder.

3. Approach and identify the patient, explain what is to be done, and enlist her cooperation.

4. Prepare and position the patient.

Provide for privacy by closing the door of the room, pulling the cubicle curtain, or using a screen.

Position the bed by lowering the siderail, if one is used, and elevating the head of the bed slightly. Position the patient by having her lie on her back with her knees flexed and elevated.

Drape the patient to avoid undue exposure. Place the bath blanket over her, have her hold the upper edge, while you fan-fold the upper covers to the foot of the bed. Raise the lower edge of the bath blanket to her pubic area and place the lower sides of the blanket over each knee, as shown in the sketch.

Remove the soiled pad or dressing. Observe the amount and type of drainage, then wrap in paper for discarding. Place the patient on a bedpan, after placing the Chux under her hips.

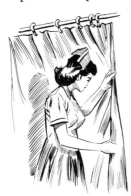

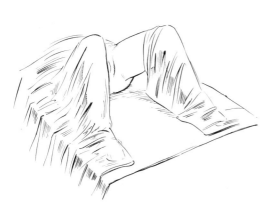

Important Steps	Key Points
5. Give the perineal care. 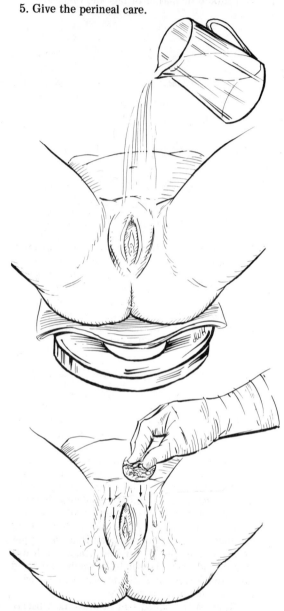	Pour warm (105°F.) tap water or prescribed solution over the perineal area to rinse off urine, fecal or vaginal drainage. Moisten several cotton balls or gauze squares with the remaining solution. Use forceps or your fingers to hold, and stroke from the pubic area down toward the rectum, then discard. *Do not make more than one downward stroke with the cleansing cotton ball.* (Cotton balls and gauze clog the plumbing, so they should be discarded by wrapping them in paper and put in the trash container, not in the bedpan.) *Note:* Some agencies use a disposable toilet cleansing tissue instead of cotton balls or squares. Follow your agency procedure. Wipe the perineum dry with fresh cotton balls, or gauze squares. (Toilet tissues may also be used in this unsterile procedure.) Use each ball, gauze or tissue only once, stroking from the pubis to the rectum, then discard it in the paper. If you wipe upward, you may bring fecal material into the wound or vaginal opening; this could lead to a serious infection. Remove the bedpan. Dry the lower perineum and the buttocks. Wrap soiled cotton balls or gauze before disposing of them in the trash. Apply the clean dressing or the pad. Fasten ends of pad to sanitary belt. Use T-binder to secure the dressings in place. (The cross-bar of the T-binder is fastened around the waist, the tail of the T passes through the legs from the back and is fastened to the waist of the binder in the front.)
6. Replace the top covers and remove the bath blanket.	Fold it and return it to the bedside stand or the storage place. Remove the Chux.
7. Remove the equipment from the patient's unit.	Wash, rinse, and dry the equipment. Store in the proper place. (In some agencies, the perineal tray is exchanged daily with clean equipment from Central Supply.)
8. Provide for the patient's comfort.	Leave signal cord within reach, raise siderail if used, adjust position of bed as desired, and leave bedside stand and personal articles within easy reach. Tell the patient when you expect to return.

Important Steps	Key Points
9. Report and record.	Record procedure on the patient's chart and report to your team leader or the nurse in charge that it has been done. Charting example: 10:30 A.M. Perineal care given. Moderate amount of lochia, a few small clots. A. Jones, NA

ITEM 3.   SELF PERINEAL CARE BY THE PATIENT

When the patient is allowed up and is able to care for herself, she should be taught to perform the procedure herself. She can assemble the necessary materials, take them to the bathroom, pour the solution, cleanse and dry herself, and apply a clean pad or dressing.

The following points should be stressed when you give instructions to the patient:

1. Be sure to have a paper or brown bag in which to wrap the soiled pad or dressing and the cotton balls or gauze used to clean and dry the perineum. All soiled material should be wrapped securely before disposing of it.

2. When cleansing or drying with a cotton ball or gauze, wipe once *from front toward the rectum* with each ball. Discard, and use clean ball for the next stroke until the entire perineum has been cleaned and dried.

ITEM 4.   PERINEAL CARE FOR THE MALE PATIENT

Perineal care may be ordered for the male patient following various types of perineal surgery. Usually the procedure is carried out by a male health worker or orderly since the male patient may be more embarrassed if it is done by a female health worker. However, not all agencies have as many male health workers as they would like, and so it may be necessary for the female health worker to carry out the procedure for a male patient, until he is able to do it for himself.

The steps of the procedure are the same as those listed in Item 2 for the female patient.

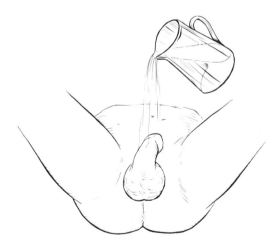

A sanitary pad would not be used for the male patient, however; his dressings would be held in place by a double-tailed T-binder. The double-tailed binder allows for proper support of the scrotum, as shown below.

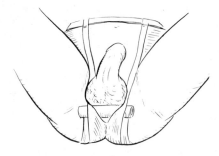

ITEM 5.   CONCLUSION OF THE LESSON

After you have practiced the perineal care procedure until you are thoroughly familiar with it and can do it skillfully, arrange with your instructor to take the performance test. You should be able to demonstrate the procedure accurately.

PERFORMANCE CHECKLIST

In the classroom or skill laboratory, your instructor will ask you to demonstrate your skill in carrying out the following procedures without reference to your study guide, notes, or other source material. You are to use the Chase doll to simulate the patient.

1. Given a woman patient who has delivered a baby a few hours ago, you are to give her perineal care in order to cleanse the perineum of discharges, and apply a clean sanitary pad without causing her embarrassment or discomfort.

2. Given a male patient who has had perineal surgery, you are to give him perineal care, apply clean dressings, and secure the dressings with a double-tailed T-binder in the proper way. State how you would attempt to reduce his embarrassment about this procedure.

3. Properly record the following notations.

   At 2:00 p.m., a patient who had a purulent, highly offensive vaginal discharge was seen by Dr. Smith, who ordered tap water perineal care to be given "Stat." The return flow was at first light yellow in color, gradually becoming clear. The offensive odor persisted throughout the treatment. The patient complained that the solution was too hot (115°F.). She said also that she would refuse to have another such treatment even if it was ordered by the doctor.

PERFORMANCE CHECKLIST

PERINEAL CARE

GIVING PERINEAL CARE TO A FEMALE PATIENT

The student will demonstrate the proper giving of perineal care to a female patient.

1. Wash hands.

2. Obtain all needed supplies.

3. Identify patient and approach her in a matter-of-fact, reassuring manner.

4. Provide for patient's privacy by closing door, pulling curtain, or using screens.

5. Position patient on her back with knees bent and elevated.

6. Drape patient with bath blanket to prevent undue exposure.

7. Remove soiled dressing or pad.

8. Place patient on bedpan with a Chux under hips and pan.

9. Pour water or solution of $105°$F. over the perineal area.

10. Use moistened cotton balls, one at a time, and stroke gently from pubic area toward rectum once with each to cleanse perineum. Use gentle strokes to avoid causing discomfort.

11. Use dry cotton balls, gauzes, or tissue to dry perineum, stroking from front to rectum one time with each ball.

12. Remove bedpan and apply clean pad.

13. Discard all soiled dressings, pads, cotton balls, etc., by wrapping them in paper before disposing of them.

14. Provide for patient's comfort by removing bath blanket, adjusting top covers, placing signal cord, elevating siderail.

15. Remove equipment from bedside and clean it before returning it to storage place.

PERINEAL CARE FOR THE MALE PATIENT

The student will demonstrate the correct method of perineal care for a male patient.

1. Wash hands.

2. Obtain all supplies.

3. Identify patient and approach him in a matter-of-fact, reassuring manner.

4. State ways which would attempt to reduce embarrassment, e.g., explanation of procedure, reasons for it, avoiding suggestive conversation or actions.

5. Provide for patient's privacy by closing door, pulling curtain, or using screens.

6. Position patient on his back with knees bent and elevated.

7. Drape patient with bath blanket to prevent undue exposure.

8. Remove soiled dressing.

9. Place Chux under hips and place him on bedpan.

10. Pour water or solution of 105° F. over perineal area.

11. Clean perineum by using moistened cotton balls and stroking gently from pubic area toward rectum once with each one.

12. Dry perineum by using dry cotton balls, gauze, or tissue, wiping from the front to rectum once with each one.

13. Remove bedpan.

14. Apply clean dressing and secure it with a double-tailed T-binder. Apply T-binder and dressing correctly to support scrotum.

15. Discard all soiled dressings, pads, cotton balls by wrapping them in paper before disposing of them.

16. Provide for patient's comfort by removing bath blanket, adjusting top covers, placing signal cord, elevating siderail.

17. Remove equipment from bedside and clean it before returning it to storage place.

NOTES

Unit 25

CARE OF THE PATIENT WITH GASTROINTESTINAL TUBES

I. DIRECTIONS TO THE STUDENT

Read the lesson carefully because it is quite complex. You will need to study every detail in order to become knowledgeable about the care of patients who require the use of gastrointestinal (g.i.) tubes of several varieties.

II. GENERAL PERFORMANCE OBJECTIVE

At the completion of this unit you will be able to employ the correct techniques for caring for patients with various gastrointestinal tubes: tubes with suction, without suction, and those used for special feedings and special laboratory tests.

III. SPECIFIC PERFORMANCE OBJECTIVES

When you have finished this unit, you will be able to:

1. Identify four kinds of tubes used in the gastric analysis procedure.

2. Assemble equipment and assist with the insertion of the various gastrointestinal tubes.

3. Feed a patient with a gastrostomy or enterostomy tube, or through the proctoclysis procedure.

4. Identify and describe the action of the four common types of suction apparatus, e.g., portable electric suction, wall-outlet suction, Gomco Thermotic Pump, and a water displacement system, with or without suction and with intermittent or continuous action.

5. Describe and be prepared to give major nursing care activities to patients with various types of gastrointestinal tubes, e.g., testing, drainage, suction and feeding.

6. Describe and record correctly and accurately the color, amount, and consistency of the intake and/or output of patients with gastrointestinal tubes discussed in this unit.

IV. VOCABULARY

burette—a graduated glass.
Cantor tube—a single long tube used for intestinal decompression. It has a mercury-weighted balloon at its distal tip to assist in stimulating peristalsis and moving the tube into the intestine. It is inserted through the nose and down the digestive tract to the intestine; the proximal end of the tube is connected to a suction machine.
decompression—removal of air or drainage from a wound, cavity or passageway.
distention—the state of being stretched out or bloated, e.g., the abdominal cavity may be distended with gas or fluid.

enterostomy (enter- = intestine; -ostomy = mouth)—a surgical operation to make a permanent or temporary opening through the abdominal wall into a part of the intestinal tract. This opening is used when feeding patients who may have a carcinoma in the digestive tract above the surgical opening.

esophagus—the muscular tube in the digestive tract which connects the oral cavity with the stomach. It is located directly behind the trachea (windpipe).

Ewald tube—a specific rubber tube with a large lumen (opening) passed through the mouth and down the esophagus to the stomach to withdraw stomach contents for various laboratory examinations. Useful in determining a disease (diagnosis).

flatus—expulsion of gas (air) rectally; if gas is expelled orally, it is called burping or eructating.

gag reflex—an involuntary *(not* controlled by the will) retching or vomiting action caused by stimulation of certain nerve endings in the back of the throat which in turn stimulate the vomiting center in the brain.

gastric—refers to stomach.

gastrostomy (gastro- = stomach; -ostomy = mouth)—a surgical operation making a temporary or permanent opening through the abdominal wall into the stomach. A tube is inserted into the opening and the patient may be fed in this manner. This procedure may be done for a carcinoma in the upper digestive tract.

gavage—feeding through a tube inserted into the stomach. The tube is inserted through the nose and down the esophagus to the stomach.

Gomco Thermotic Pump—a special electric suction machine commonly used with various gastrointestinal tubes.

Jutte tube—special rubber gastrointestinal tube which has a fine wire tip over the distal end.

lavage—washing out of a cavity, e.g., gastric lavage is to wash out stomach contents and is used in emergency cases such as that of a child swallowing a poisonous fluid.

Levin tube—a long plastic or rubber single-lumen tube inserted through the nose or mouth to the stomach and used to drain off stomach fluids and to keep the stomach decompressed (free of gas).

medulla—lower portion of the brain stem, the enlarged portion of the top of the spinal column inside the cranium (8 bones of the skull).

Miller-Abbott tube—the most common double-lumen g.i. rubber tube used to drain or decompress the small intestine. It has an inflatable rubber bag on the distal end which helps stimulate peristalsis (involuntary wavelike motion of digestive tract) when in the small intestine. It is inserted through the nose down the esophagus, through the stomach, and into the intestine. The proximal end of the tube is connected to a suction machine.

naso-gastric tube—a rubber or plastic tube inserted through the nose (naso) down to the stomach (gastro).

nausea—inclination or desire to vomit.

peristalsis—involuntary wavelike motion of the digestive tract that moves food through the digestive tract (alimentary canal).

Rehfuss tube—a gastrointestinal drainage tube that has a small metal tip on its distal end. It is inserted through the nose down to the intestine.

suction—to suck up (or draw up) by means of reducing air pressure.

Wangensteen suction—an early type of water-displacement suction apparatus used with various gastrointestinal tubes for g.i. drainage.

V. INTRODUCTION

Gastrointestinal intubation is the insertion of a specified tube through the nose (naso) or throat into the stomach (gastro) or the intestine. The primary reasons for this relatively common procedure are:

1. To drain the stomach or intestinal tract by means of some kind of suction apparatus. It is used to prevent postoperative vomiting, to prevent postoperative obstruction (blocking) of the intestinal tract, and to prevent gas formation in the stomach or intestine after an operation.

2. For diagnosis (to identify a disease, to determine the cause of a pathological condition).

3. To wash out the stomach contents, e.g., after taking a poison.

4. To provide a route for feeding one who is unable to take food by mouth.

There are usually three markers (black rings) on the distal end of each of the tubes to indicate how far the tube has been inserted: 1 band = stomach, 2 bands = pylorus, and 3 bands = duodenum.

ITEM 1. LEVIN TUBE

This is the most commonly used tube for gastric (stomach) intubation and suction. It is designed to empty (decompress) the stomach of its contents (food, blood, gas, or other drainage). The Levin tube is about 3 feet long; its tip is solid, but there are a number of holes along the side of the tube for about the first 6 to 9 inches. The other end of the tube is open and is usually connected to one of several types of suction equipment (to be discussed later in this unit).

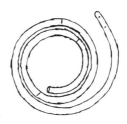

Insertion of Gastric Tube for Drainage Purposes

The most common one used for this purpose is the Levin tube.

To assist the nurse, technician, or doctor during the procedure, you must know what the procedure is. *At this time you will not be expected to insert the tube;* however, you will need to practice getting the patient and supplies ready and know the steps of the procedure so you can assist as necessary.

Important Steps	Key Points
1. Prepare equipment.	Wash your hands and clear a place for the equipment on the bedside stand. If a *rubber Levin tube* is used, you will need to cool it and make it stiff for insertion through the nose by placing it in a pan of chipped ice until thoroughly chilled (15 to 30 minutes). Generally, the *plastic Levin tube* is now used. It is stiff enough for insertion and will not have to be chilled. However, if for any reason it is not stiff enough, it can also be chilled in a pan of chipped ice. Assemble an emesis basin, tissues, a lubricant for the tip of the tube (to ease insertion), a 20 to 50 cc. aspirating syringe, some adhesive tape, and a fresh glass of water. In some agencies, you will obtain these items separately for the patient; in other agencies a special tray may be ordered which includes the tube, lubricant, and aspirating syringe.

Important Steps

Key Points

2. Approach the patient, explain what you are going to do, and enlist his cooperation. Wash your hands.

Check the identification bracelet to be sure you have the correct patient.

The patient may be in pain and very frightened. You need to help reassure him that the nurse or doctor will be gentle with him and that you will tell him exactly what is being done.

The purpose of passing the tube may be to prepare for some gastric studies, as a means of feeding, or to relieve distention in the stomach caused by gas, bleeding, etc. Ask the charge nurse what the purpose of the specific procedure is. Then explain the purpose to the patient. Explain that the passage of the tube is painless but that it could cause gagging as it passes down the back of the throat. However, tell him to breathe deeply and he is less likely to become nauseated and vomit.

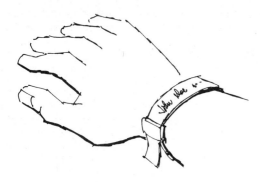

3. Position the patient.

Usually Fowler's position is assumed if possible. This enables the tube to move down the digestive tract with the help of gravity. It is also easier for the patient to spit out vomitus if this becomes necessary. The patient can be in the supine position, however, if his condition warrants it.

4. Give basin and tissues to the patient.

Hand the emesis basin and tissues to the patient if he is able. Otherwise place the emesis basin close beside his face with the tissue near the pillow.

5. Measure tube for insertion distance.

The nurse or doctor who is inserting the tube measures the distance from the patient's nose to the proximal earlobe and then down to the umbilicus (navel). This is roughly the distance from the lips to the stomach. Mark this distance on the tube by placing a piece of tape at that point.

6. Take working position and lubricate the tip of the tube.

The worker who is inserting the tube will stand at the right side of the patient; the tip end of the tube will be grasped in the right hand; and the left hand will hold the remaining tube. (Reverse hand positions if left-handed.)

The tip end of catheter (tube) is lubricated; water can be used. It moistens the tube and permits easier insertion. If the tube should get into the lung, the water on the tip end of the tube is less likely to irritate the lung tissue than would an oil-base lubricant. (Follow your agency procedure.)

7. Instruct patient to open his mouth and hold glass of water.

Tell the patient to swallow a mouthful of water as the tube is passed down the esophagus to the stomach (bend head forward so chin rests on neck). If patient is unable to hold water and emesis basin, you may need to do this for him.

Important Steps	Key Points

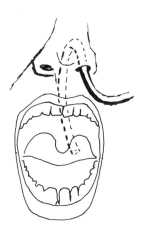

The tube is passed in one of two ways:

Through the mouth: Pass tube over the top and middle of the tongue toward the back of the throat.

Through the nose: Pass tube gently up one nostril. (Use the one which seems to be free of blockage or obstruction. Each side of nose will need to be tested; usually one side is easier to use.) You can check the position of the tube as it passes down the back of the patient's throat, having him open his mouth and holding down his tongue with a tongue depressor (see accompanying diagram). The tube will be rotated very gently and slowly between index finger and thumb for ease of insertion.

U
N
I
T
25

8. The tube is pushed slowly, gently, but firmly into the stomach.

If the tube is pushed too fast, it will stimulate the nerve endings in the back of the throat and they in turn will stimulate the center in the medulla of the brain which causes the patient to vomit. Continue to have him swallow water as the tube is passed; this sets up the peristalsis in the esophagus. He may prefer to suck on ice chips (if permitted) rather than drink water. Try to keep patient relaxed by talking quietly and reassuringly. Take your time.

9. Check to see if the tube is in the stomach.

Since the stomach always has a little gastric juice in it, it is relatively simple to check whether the tube is in the stomach. Apply the aspirating syringe to the exposed end of the tube; pull the plunger back. This action should pull the gastric juice up through the tube into the syringe. If gastric juice is not obtained, it must be determined if the tube is in the trachea (the breathing passageway which lies directly in front of the esophagus). You should have the syringe ready to hand to the doctor or nurse, as well as the emesis basin in which the aspirated contents can be placed. Hold the syringe and emesis basin conveniently for the doctor or nurse.

10. Test to see if the tube is in the trachea.

Patient may become apprehensive at this point. You can reassure him that all is well and that the procedure will be finished soon.
The doctor or nurse will place the free end of the tube in water; if it bubbles, this usually indicates it is in the lung and must be removed at once.

Or

Hold the free end of tube near your ear; if there is a crackling sound, the tube is in the lung and should be removed immediately.

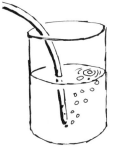

Important Steps	Key Points

Key Points (continued)

Or

Ask the patient to hum. If he *can* hum, the tube is in the esophagus, which is the correct placement. If he *cannot* hum, the tube is improperly placed and should be removed at once.

If the patient becomes cyanotic (blue) or dyspneic (has difficulty breathing), the tube is probably in the trachea. It must be *removed immediately.*

11. Secure the tube to the patient's face with adhesive tape.

When it is determined that the tube is in the stomach, the exterior tip of the tube is taped to the patient's face (the tube will have to be removed and reinserted if it inadvertently went into the trachea). Usually the tip of the tube is taped to the forehead; this will keep the tube out of the patient's way as he moves.

12. Attach free end of tube to suction machine.

The doctor may order a suction to be attached to the tube (to pull out contents from stomach in order to keep it free of gas and drainage). He will state whether he wants continuous or intermittent (off-and-on) suction and will indicate the degree of pull he wants. *Call charge nurse if there is no suction action.*

The free end of the tube is clamped and pinned with a safety pin around the tube, securing it to the patient's gown. Plenty of room should be provided for the patient to move about freely without pulling on the tube.

The tube may also be used for gastric feeding.

13. Prepare to irrigate tube.

The order to irrigate will be issued by the doctor. Irrigation of the tube is done to keep the lumen (opening) of the tube open to permit clear passage for drainage through the tube. Irrigations are usually ordered at stated intervals or PRN (whenever necessary). Besides keeping the lumen open, this prevents gas from accumulating in the stomach which could cause considerable discomfort to the patient.

A. Assemble irrigating equipment.

Obtain a clean aspirating syringe, irrigating solution, and a receptacle for returned solution (an emesis basin will suffice). You may be responsible for getting the equipment ready for the doctor or nurse.

B. Disconnect the tube from the machine and draw up the irrigating solution.

Usually the next four steps are done by the doctor or nurse; however, you should be ready to assist if needed.

Disconnect the tube from the suction machine and secure end of tube attached to machine on its holder.

Hold Levin tube between middle fingers of left hand; also hold plunger of syringe between

Important Steps	Key Points
	index finger and thumb. With your right hand, pull the plunger of the syringe and draw up 15 to 30 cc. of irrigating solution.
C. Attach filled syringe to the free end of the Levin tube and then irrigate.	Inject 10 to 15 cc. of solution slowly into the tube. Pull back on plunger to withdraw fluid. Work *gently* and *slowly* to prevent injury to the sensitive mucous lining of the stomach. The process of injecting and withdrawing solution is repeated until the lumen is clear. *Note:* If fresh bleeding is apparent, the procedure will be stopped immediately and the doctor notified at once if he is not present.
D. Observe contents of the irrigating solution.	The color, odor, consistency, and amount (absence or excess) must be noted and accurately recorded on the patient's chart.
E. Remove syringe from the tube and attach the tube to the suction machine again.	Clean and tidy the bedside unit and equipment. The tray used for irrigation may be reused. However, it is usually exchanged PRN.
14. Leave the patient comfortable.	Because the process of draining the patient's stomach continues over a period of time, he usually is NPO (since everything he would take by mouth would come right back through the tube). The patient therefore loses tissue fluids rapidly and becomes dehydrated. Thus it is important for him to receive intravenous feedings to replace liquid and chemical losses.

There are two other helpful means of unclogging the tubing which are essential to follow:

A. Gently move the tubing in and out slightly.	Occasionally one of the eyelet openings at the distal end of the tube adheres to the wall of the stomach; by pulling the tube away from the lining of the stomach, the tube is permitted to drain fully again.
B. Gentle "milking action" of the tube may free the blocking. (Hold tube securely in place while milking.)	Some thick material may stop up the lumen of the tube between the nose and the drainage bottle. Gently squeeze the tubing between your palm and fingers. Move gently and carefully along the tubing in this manner until suction is restored.
15. Report and record.	Completion of treatment with description of stomach contents. Charting example: 10:30 A.M. Levin tube inserted. Tubing irrigated with NaCl solution, solution returned clear. Many gas bubbles noted. Felt relief immediately. Attached to low suction. A. Brown, RN

UNIT 25

One of the most uncomfortable aspects of this procedure is the constant irritation of the tube at the back of the throat. Therefore, the doctor may permit the patient to suck on ice chips or throat lozenges or hard candy to keep his throat as well as the tube slightly moist. The nose may also become tender, sore, and cracked; good hygiene must be given not only to the nose but also to the throat. Frequent opportunities to cleanse his mouth are comforting to the patient as well as an excellent way to prevent infections from the tube's continuing irritation.

Because the patient is usually very ill and apprehensive, you must keep his environment quiet, clean, tidy, and well-ventilated. The patient often is super-sensitive to odors—so his room and belongings must be kept immaculately clean and sanitary. Unsavory stimuli in his environment can cause him to become nauseated and vomit.

Answer his light promptly. Check on him frequently.

ITEM 2.   INSERTION OF INTESTINAL TUBES FOR DRAINAGE PURPOSES

In this procedure, you will again be assisting the doctor or nurse to insert the tube. However, you need to know the procedure and be ready to help as needed. Stand opposite the doctor or nurse; talk reassuringly to the patient.

Miller-Abbott Tube. This is a long double-lumen rubber tube used for draining the small intestine. One of the lumens supplies the drainage passageway; the other supplies an air-passage to inflate the balloon at the distal end of the tube. The inflated balloon in the small intestine stimulates peristalsis (the wavelike movement of the digestive tract).

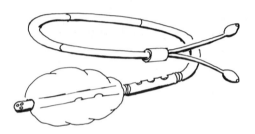

The procedure for inserting this tube is the same as the procedure for insertion of the Levin tube.

Important Steps	Key Points
1. After the tube reaches the stomach, inflate the balloon.	The doctor or nurse will use a sterile syringe and needle to inject 5 to 10 cc. of air (or mercury) into the outlet connecting the air passageway to the balloon. The inflated (and weighted, if mercury is used) tube then passes into the small intestine.
2. Place the patient in *right Sims'* position. 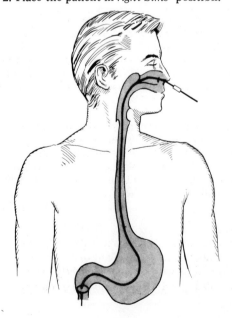	This makes the passage of the tube faster and easier by helping the peristaltic action and gravity to move the tube from the stomach to the small intestine. The tube should not be secured until it is finally inserted into the small intestine. This can be determined by the ring markings on the outside of the tubing as well as by the appearance of the drainage. When the tube reaches the intestines, it is attached to a suction machine. The tube is secured to the patient's face with adhesive tape and pinned to his gown to permit freedom of movement. Removal of this long tubing should be done slowly—a few inches every 5 minutes or so. Rapid removal can stimulate the gag reflex and the patient may vomit unnecessarily. The same precautions are observed when using this method as for patients using a Levin tube.

Important Steps	Key Points

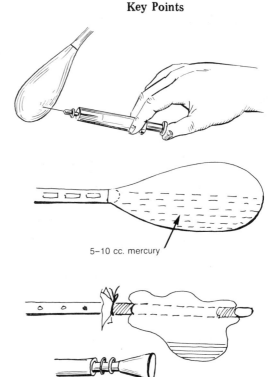

5–10 cc. mercury

Cantor Tube. This is another type of intestinal drainage tube. It has a small inflatable bag sealed to the distal end of the tube. Before insertion of this tube through the nose, the inflatable (balloon) bag is injected (with needle and syringe) with 5 to 10 cc. of mercury. This will make the tip end of the tube somewhat bulky for insertion, and therefore it must be well-lubricated. The principle of operation is the same as for the Miller-Abbott tube. The proximal end of the tube is attached to a suction machine. The drainage holes in the tube are proximal to the balloon-bag.

Harris Tube. This is another long, single tube used for intestinal suction and drainage. It is similar to the Cantor tube, except that the inflatable balloon is tied to the distal end of the tube (it has 4 cc. of mercury in it). The holes that allow the drainage to be sucked into the tubing are proximal to the balloon-bag. The well-lubricated tube is inserted through the nose, using the Levin tube procedure.

The nursing care and observation of the equipment and drainage are the same as for other patients with gastrointestinal suction and drainage.

ITEM 3.   INSERTION OF TUBE FOR REMOVAL OF GASTRIC CONTENTS FOR DIAGNOSTIC STUDY

Each agency has available a gastric analysis tray which is usually obtained from the supply department. Items found on the tray would include a stomach tube (Levin, Rehfuss, Jutte, or Ewald), a tube clamp, lubricant, towel, aspirating syringe, and several specimen bottles (the number will vary depending on the examination to be done). Your agency laboratory manual would give the specifics.

The various tubes mentioned above are named in your vocabulary list. If you have forgotten what they are, review the vocabulary before proceeding with the lesson. Diagrams continue on the next page.

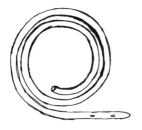

Levin tube.

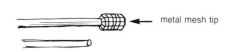

metal mesh tip

Jutte tube.

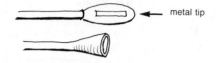   metal tip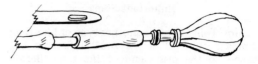

Rehfuss tube.   Ewald tube.

ITEM 4.   INSERTION OF TUBE FOR GASTRIC ANALYSIS

The procedure for insertion of a tube for gastric analysis follows the procedure for intestinal drainage. Usually this will be done by the nurse, the doctor, or a laboratory technician. You will need to be available to assist and to reassure the patient.

Important Steps	Key Points
1. Wash your hands and prepare the equipment.	Obtain a Gastric Analysis Tray from supply. Assemble the equipment for easy access on the bedside stand. Place it conveniently near the patient's head (on the side you are working).
2. Approach and identify the patient; explain the procedure.	Explain that a tube will be inserted through the nose or mouth (see your agency preference). Although the passage of the tube is painless, some people gag when the tube passes down the back of the throat. Slow, deep breathing and swallowing help to minimize gagging.
3. Position the patient.	
4. Give basin and tissues to the patient.	
5. Measure tube for insertion distance.	
6. Take working position and lubricate the tip of the tube.	
7. Instruct patient to open his mouth, hold glass of water, and swallow a mouthful.	
8. The tube is pushed slowly, gently, but firmly into the stomach.	
9. Check to see if the tube is in the stomach.	
10. Withdraw gastric contents.	The plunger is pulled back to obtain at least 10 cc. of gastric contents.
11. Place specimen in labeled specimen jar.	Each specimen jar must be labeled with patient's name, room number, hospital number, time, date, and whether it is specimen 1, 2, or other. The number and times specimens are to be collected will depend on what the purpose of the test is. Check your laboratory manual for the specific requirements of your agency. You may be asked to take care of the specimen. If you do not remember the procedure for labeling and recording a specimen, refer to the units on urine and bowel elimination.

Important Steps	Key Points
12. Make the patient comfortable.	The tube may be left in temporarily until all needed specimens have been collected; then it will be removed. Reassure the patient; ask if there is anything needed. Be sure to check this patient frequently because he may become quite apprehensive. Also, the tube is very annoying and irritating. Tidy the work area so that it is neat and clean. Return all used supplies to the proper place when the procedure is complete.
13. Record on the patient's chart.	Record the time, amount, color, and consistency of the specimen. Charting example: 6:30 A.M. Gastric specimen obtained via the Ewald tube. Specimen 1 contained 10 cc. foul-smelling, dark-brown liquid. Odor somewhat like feces. Specimen to laboratory stat. A. Brown, RN
14. Send or take specimen to laboratory.	Include physician's order and/or the laboratory requisition with each specimen. Specimens must go to the laboratory at once for correct interpretation.

U
N
I
T
25

ITEM 5. SPECIAL FEEDING METHODS: GASTRIC GAVAGE, GASTROSTOMY AND ENTEROSTOMY FEEDINGS

Gastric gavage is a feeding given through a tube inserted through either the mouth or nose into the stomach. Patients who receive this type of feeding are unable to take foods orally (by mouth). Patients of any age may be fed in this manner, from the very small infant to the elderly geriatric patient.

The feeding can be given continuously over a 24-hour period by means of a special Murphy drip method, or it can be given at prescribed intervals, e.g., q.i.d., four times a day, or q.4 h. (every four hours).

Gavage feedings are specially prepared formulas made in the Diet Kitchen. They vary in nutritive value, and therefore the physician prescribes not only what caloric value he wants but also the volume of fluids and frequency to be given in a 24-hour period. The determination will depend on the patient's disease, age and weight.

The *gastrostomy* feeding may also be used. In this case a small incision is made in the upper left abdominal wall directly into the stomach. A gastrostomy tube (catheter with a large lumen) is inserted into the opening. The area is sutured (sewn) to close the surgical wound and also to secure the catheter to prevent it from slipping out of the incision. In about 10 days the wound is healed and the tube can be taken out and reinserted p.r.n.

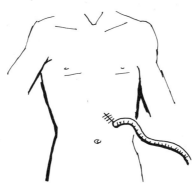

The *enterostomy* (surgical formation of a permanent opening into the intestine through the abdominal wall) may be used as a method of feeding when the patient is unable to be fed through the stomach because of advanced carcinoma (cancer) of the stomach or major gastric surgical procedures or complications. The feeding tube is inserted into the stoma and the technique of feeding follows exactly that for the gastric feeding. If you have forgotten what a stoma is, review the unit on bowel elimination.

Although you will not be doing the initial insertion of the tube, you probably will be responsible for giving the periodic feedings if you are assigned to the patient. You must therefore understand the procedure and demonstrate concern, support, and the ability to perform the task easily, correctly, and quickly.

Important Steps	Key Points
1. Wash your hands and prepare the equipment.	The tray for the feeding procedure can be obtained from the supply department. The formula (feeding) is obtained from the Diet Kitchen. It is usually then stored in the refrigerator on the nursing unit, although it is ordered daily, like any other diet. Take the equipment to bedside and place it conveniently on the bedside stand or overbed table.
2. Approach and identify the patient, explain what you are going to do, and enlist his cooperation.	Some of the patients receiving this type of feeding may be unconscious, and therefore will not be able to cooperate. Check your patient's identification bracelet to be sure you have the correct person.
3. Position the patient.	Use the same position as that for the gastric intubation procedure. However, for enterostomy and gastrostomy feedings, the patient should be in a dorsal recumbent position.
4. Hand the basin and tissues to the patient.	Same as in gastric intubation procedure.
5. Measure tube for insertion.	Same as Step 5 of gastric gavage procedure. However, the gastrostomy and enterostomy tubes are inserted directly into the special openings in the abdomen. These tubes are usually 12 to 18 inches long.
6. Insert tube.	Follow previous procedure. If tube is already in place, check before you begin feeding to see if the tube is still in the stomach or in the intestine.
7. Pour an ounce of water into funnel, syringe or burette.	The syringe, funnel or burette is attached to the free end of the tube. The room-temperature water is used to see that the tube is open. *Note:* If the tube is inserted each time it is used, this step would be omitted.

Important Steps	Key Points

8. Pour warmed formula (105°F.) into the equipment.

Formula should be given slowly; gravity pull will draw it in. You can regulate flow by raising and lowering the receptacle as demonstrated in the adjacent diagram.

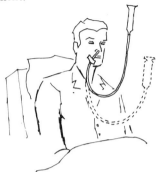

Regulating formula flow.

9. Keep level of formula no lower than neck of syringe.

If you allow the formula level to fall below the neck of the syringe, air will enter the tubing and then the stomach. This can cause great discomfort because of distention of the stomach. Continue adding formula to the syringe until the prescribed amount is given.

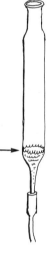

10. Pour 1 to 2 ounces of water in syringe to clear tube.

When the formula feeding is finished, pour in fresh water to clear the tube. Again, be sure to keep the liquid above the neck of the syringe to prevent air bubbles from collecting in the system or in the patient's stomach. (This step will be eliminated if the tube is removed after each feeding.)

11. Clamp tubing.

If tubing is removed, clamp it tightly between your right index finger and thumb to prevent the tube from dripping as it is removed. If the tubing is left in, close it (with clamp or medicine dropper which comes on your tray) before removing funnel, syringe or burette to prevent backflow of the formula.

With clamp.

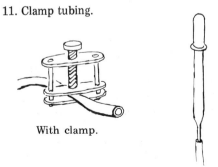

With medicine dropper.

Important Steps	Key Points
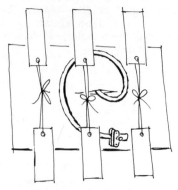	For gavage: Secure the end of the tube with tape to the patient's forehead. Be sure to avoid irritating the skin area and keep it clean and dry.
Secure under bandage.	For gastrostomy and enterostomy: Secure end of tube under the dressing on the abdomen.

12. Give oral hygiene and nose care (for gavage only).

If tubing is left in the mouth, be sure that the nose is kept moist, clean and free from crusts. Sometimes the tubing is left connected to a large flask which may be hung on an IV pole at the head of the bed.

13. Make patient comfortable.

A person undergoing this procedure needs extra reassurance, kindness, and patience. It is possible that he will have to be fed by this means for a long period of time. You may need to teach the patient and his family how to accomplish this feeding procedure. Be sure to stress *safety* technique of checking to make sure that his tube is not in the lung. Stress importance of cleanliness of the equipment, the patient, and the environment to his peace of mind and its importance as a preventive measure against infection.

Be sure to tell the patient when you expect to return, and keep your word.

14. Record on patient's chart.

Record amount of formula, how taken, and any other comments about the patient's reaction. Charting example:

8:00 A.M. Gastric feeding given. 200 cc. formula taken without difficulty. A. Brown, RN

ITEM 6. PROCTOCLYSIS OR FEEDING OF FLUIDS OR NOURISHMENT INTO THE COLON

This method, although seldom used now, is another way of giving patients fluids and nourishment when any of the previously described methods are inappropriate. The fluids are given slowly, drop by drop, over a long period of time, through a special drip tube (Murphy drip) attached to the catheter or tubing. The tubing and Murphy drip can be connected to the gastrostomy or enterostomy stoma, or they can be attached to a rectal tube, and the feeding given rectally. If the nourishment is given rectally, the treatment should be preceded by an enema to cleanse the colon in preparation for the proctoclysis.

The procedure for giving the proctoclysis is similar to other tube feedings. The rectal tube (18 to 22 French catheter) is lubricated and then inserted about 4 to 5 inches into the rectum. It is taped in place by looping tape around the tube once and attaching the tape to each side of the buttocks. The flask for holding the feeding is attached to the tubing and the Murphy drip, and then attached to the free end of the rectal tube. The flask is hung on an IV pole adjusted to a height of 12 inches above the mattress. (See following diagram.)

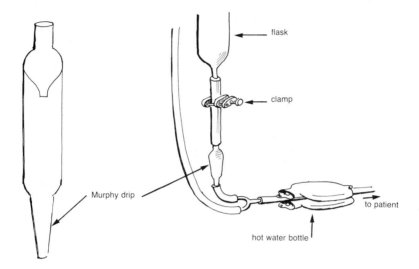

Since the feeding must be at a temperature of 105°F. to facilitate absorption, place hot water bottles around the tubing (near the rectal area). Hold them in place by wrapping a bath towel around the hot water bottles and securing with tape or safety pins. It would not help to place the hot water bottles around the flask (and not in the tubing) because the fluids would then cool as they passed through the tubing. The rate of flow of the fluid will be adjusted to the doctor's order, depending on the amount of feeding the patient is to receive over the stated period of time.

ITEM 7. GASTROINTESTINAL DRAINAGE WITH AND WITHOUT SUCTION

A. Drainage Without Suction

Let us discuss common methods of draining secretions from incisions without suction.

The *Penrose drain*, a tube frequently employed, is a flat, soft rubber drain available in various widths from ¼ inch to 2 inches. The physician inserts one end of the drain into the wound in the designated site, using strict aseptic technique. The free end of the tube resting on the skin may be held securely in place with a stitch of surgical suture or a safety pin. The tube is covered with sterile padding (dressing) to catch the drainage. The dressing is changed PRN. Care must be taken not to dislodge the tube when changing the dressing (usually done by the doctor or nurse) using strict aseptic technique to prevent infection. Careful observation of the amount, color, odor, and consistency of the drainage is vital to the physician's planning of the medical care for his patient. Therefore, the observations and recordings must be accurate.

A *cigarette drain* is a Penrose drain with a gauze bandage pulled through the lumen acting as a wick, like tobacco in a cigarette. It may be used as the doctor deems necessary. The same precautions are to be taken in placing, caring for, and removing the cigarette drain as were described for the Penrose drain.

A *T-tube rubber drain* is commonly used to drain bile from the liver into the intestine—often following a cholecystectomy (surgical excision of the gallbladder). Care must be taken not to dislodge the catheter. Since a large amount of bile may be excreted in 24 hours, the T-tube may be attached to an external tubing system which empties into a drainage bag or bottle attached to the patient's bedside. T-tubes can be used any time the physician indicates the need.

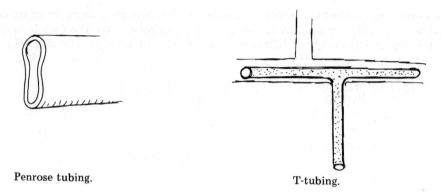

Penrose tubing.

T-tubing.

Urethral catheters may also be used to drain surgical incisions. The size of the lumen must be large enough to accommodate the drainage, e.g., a large lumen is used if a large amount of thick fluid is to be drained. Since catheters come in varying sizes, the actual size is selected on the basis of the need. The choice is usually made by the physician.

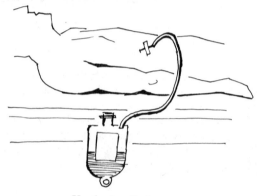

Urethral catheter
in abdominal incision.

B. Drainage With Suction

Wound drainage can also be accomplished by connecting various tubes to different types of suction machines (special machines which suck or withdraw contents from a cavity by means of decreasing air pressure). Suction can be maintained on a continuous basis or intermittently (on and off) as the doctor orders. There are four general types of suction apparatus that you should know about:

(1) A *portable electric suction machine* is a common piece of equipment. It has a gauge on it which permits regulation of the amount of suction you wish to use. It is particularly useful when the drainage becomes thick and viscous.

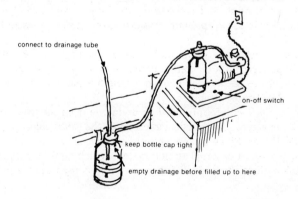

connect to drainage tube

on-off switch

keep bottle cap tight

empty drainage before filled up to here

Your main responsibility will be to see that the drainage bottle does not overflow; it would back up into the vacuum bottle and when that is full, into the motor. The repair in such a case is costly, and sometimes impossible. Therefore, you must check frequently for the amount of drainage, how well the suction is working, and the general comfort of your patient.

(2) Most health agencies now have suction outlets in the wall at the head of the patient's bed. This avoids having to clutter the patient's room with extra equipment, thereby helping to keep the surroundings neat and tidy. These wall-suction units are particularly useful in special care units, i.e., ICU, CCU, and others. Occasionally there is a problem of maintaining enough suction in the entire system (supplying all patients). Some physicians are therefore reluctant to use this system. Again, your responsibility will be to see that the drainage bottle does not overflow.

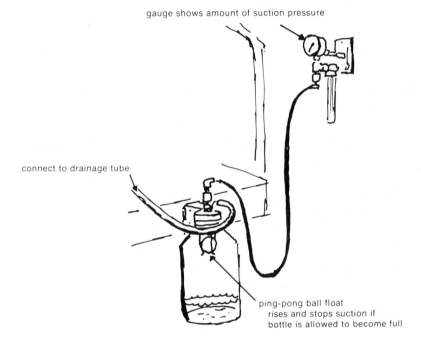

gauge shows amount of suction pressure

connect to drainage tube

ping-pong ball float
rises and stops suction if
bottle is allowed to become full

(3) Another type of suction machine which is often used is the *Gomco Thermotic Pump.* This is an electric pump (without a motor) which provides intermittent suction through alternating air pressure by expanding and contracting the air. The Gomco suction can be regulated by a "low" or "high" pressure button (the amount of pressure will be ordered by the physician). You will see this type of machine used most often with patients who have either gastric or intestinal suction tubes.

The nursing measures that must be observed include special mouth care given frequently to these patients. Since they are NPO, the mouth becomes very dry, tastes bad, and the lips may become cracked. (These are ideal locations for pathogens to set up housekeeping.) To keep the mouth and lips moist, swab the oral cavity with a cotton swab which has been moistened in equal parts of glycerine and lemon juice. This liquid comes prepackaged for use in most agencies; if not, you can mix the solution, which is very refreshing to the patient. Mouthwash may also be used if the patient is able to spit the liquid out; he must not swallow it.

The nostrils (external openings of the nares or nose) often become dry and tender. Keep them moist with a thin coating of glycerine and lemon juice.

Again, close observation of the drainage bottle contents is important to prevent overflow. Check the workings of the machine frequently to be sure it is pulling the drainage from the cavity (stomach or intestine). As the pressure alternates, the red light and the green light alternate on the operating unit.

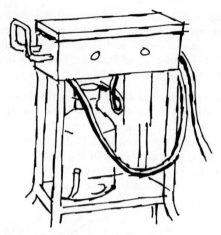

(4) The fourth type is a *two-bottle water displacement system* designed to create suction (an early type of suction apparatus). One of the earliest models was the Wangensteen Suction machine. There have been several adaptations to the basic system, but most hospital personnel still continue to use the term Wangensteen Suction when they refer to a water replacement system of suction. The figure shown below illustrates a modification but demonstrates the main principles. When the top water bottle is empty, the bottom bottle is rotated in the frame to the top position. The two water bottles are supported in the metal frame, and the entire frame is rotated so that the bottles exchange positions. It is vital that you check frequently that the water level in the top bottle never goes below the neck of the bottle; if it did, the suction would be lost and the draining stopped.

The water drains to the bottom much as the sand drains in a 3-minute egg timer. The draining water produces a suction in the drainage bottle which in turn causes the drainage to be drawn into it. Because of the nature of this suction operation, all bottles must be absolutely airtight to assure keeping enough constant suction to withdraw the drainage fluids. Of course, airtight connections are essential for proper operation of any and all suction systems.

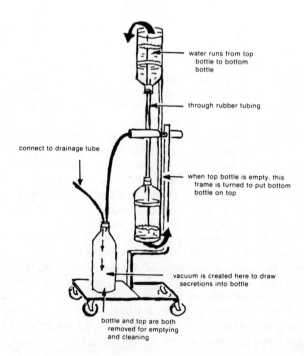

Note: The water replacement system is an excellent example of Bernoulli's Principle: as a gas or liquid flows, it enters a constricted area, and the velocity increases. As it moves out the other end of the constriction, the velocity decreases. This raises the pressure in the lower bottle on the frame, creating a vacuum in the suction bottle.

ITEM 8. EMPTYING AND MEASURING THE CONTENTS OF DRAINAGE BOTTLES

Important Steps	Key Points
1. Wash your hands, approach and identify the patient, explain the procedure to the patient, and turn off suction momentarily.	This will break the suction in the system, allowing easy removal of the rubber stopper on the drainage bottle.
2. Remove rubber stopper from bottle top.	Unclamp holding bracket if there is one.
3. Pour contents into graduate.	Measure the contents and record the time, amount, color, odor, and consistency after re-assembling system.
4. Rinse graduate and drainage bottle.	Dry the outside of the drainage bottle with paper towels and then discard them in the wastebasket.
5. Replace rubber stopper on top of cleaned drainage bottle.	Make sure it is airtight and is held in place with the clamps securely tightened.
6. Turn the switch back to "on" position on suction machine.	This will re-establish the suction system. Observe the flow of drainage for a few minutes. Tell the patient when you will return.
7. Make the patient comfortable and record the amount of drainage on the chart of I and O sheet.	

You have now learned about drainage systems with and without suction. You have also learned about continuous and intermittent suction equipment, and you have become acquainted with four common types of suction apparatus and how to empty the drainage bottles.

You will be expected to be familiar with these various types of equipment, all of which are used with the gastrointestinal tubes that were discussed earlier in this lesson. When you take care of patients with the various gastrointestinal tubes, you should remember the following:

(1) Demonstrate kindness, gentleness, and quiet concern for their comfort.

(2) Give meticulous and frequent oral hygiene and nose care.

(3) Provide for freedom of movement, as much as possible, by securing the suction tubing to the clothing or skin to permit maximum activity.

(4) See that the patient does not lie on the tubing; do not permit the tubing to be kinked because the suction will stop as will the fluid drainage.

(5) When you are checking to see if the suction machine is operating satisfactorily, first check to see that it is properly attached to the patient and the wall outlet, that the machine is turned on, and that the tubes are not kinked. If you have checked all these points and made sure that the drainage bottle is not overflowing, but the machine is *not* working, report stat (at once) to your team leader. This can be crucial to the well-being of your patient because there may be a plugged tube.

(6) Observe, report, and record the contents of the drainage bottles accurately. Report and record unusual contents promptly to your charge nurse.

These patients will provide a challenge to nursing care. They often relax if you give an extra backrub, straighten or change bed linens PRN. Your quiet, observant attention to details when caring for these patients can hasten their recovery.

VI. ADDITIONAL INFORMATION FOR ENRICHMENT

Your instructor will provide you with a list of reading materials if you wish to learn more about the subject of gastrointestinal tubes.

POST-TEST

True or false: Mark "T" for all true statements and "F" for all false statements.

_T_ 1. Observe drainage often for signs of bleeding.

_F_ 2. Give the patient sips of water frequently to combat dehydration.

_T_ 3. Check the Levin tube frequently to be sure tube is open and draining freely.

_T_ 4. Oral hygiene is important while a patient has a Levin tube in order to prevent crusts or blisters from forming in patient's mouth.

_T_ 5. Offer cracked ice or throat lozenges to patient in order to avoid irritation and infections of the mucous membrane.

_T_ 6. Gastric suction may be used to decompress the stomach.

Complete the following statements.

7. List four reasons for insertion of a gastrointestinal tube.

(a) prevent post-op vomiting

(b) wash out stomach

(c) diagnosis

(d) gas formation prevention

8. Explain how to measure gastric materials from suction jar.

turn off suction momentarily, remove rubber stopper from top of drainage bottle. Pour contents into graduate, measure contents, rinse graduate + drainage bottle, replace stopper on top of drainage bottle, turn suction back on. Record contents on chart.

9. Name the four common tubes used in a gastric analysis examination.

(a) Levin   (c) Jutte

(b) Rehfuss   (d) Ewald

10. Name and describe the action of four common suction apparatus.

(a) Portable, electric suction machine gauge permits regulations of amount of solution

(b) Two bottle - water displacement system, drains from top to bottom bottle, creates suction bottles are attached

(c) Wall suction in pt. room gauge permits regulation of amount of suction

(d) Homes Thermatic pump electric pump, alternating air pressure by expanding + contracting air.

11. List at least four nursing measures you would use in caring for patients with a gastrointestinal tube.

(a) _good oral hygeine + nose care_

(b) _Give kindness, gentleness, comfort_

(c) _Provide freedom of movement_

(d) _Maintain open lumen so fluid will continue to drain. observe, record & report contents of drainage_

12. List three reasons for draining the stomach or intestinal tract postoperatively.

(a) _Prevent post op vomiting_

(b) _Prevent intestinal obstruction_

(c) _Prevent gas formation_

POST-TEST ANNOTATED ANSWER SHEET

1. T   (p. 503)

2. F   (p. 503)

3. T   (p. 504)

4. T   (p. 504)

5. T   (p. 517)

6. T   (p. 498)

7. (a) Prevent post-op vomiting, intestinal obstruction, gas formation. (p. 498)

   (b) For diagnosis. (p. 499)

   (c) Wash out stomach (lavage). (p. 499)

   (d) To provide a feeding route when food can't be taken orally (gavage). (p. 499)

8. Turn off suction momentarily, remove rubber stopper from top of drainage bottle. Pour contents into graduate, measure contents, rinse graduate and drainage bottle, replace stopper on top of drainage bottle, and turn suction back on. Record contents on chart. (p. 515)

9. (a) Levin tube

   (b) Rehfuss tube

   (c) Jutte tube

   (d) Ewald tube (p. 505)

10. (a) Portable electric suction machine; gauge permits regulation of amount of suction. (p. 512)

    (b) Wall suction in each patient unit; gauge permits regulation of amount of suction. (p. 513)

    (c) Gomco Thermotic pump: electric pump which provides intermittent suction through alternating air pressure by expanding and contracting air. (p. 513)

    (d) Two-bottle water displacement system: an early suction apparatus, drains water from top bottle to bottom bottle and creates suction; bottles are switched from top to bottom and back again. (p. 514)

11. (a) Demonstrate kindness, gentleness, comfort.

    (b) Give oral hygiene and nose care.

    (c) Provide freedom of movement. (p. 515)

    (d) Maintain open lumen so fluid will continue to drain. Observe, record and report contents of drainage.

12. (a) Prevent postoperative vomiting.

    (b) Prevent intestinal obstruction. (p. 498)

    (c) Prevent gas formation.

NOTES

PERFORMANCE TEST

1. Given a patient with a feeding tube, you will assemble the equipment, prepare the patient (or the mannequin, Mrs. Chase), and give a feeding of 50 cc. of water following the procedure outlined in the lesson, maintaining safety precautions. You will practice recording the activity on the nurse's notes.

2. Given a patient with a gastric suction apparatus and a three-fourths full drainage bottle, you will empty the bottle and reattach it to the suction machine using the procedure which you have just learned. Upon completion of the bottle change, you will record the output on the appropriate records.

PERFORMANCE CHECKLIST

CARE OF THE PATIENT WITH GASTROINTESTINAL TUBES

GAVAGE

The student will demonstrate the proper care of a patient with gastrointestinal tubes.

1. Wash hands and prepare equipment.

2. Approach and identify patient.

3. Position patient (Fowler's).

4. Hand emesis basin and Kleenex to patient.

5. Pour 1 ounce water, room temperature, into funnel to check that tubing is *patent.*

6. Pour warmed formula (105°) into syringe.

7. Regulate flow by raising and lowering feeding tube.

8. Keep level of formula above neck of syringe to prevent air from entering stomach.

9. Continue giving formula until prescribed amount has been given.

10. Pour 1 to 2 ounces water to clear tube.

11. Clamp tube; remove funnel from tube.

12. Secure distal end of tube.

13. Give oral hygiene and nose care.

14. Leave patient comfortable (position in good alignment, call cord and bedside stand nearby; tell patient when you will return).

15. Chart activity.

REMOVAL AND REPLACEMENT OF DRAINAGE BOTTLE

The student will demonstrate the removal and replacement of drainage bottle.

1. Wash hands.

2. Identify patient.

3. Explain procedure to patient.

4. Turn off suction.

5. Remove stopper from bottle.

6. Pour contents of jar into graduate cylinder.

7. Attach new drainage jar to the apparatus.

8. Replace rubber stopper.

9. Turn on suction machine (put in operation for several minutes).

10. Measure and record volume, color, odor, and consistency.

11. Rinse and dry materials used.

12. Provide for patient comfort and safety.

13. Inform patient of time of return.

Unit 26

THE CARDINAL SIGNS: TEMPERATURE, PULSE, RESPIRATION, AND BLOOD PRESSURE

I. DIRECTIONS TO THE STUDENT

Proceed through this lesson. When you have finished, practice taking temperature, pulse, respiration, and blood pressure with other students in the skill laboratory and in the presence of your instructor.

You will need the following equipment:

1. Graphic chart

2. Pen and ruler

3. Watch with a second hand

4. Thermometer (glass or electric)

5. Sphygmomanometer (blood pressure cuff)

6. Stethoscope

II. GENERAL PERFORMANCE OBJECTIVE

After completing this lesson, you will be able to obtain an accurate temperature, pulse, respiration, and blood pressure on adults and children, and record readings correctly on the patients' charts.

III. SPECIFIC PERFORMANCE OBJECTIVES

Following this lesson you will be able within stated time limits accurately to:

1. Take and record the body temperature of an adult and a child by use of a glass or electric thermometer orally, rectally, or axillary.

2. Take and record an apical and radial pulse.

3. Count and record the patient's respirations.

4. Take and record blood pressure.

5. Recognize deviations from normal vital sign patterns.

IV. VOCABULARY

A. Temperature

axilla—the armpit.
centigrade—a thermometer scale used to measure heat; it is divided into 100 degrees ($^\circ$) from the freezing point of water at 0°C. at the bottom, and the boiling point at

100°C. at the top. This is used mainly in Europe and Latin America. Scale is recorded as 100°C., or 100 degrees centigrade.

enzyme—complex substance, produced by living cells, which acts on other substances, causing them to split up into simpler substances, e.g., those found in the digestive juices.

Fahrenheit—a thermometer scale used to measure heat; the freezing point of water is 32°F., and the boiling point is 212°F. This scale is recorded as 32°F. (32 degrees Fahrenheit) and is used chiefly in the U.S. and England. Medically, a thermometer is a glass or electric instrument used to measure the body temperature.

febrile—feverish, pertaining to fever.

fever—pyrexia, or elevation of temperature above normal, which is 98.6°F. (98.6 degrees Fahrenheit) for the average person.

metabolic—refers to metabolism; the transformation of a substance taken into the body to become tissue-building substances, and the excretions of the remaining waste substances. In short, it involves all the chemical reactions needed to keep the body tissues living and functioning.

mucosa—mucous membrane which lines body passages and cavities communicating with the air, and which secretes mucous.

B. Pulse

arrhythmia—irregular heart beat.

bradycardia—slow heart action; generally a rate below 60 per minute for an adult and below 70 per minute for a child, and is seen in uremia, jaundice, fractured skulls, and stroke.

tachycardia—abnormal rapidity of heart action, usually over 100 per minute for adults at rest, and over 200 in infants, and is seen in patients with heart diseases, goiter, and those in shock.

thready—a pulse beat that feels weak and feeble; it can hardly be felt.

bounding—a rapid, big pulse.

C. Respiration

apnea—absence of respirations.

Cheyne-Stokes—a type of irregular or arrhythmic breathing. At first it is slow and shallow; then it increases in rapidity and depth until it reaches a maximum. It then decreases gradually until it stops for 10 to 20 seconds; then repeats the irregular rhythm.

deep breathing—large amount of air taken in.

diaphragm—a musculomembranous wall separating the abdominal cavity from the thoracic (chest) cavity.

dyspnea—difficult breathing; breathing hard, as though one had just climbed a stairway. It is usually rapid, labored and noisy. Long periods of dyspnea are very tiring for the patient.

hyperpnea—an increased respiratory rate or breathing which is deeper than usual while resting; frequently occurs after exercise.

hyperventilation—to increase (hyper) ventilation by breathing excessively fast.

orthopnea—respiratory condition in which breathing is possible only when person sits or stands in an erect position. (This condition is seen in some severe cardiac or pulmonary diseases.)

shallow breathing—small amount of air taken in.

V. INTRODUCTION

The cardinal or vital signs are those that are the first means of assessing a patient's condition. Mechanisms in the body that govern these signs are so finely adjusted that departure from normal rates is looked upon as a symptom of disease. The variations of certain vital signs are so typical of certain diseases or stages of a disease that the medical care plan and diagnosis can be entirely dependent on these signals. These vital signs include the patient's body temperature, pulse, respirations and blood pressure.

ITEM 1. BODY TEMPERATURE

A. Importance of Taking Body Temperature

We are concerned with body temperature because a definite temperature range is required for efficient cellular functioning and proper enzymatic activity. The body temperature represents a balance between heat produced in the tissues and the external environment, and the heat lost to the environment. Fevers (high temperatures) indicate a disturbance of the heat-regulating centers.

In the human being (a warm-blooded animal), when the balance between heat produced and heat lost is in equilibrium (balance), the average body temperature reading on a thermometer is 98.6 degrees Fahrenheit (98.6°F.) or 37 degrees centigrade (37°C.); 1° centigrade equals 1.8° Fahrenheit or 36.9°C. equals 98.5°F. Changes in the temperature range between 36° to 38°C. (97.6° to 99°F.) are within normal or average range. Heat is lost by the body through excreta (feces, urine), expired air, and perspiration (cooling through evaporation).

Note: In the warm-blooded animal the normal body temperature is set at a specific level; the control system attempts to maintain this level at all times. However, in the cold-blooded animal (snake, fish) temperature varies with the surrounding environmental temperature.

Whether the patient's temperature is taken orally (by mouth) or rectally (by rectum) is usually dependent on the patient's condition and his physician's order. Rectal temperatures should be taken when oral measurements are contraindicated because of questionable accuracy or discomfort, e.g., mouth breathing due to nasal congestion, nasal surgery, nasal tubes, or when the patient will not keep his mouth closed over the thermometer (e.g., children often will not). Oral temperatures should be taken when there is a question of accuracy or discomfort, as with rectal or perineal surgery. Axillary temperatures are taken when oral or rectal temperatures are contraindicated, or upon agency procedure.

Oral temperatures *should not* be measured within 30 minutes following the intake of hot or cold foods or fluids, or when the patient has been smoking or chewing gum because these actions will produce a temporary incorrect reading. In other words, you would be getting a temperature recording of the mouth, not the body temperature.

Body temperature should be evaluated in relation to:

1. Patient's usual body temperature. Some people run a "low-normal" or a "high-normal" temperature consistently. This then is the normal body temperature for those people, e.g., some individuals' normal temperature may be recorded as 97.6°F.

2. Time of day. The body temperature upon awakening is generally in low-normal range due to inactivity of muscles. Conversely, the afternoon temperature may be high-normal due to metabolic processes, activity, and the temperature of the atmosphere.

3. Environmental temperature. As you may expect, the body temperature is lower in cold weather and is warmer in hot weather.

4. Phase in menstrual cycle and pregnancy. Body temperature drops slightly just before ovulation (the normal monthly ripening and rupture of the mature Graafian follicle), and then may rise to one whole degree above normal during ovulation. Within a day or two preceding the onset of the next menstrual period, the temperature drops again. During pregnancy, the body temperature may consistently stay at high-normal due to an increase in the patient's metabolic rate.

5. Amount of physical exercise. Physical exercise calls for the use of large muscles which create greater body heat by burning up the glucose and fat in the tissues.

(Muscle action generates heat.) You know that when you are cold, you exercise to warm up. Also, chattering or shivering (contracting of certain muscles) are ways in which the body tries to keep its temperature balanced. The reverse is true in hot weather; we tend to become inactive since muscle exercise generates heat.

6. Age of the patient. In old age, the loss of subcutaneous tissue (tissue directly under the skin) and decrease of blood flow due to arterial changes may cause the temperature to be lower and may cause less tolerance for cold weather. The muscle activity of older patients is limited, and therefore less heat is produced. At birth, heat-regulating mechanisms are generally not fully developed, so there may be marked fluctuations in body temperature occurring during the first year of life.

7. Emotional status of the patient. Highly emotional states (e.g., crying) cause an elevation in body temperature. The emotions increase the activity of secreting glands and thereby increase the heat production.

8. Diseased condition of the patient. Toxins from some infective agents, some pathogenic diseases, or some chemical reactions may produce elevated body temperatures or fevers. The fever is a protective defense mechanism the body employs to fight germs and their toxins.

9. Method of measuring body temperature. A rectal temperature usually measures slightly higher than oral, and an axillary temperature measures lower than oral.

10. The course of a fever can be observed on the recorded temperature graph in the patient's chart. There are three distinct stages in a fever:

   a. The *onset* (when temperature begins to rise). It can be sudden and violent as in pneumonia or it can be slow and gradual as in typhoid fever.

   b. The *fastigium* or *stadium*. (Fastigium is a Latin word for roof; stadium is a Greek word for the distances in a race.) This is the period when the temperature remains at a high, constant level.

   c. The *subsiding* stage, or the period of temperature returning to normal. It can fall slowly over a period of days or abruptly; in the latter case it is called the *crisis*. The crisis used to be a very significant point in the recovery or death of a pneumonia patient. However, today with the advent of powerful drugs used to combat pneumonia, the temperature now drops more gradually.

11. Fevers are classed according to certain characteristics:

   a. *constant fever*—the temperature is continuously elevated; usually there is less than one degree of variation within a 24-hour period.

   b. *intermittent fever*—the alternate rise and fall of the temperature, e.g., low in the morning, high in the afternoon, or low for 2 to 3 days followed by a high temperature for 2 to 3 days.

   c. *remittent fever*—the falling of a high temperature, usually in the morning, rising later in the day. The significant fact is that the temperature never falls to normal in this type of fever until recovery occurs.

B. Equipment Used in Measuring Body Temperature

Clinical Thermometers. The self-registering Fahrenheit clinical thermometer is the instrument used in the United States. The clinical thermometer is a glass bulb containing mercury and a stem in which the mercury can rise. On the stem is a graduated scale representing degrees of temperature, the lowest registered being 95°F. (35°C.) and the highest 110°F. (43.3°C.) because body temperatures below and above these points are rare. In other words, the range on a Fahrenheit thermometer scale is 95° to 110°F. The range on a centigrade thermometer scale is 35° to 43.3°C. An arrow on the scale marks normal temperature at 98.6°F. The long lines on the scale represent full degrees, but only the *even numbers are written.* The short lines on the scale represent two-tenths (2/10) of a degree. Temperatures are recorded using an even number to represent tenths, e.g., 99.2°F. or 99.4°F., but never 99.3°F. or 99.5°F.

Mouth (oral) thermometers with long, slender bulbs register more rapidly than rectal thermometers with short, fat bulbs because there is a greater glass surface surrounding the mercury; therefore, the heat expands this mercury more rapidly. In the short bulb, there is less glass surface over the mercury and it takes longer to heat the mercury to make it rise in its column (mercury expands with heat). The slender bulb must *not* be used in the rectum because it is likely to puncture and injure the mucosa. However, both mouth and rectal thermometers are made with short, fat bulbs and are less easily broken than the slender type. The oral thermometer is used to take either an oral or axillary temperature.

The portable battery-operated electric thermometers register body temperature in 10 seconds or less. They usually have an "on-off" button or an area to be pressed to activate the battery. They require a warming-up period, which consists of activating the battery and placing the tip of the probe against your finger to activate the gauge, which comes in two types: digital, on which you press your finger (digit) to the "on" button to indicate the degree on a scale with a needle, much as a weight scale indicates pounds; and numerical, which has a scale like that on the clinical glass thermometer. The probe, oral or rectal, consists of a totally disposable unit or is covered with a plastic sheath which is changed and then discarded after each use.

U
N
I
T
26

A. Measuring the Temperature with an Oral Thermometer

Important Steps	Key Points
1. Wash your hands. Approach the patient; explain what you are going to do.	Identify the patient by checking his identification band. Determine his condition: can he cooperate and safely use an oral thermometer? If not, you may need to take a rectal or axillary temperature (these procedures will be described later).
2. Obtain equipment. 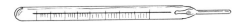 Oral thermometer.	In some agencies the patient is issued his own thermometer on admission. It is usually stored somewhere in the patient's room. In other agencies the thermometers come on a tray daily from the supply room. Remove the thermometer from the container. If it is stored in an antiseptic solution, you must *always rinse* it under cold water to remove the solution before placing the thermometer in the patient's mouth. Remember: do not use hot water to rinse because it will cause the mercury to expand and it could break your thermometer. If you are using an electric thermometer, assemble the monitoring kit and the supply of disposable covers for the probe. Place clean cover on probe and push "on" button to warm up the machine.
3. Check the level of the mercury in the thermometer.	If the mercury is above the 96°F. mark, it will need to be shaken down.

Important Steps	Key Points
4. Shake mercury down.	Hold thermometer securely at the top end between your right thumb and index finger (reverse if you are left-handed). Shake thermometer in a quick downward flip and with a twisting motion of the wrist. See diagram. Usually this will take some practice. Shake down to 96°F. or lower.

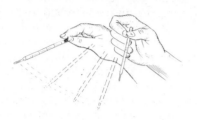

5. Place thermometer in patient's mouth.	Ask patient to open his mouth and place the thermometer slightly to one side of his mouth under his tongue. By placing the thermometer deep in the mouth, it will be surrounded by tissue which is rich in blood supply, thus enabling an accurate temperature reading. Remind him to keep his lips closed tightly; this will prevent the cooler outside air from influencing the temperature recording.

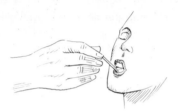

6. Leave thermometer in place for accurate recording.	When using the glass thermometer leave in place for 3 to 5 minutes. Keep the electric thermometer in place for 10 to 20 seconds. Be sure to warn the patient not to bite down on the glass thermometer; it might break and he could swallow the broken glass or mercury.

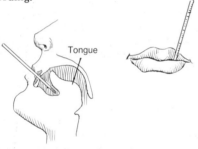

Tongue

7. Remove thermometer.	Again, hold top end of thermometer between your thumb and index finger. Wipe thermometer off with tissue. Wipe from top end to bottom to avoid taking the patient's germs up to your fingers.
8. Read the thermometer.	Hold thermometer at your eye-level. Rotate the thermometer toward you until you can clearly see the column of mercury. Observe the marking (calibrations) on the scale which is even with the top of the mercury column. Remember: each of the long lines represents a full degree (only the even-numbered degrees are numbered, i.e., 96°, 98°, etc.). The four short lines alternating with the long lines represent 2/10 of a degree.

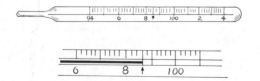

If the mercury column ends at one of the small lines, look to see which long line is immediately below it (nearer the patient's mouth). That will tell you the degree, e.g., 98°F.; then if the mercury level was at the second small line above the 98°F. mark, the patient's temperature would be 98.4°F.

Important Steps	Key Points
9. Replace thermometer in holder.	Check to see that thermometer is not broken (if it is, replace it immediately using your agency procedure). Shake mercury down to 96°F. Return it to the holder. Holders without antiseptic solution (dry method) are recommended. Wash your hands.
10. Record temperature.	Note it immediately on your work sheet (it may be on the composite temperature board for all the patients on the unit). Since you will be taking several readings, you will forget it if you don't record immediately. This information will be transferred to the patient's chart when you have charting time.

Cleansing of thermometers is determined by agency procedure. If you are using an individually issued thermometer, the cleansing you gave after taking the thermometer out of the patient's mouth will be sufficient inasmuch as he is the only one using it. If the agency returns them to the processing area after each use, you will need to wash the thermometer in *cold* running water and soap before returning it to the stock tray for reprocessing. Follow agency procedure.

With the electric thermometer, you will usually be using a disposable plastic sheath over the actual thermometer (probe) unit; this can be discarded in the wastebasket immediately after use.

Do not store oral and rectal thermometers together; they can easily be confused. It would be totally unsanitary to place a rectal thermometer in a patient's mouth by error!

B. Taking the Temperature with a Rectal Thermometer

Important Steps	Key Points
1. Wash your hands, approach and identify the patient.	Generally you will take rectal temperatures in special cases, e.g., patients who are confused, comatose adults, children, or those with an oral injury or disease. Always explain the procedure if the patient is conscious.
2. Obtain equipment.	Rectal thermometers will also probably be stored in the patient's room. Shake mercury down to 96°F. or below. You will need some type of lubricant (mineral oil, K-y jelly, etc.) with which to lubricate the bulb end of thermometer for smooth, comfortable insertion into the rectum. If it is not lubricated well, it may be irritating to the mucous lining of the muscles and stimulate the rectum to expel (push out) the thermometer. Do not **dip** thermometer into a jar of lubricant because you will contaminate (infect with pathogenic organisms or other impurities) the contents of the jar. Instead, use a tongue depressor to take the amount of lubricant you need and place it on a piece of gauze. Then put the tip of the thermometer in the lubricant. Use the gauze to spread it over the entire tip. Hold thermometer at the top end as described in the previous section.

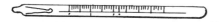

Rectal thermometer.

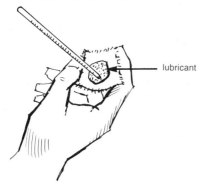

lubricant

Important Steps	Key Points
3. Position patient in Sims' position.	This will make the anal opening clearly visible for ease of insertion. Drape upper bed covers to expose only the rectal area. Maintain the patient's modesty and warmth.
4. Insert thermometer in rectum. 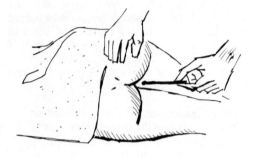	With left hand lift upper buttock slightly so you can see anus clearly. Holding thermometer in your right hand (reverse if you are left-handed), insert lubricated bulb end into rectum about 1½ inches. Ask patient to take a deep breath; this will relax the rectal sphincter and make for easier insertion of thermometer.
5. Hold thermometer in place.	If the patient moves about and you are not holding the thermometer securely, it could easily move inside the patient. Removal of a thermometer after it has gone inside the patient's rectum may even necessitate taking the patient to surgery. You must prevent this from happening.
6. Leave thermometer in for the required length of time for accurate reading.	Leave the glass thermometer in for 3 to 5 minutes, as in the previous procedure. The electric thermometer will record in 10 to 20 seconds. *Note:* The presence of fecal matter in the rectum would probably increase the rectal reading because of the heat produced by the decomposition process of waste products; therefore, be sure the rectum is free of feces.
7. Remove thermometer and read.	Wipe thermometer clean with gauze or tissue. Read it in the same manner as you would an oral temperature. The rectal temperature is usually 1½ degrees higher than the oral temperature because it is in a closed cavity and not exposed to outside air, which could lower the temperature (e.g., when the patient opens his mouth while having his oral temperature taken). Wash your hands.
8. Record temperature.	Record immediately on work sheet. Chart temperature on graphic sheet. All temperature recordings on the graphic sheet are oral temperatures unless otherwise designated. Therefore, when recording a rectal temperature, you chart this sign ® over the temperature reading to designate that it was taken rectally, e.g., ® 98.6° F.

C. Measuring the Temperature by the Axillary Method

Important Steps	Key Points
Steps 1 through 4: Use same procedure as for taking oral temperatures.	
5. Place thermometer in patient's axilla (armpit).	Be sure axilla is dry. If wet, pat dry gently—excessive rubbing will generate heat. Place thermometer in center of armpit. Have patient hold his arm tightly against his chest; the arm can rest on his chest.

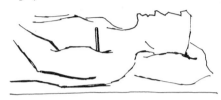

U
N
I
T
26

6. Leave thermometer in place for *10 minutes.*	This is the least satisfactory way to take the temperature and is done when the temperature cannot be taken orally or rectally. The axillary temperature is about one degree lower than the oral temperature. This is true because the arm cannot be held tight enough to avoid air contact which produces some cooling effect.
Steps 7 through 10.	These are the same as in the oral temperature procedure, except that when charting an axillary temperature on the graphic record, write Ⓐ over the temperature reading to indicate that it was taken by the axillary method, e.g., Ⓐ 97.6°F.

ITEM 2. PULSE

Every time the heart beats, it sends blood through the arteries. The pulse is the resultant throb of the heartbeat in the artery, or contraction of the left ventricle (lower left chamber of the heart). The pulse can be felt wherever a superficial (beneath the skin) artery can be held against firm tissue, such as a bone. The pulse is felt most strongly over the:

1. Radial artery in wrist at the base of the thumb.

2. Temporal artery just anterior to or in front of the ear.

3. Carotid artery on the front side of the neck.

4. Femoral artery in the groin.

5. Apical pulse over the apex of the heart.

If the pulse is difficult to find in these areas (e.g., in infants and the obese or in the case of some cardiovascular diseases), the physician may order an apical pulse. The apical pulse is one that is taken by use of a stethoscope over the apex (tip) of the heart.

You may also be requested to take *both* a radial and an apical pulse to see if there is a difference in the rates. If there is a significant difference, it may indicate some disease of the person's blood vessels.

In general, the heart rate has an inverse relationship to the blood pressure and to the size of the individual, e.g., a rapid pulse usually accompanies a low blood pressure. The average pulse rate for a newborn is 130 to 140 beats per minute, while the average pulse rate for an adult at rest is 70 to 80 beats per minute. Exercise, fever and digestion are some of the things that may cause an accelerated (faster) pulse rate. Because of the increase in metabolic rate in pregnancy, the pulse rate may be up to 100 beats per minute, which is generally considered the upper limit of normal during pregnancy.

A temporary increase in pulse rate may be due to fear, anger, physical exercise, anxiety, and elevated body temperature. A prolonged rapid rate may be indicative of hemorrhage or heart disease. A rapid pulse rate is called *tachycardia*. Some drugs, brain disorders or cardiac diseases cause a slow pulse rate called *bradycardia*.

The strength of the pulse is equally as important as the rate of the pulse. With moderate pressure of the first two or three fingers on the vessels, a strong pulse would beat regularly and with good force. There are several ways in which a pulse may be described. Most of the common ways are:

1. Strong and regular: even beats with good force.

2. Weak and regular: even beats with poor force.

3. Irregular: both strong and weak beats occur within a minute.

4. Thready: generally means it is of weak force and irregular.

In taking a pulse, you are interested in the *rate* of the beats (the number per minute), the *force* of the pulse beat (strong or weak and regular or irregular), and the *rhythm* of the beats (normal rhythm has the same interval between the beats).

What does your own pulse feel like? Place your first two fingers over your radial artery with enough pressure to feel your pulse. How does it feel?

A. Equipment Used in Measuring Pulse

For taking all pulses you will need a watch with a secondhand, a pad, and a pen. For taking an apical pulse you will need a stethoscope in addition to the other items. A stethoscope is an instrument used to detect and convey the sounds produced in the body (i.e., heart, lung, etc.). Ordinarily it consists of Y-shaped rubber tubing connected to a plastic or metal ear piece at the top of the Y and either a flat disc or cone diaphragm at the bottom of the Y. The ear pieces fit snugly into the outer ear (or the external auditory meatus). The ear piece is usually bent slightly forward; this part goes toward the front of the ear. When using the cone-shaped body piece, the free end goes against the patient's skin.

In the disc-type instrument the free, flat diaphragm side lies against the patient's skin, and is placed over the tip (apex) of the heart near the midline of the chest to the left of the sternum (breast-bone).

Alcohol, aqueous Zephiran, or a similar antiseptic solution should be used to cleanse the ear pieces before and after you place them in your ears, and to cleanse the disc or cone diaphragm to prevent the spread of infection. *Never* place a stethoscope back in the equipment area unless you have cleansed both the disc (cone) and ear pieces. You could transmit an ear infection to the next user, or contract an ear infection from a stethoscope that has not been correctly cleaned after use.

B. Measuring the Pulse (Radial, Temporal, Femoral)

Important Steps	Key Points
1. Wash your hands, approach and identify the patient, and explain what you are going to do.	Of course, this is a part of taking the vital signs, so you will probably already have explained to the patient what you are doing. The pulse can be taken separately, however. See that the patient is settled in a comfortable supine position.

Important Steps	Key Points
2. Place your three middle fingertips over the radial artery in the wrist at the base of the thumb.	Sometimes it is helpful to place the patient's arm comfortably across his chest while you are counting his pulse. Do not start counting immediately since the movement of the arm creates some exertion. Place your fingertips flatly and lightly on the radial artery. (Do not use the end of your fingers because you might poke or scratch the patient with your fingernails.) If you press too hard, you will obliterate (close off) the artery and you will feel no pulse. Do not use your thumb to take the pulse; you will probably feel your own pulse in your thumb and not the patient's.

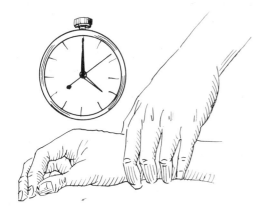

3. Count pulsations.	Count each beat for one full minute. (Use the second hand of your watch to observe the 60 seconds.) As you count, note the regularity or irregularity, and the strength of the beat. You may need to count for the second minute to be sure you counted correctly. Average pulse rates are: For infants: 115-130 beats/minute. For adults: 70-80 beats/minute. For elderly: 56-60 beats/minute. For adult female: 76-80 beats/minute. For adult male: 72 beats/minute.

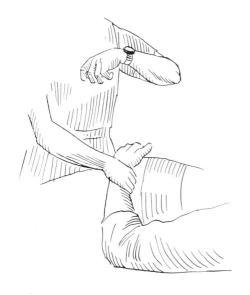

C. Measuring an Apical Pulse Rate

1. Wash your hands, approach and identify the patient, and explain what you are going to do.	Gain his confidence. Explain that you can hear the pulse beat more accurately through the stethoscope than you can feel it with your finger.
2. Position the patient and obtain the stethoscope.	The supine position is best for taking the apical pulse. (The head of the bed may be slightly elevated if it is more comfortable for the patient.) Obtain stethoscope from storage area. Wipe ear piece and diaphragm clean with antiseptic gauze (some are prepackaged).

Important Steps	Key Points
3. Drape patient.	Expose the chest area just enough to see the area over the apex of the heart. Fold top bedding to bottom of ribs. Fold patient's gown toward his head, exposing an area of about 12 square inches.
4. Warm diaphragm in your hand.	The metal is cold, and you must avoid startling the patient by placing a cold object on his chest (this would momentarily increase the heart rate). Place the diaphragm over the apex of the heart just to the left of the sternum (breast-bone).
5. Insert ear pieces into your ears.	If the ear pieces bend forward a bit, they should be placed in your ears so that the forward bend is anterior (in front of) the ear. (Some of the newer disposable stethoscopes have straight earpieces—much like earphones used on airplanes; in that case put them in your ear so they are as comfortable as possible.)
6. Listen for heart beat. 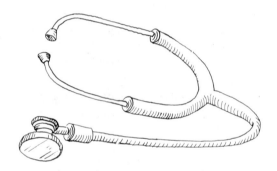	If you are unable to hear a beat, move the diaphragm around on the anterior, lower left quadrant of the left chest until you pick up the sound. Count the beats for a full minute (observe second hand on your watch for the correct time). Note the rate, rhythm, and the strength of the beat for recording later on the chart.
7. Remove stethoscope from ears and chest.	Straighten patient's gown and bed linen.
8. Wipe ear pieces and diaphragm with antiseptic wipe.	This will help prevent the spread of infection from worker to worker, or patient to patient. Replace stethoscope in storage area. Leave patient comfortable.
9. Record on patient's chart.	The apical pulse is usually recorded in the nurses' notes, i.e., 8 A.M. apical pulse rate was 60. Pulse was strong and regular. J. Jones, S.N

ITEM 3. RESPIRATIONS

The respiratory system in the human body provides for the exchange of oxygen and carbon dioxide between the atmosphere and the circulating blood. During inspiration (inhalation of air), the diaphragm (large flat muscle separating the chest and abdominal cavity) descends (or lowers) as it contracts, and the rib cage is lifted upward and outward; the lungs therefore have room to expand. During expiration (exhalation of air), the diaphragm ascends (rises) as it relaxes and the rib cage is drawn downward and inward.

To some degree, an individual can control the rate and depth of his respirations. Emotional stress, exercise, and cardiorespiratory diseases all affect the respiratory rate. For example, when a person cries, his respiratory rate becomes rapid and shallow.

The average respiratory rate for infants is 30 to 50 respirations per minute, while in an adult the average rate is 16 to 20 per minute. If an adult does not breathe at a minimal rate of 10 respirations per minute *and* in sufficient depth, you may note some of the following symptoms as a result of low oxygen supply in the blood:

1. Cyanosis or skin color changes particularly around the mouth and in nailbeds.

2. Confusion, dizziness, and a change in the level of consciousness.

3. Apprehension and restlessness.

Respirations are generally described as follows:

1. Rapid, shallow.

2. Very slow or very deep.

3. Regular, both in rate and depth.

4. Irregular (Cheyne-Stokes): hyperpnea (deeper than usual) followed by a period of no breathing or apnea.

5. Dyspnea, which is labored or difficult breathing usually with pain.

6. Orthopnea: breathing possible only when person sits or stands in erect position.

A. Equipment Used in Measuring Respirations

A watch with a second hand, a pad, and pencil are the only necessary equipment for this procedure.

B. Measuring the Respirations

For an accurate accounting of the respirations, the patient should be at rest and unaware of the counting process. Since this is difficult to do with children who are hospitalized, their respiration rates are generally taken when they are sleeping. If an adult patient is aware that you are counting his respiration, he may voluntarily breathe faster or slower.

The most satisfactory time to count respirations is after the patient's pulse count. When you have taken his pulse, continue to hold his wrist as though taking the pulse and count or feel the times his chest and/or abdomen rise. (You can also see the rise and fall of the chest.) Remember to count the rise and fall of the chest and abdomen as one respiration. Respiration includes both the inspiration and expiration. Check your wristwatch for accurate timing. Counts for 30 seconds are acceptable but then you must multiply by two to obtain a full minute's rate. Respirations are recorded as the number in a full minute. If there appears to be an abnormality in the rate or depth, count for a full minute.

ITEM 4. BLOOD PRESSURE (B/P)

Blood pressure may be defined as the pressure exerted by the blood on the wall of any vessel. The blood pressure is recorded by two numbers on the sphygmomanometer (blood pressure apparatus) representing the *systolic pressure* or the highest point reached by the contraction of the heart, and the *diastolic pressure*, which is the lowest point to which it drops between beats. Blood pressure varies with age, sex, altitude, muscular development, and fatigue. Generally it is lower in women than in men, lower in childhood and higher in advancing age.

Normal systolic pressure in adults is from 110 to 146 mm. of mercury. The normal diastolic pressure range for adults is from 60 to 90 mm. of mercury (mm. is the abbreviation for millimeter, which is a unit measurement of length in the metric system: 1 mm. = 0.0394 inch). The average systolic and diastolic pressures for infants are 58/40 mm. (diastolic) to 80/50 mm. (systolic).

Blood pressure is best measured by checking a large artery. The most commonly used is the brachial artery, which runs from the shoulder to the elbow. A patient's position, emotional state, heart condition, vessel condition, amount of circulating blood, and the muscular strength of his heart are some factors that affect his blood pressure.

A. Equipment Used in Measuring Blood Pressure

A stethoscope, a sphygmomanometer, a pad, and a pencil are required for this procedure. The sphygmomanometer is a broad rubber bag or cuff about 6 inches wide and 24 inches long, covered with cloth. It has two rubber tubes extending from the rubber bag (or bladder): one tube connects to the rubber tubing extending from the base of the mercury column on the sphygmomanometer and the other connects to a rubber bulb air pump. The cuff may be snapped, stuck, or tucked in to stay in place, depending on the kind your agency uses.

B. Measuring Blood Pressure

Important Steps	Key Points
1. Wash your hands, approach and identify the patient, and explain what you are going to do.	Bring the equipment with you (stethoscope, sphygmomanometer, paper and pencil).
2. Position patient and equipment. 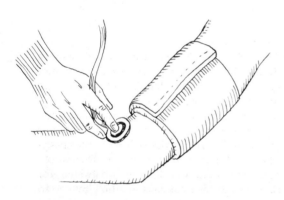	The patient is usually more relaxed when lying in the supine position, but the sitting position can also be used. Place his arm in a comfortable outstretched position on the bed or chair arm. Place B/P equipment on bedside stand near patient or on B/P standard at bedside. (Some agencies supply a wall-mounted B/P apparatus just above the head of the bed.) Positioning is important for accurate measuring.
3. Wrap B/P cuff around patient's arm. 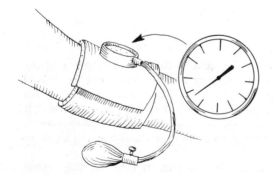	Either arm can be used. Place top edge of cuff 2 inches above elbow. Wrap cuff neatly around the arm so that each layer is directly on top. (If there is a gauge attached to the cuff, be sure that it faces you so you can easily read it.) Otherwise, place gauge on flat surface where you can clearly read the scale. Secure distal cuff end with tape, snaps, or adhesive (whichever is used by your agency).

Important Steps	Key Points
4. Attach tubes from B/P cuff.	One tube goes to the air pump bulb, the other to the gauge tubing.
5. Place stethoscope earpieces in your ears.	Ask the patient to make a fist, open and close it a couple of times, then hold the fist. With your left fingertips, feel for the brachial artery.

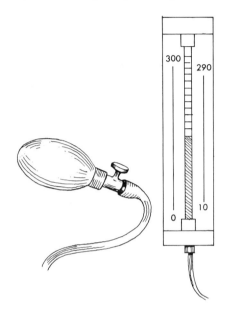

Stethoscope—an instrument used in auscultation (listening) to convey to the ear sounds produced in the body.

6. Place stethoscope (diaphragm) disc or cone over brachial artery.	The brachial artery is usually easy to find; it is located in the center of the anterior elbow area.

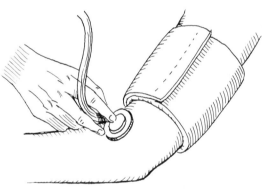

7. Close valve on air pump.	With right thumb and index finger, turn the thumbscrew on the air pump bulb in a clockwise direction until it is tight.

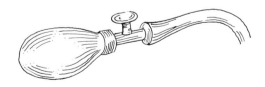

8. Pump air bulb with right hand.	The rubber bag on the B/P cuff will inflate (fill with air). As you pump, the column of mercury will rise in the sphygmomanometer. Pump until it reaches 180 mm. of mercury or about 10 degrees higher than the last beat you hear with

U
N
I
T
26

Important Steps

Key Points

the stethoscope. Tell the patient his hand might tingle a bit because the B/P cuff is temporarily constricting the flow of blood in the arm.

9. Open the valve on the air bulb. Release the pressure slowly to let the mercury column descend.

When taking the B/P you will have to *watch* the mercury column very carefully while you also *listen* to the sounds through the stethoscope.

10. Note the line at which the first beat is heard on the sphygmomanometer gauge.

As the mercury column descends (because air is released from the B/P cuff which was constricting the blood vessels in the arm), you will *see* the mercury begin to fluctuate as well as *hear* the pulse beat. Note the exact numerical line on the scale where you first hear a clear beat—this is the *systolic reading*. It is the point at which the greatest force is exerted by the heart and the greatest resistance is put forth by the arterial walls.

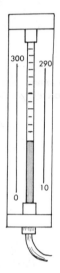

11. Continue to open the valve slowly until all air is removed.

As the mercury descends, the heart beat becomes louder and clearer, then almost immediately becomes soft and quiet. Note the number on the gauge as the last clear sound is heard—this is the *diastolic reading*. It is the point of the greatest cardiac relaxation. Agencies differ as to whether it is the last clear beat or the last beat that is heard that is recorded as the diastolic beat (check your agency procedure).

12. Repeat the process to check your accuracy.

Pump air into B/P cuff above the 180 mm. mark, as in Step 8. Proceed through succeeding steps, carefully checking the level on the B/P scale at which you hear the first and last pulse beats. (They should be the same as your first reading; if not, remove all air from B/P cuff and inflate it again for the third reading.) You must open the valve slowly, observe the mercury column closely, and listen to the pulse beats carefully. This part of the procedure is difficult and will take much practice. The first sound you hear (systolic pressure) is written as 130/   ; the last sound you hear (diastolic pressure) is recorded as   /80. Thus the final and complete B/P would be recorded as B/P 130/80 on the patient's chart.

Important Steps	Key Points
13. Remove cuff from patient's arm.	Remove stethoscope ear pieces from your ears. Be sure that all the air is removed from the B/P cuff before taking it off.
14. Fold B/P cuff and return it to storage.	Return folded cuff, stethoscope, and sphygmomanometer to storage area. Remember to clean stethoscope pieces and stethoscope diaphragm with an antiseptic wipe before returning it to storage as an infection control precaution.

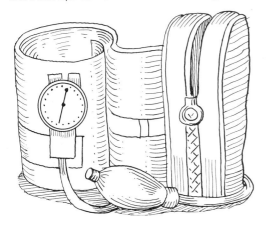

U
N
I
T
26

15. Record on patient's chart.	Describe any unusual aspects of B/P (extremely strong, weak or faint, very high or very low readings). If B/P is abnormal, report at once to the charge nurse; she will relay the information to the physician if indicated.

Note: It is difficult to obtain blood pressure readings on some people. When you have trouble, *do not hesitate* to ask for assistance or confirmation of your reading. Even after you have been in the business many years, you may still find the need to have assistance occasionally. It is more important to get a correct reading to ensure that the patient can be correctly treated than for you to be embarrassed about asking for assistance. |

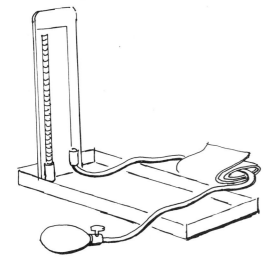

VI. ENRICHMENT

For further information on the cardinal signs, read the materials listed in the bibliography, which you instructor will give you.

POST-TEST

A. Define the following:

1. febrile: _having a fever or is feverish_

2. bradycardia: _slow heart action_

3. tachycardia: _fast heart action_

4. apnea: _lack of breathing_

5. hyperventilation: _over breathing fast + hard_

6. orthopnea: _only being able to breath sitting or upright_

7. apical pulse: _over the end of heart_

8. Fahrenheit: _a thermometer used to measure heat_

9. stethoscope: _used to measure B/P._

10. diastolic pressure: _lowest pressure it drops during beats_

B. Complete the following:

1. Temperature, pulse, respiration, and blood pressure are known as _Cardinal_ or _vital_ signs.

2. _98.6_°F. or _37_ °C. are the average adult body temperatures.

3. List three things that can either raise or lower body temperature.

   (1) _Some type of infection_

   (2) _Emotional traumas_

   (3) _time of day_

4. List two conditions which make it necessary to take ℞ temperature in adults.

   (1) _nasal surgery_

   (2) _patients who won't keep mouth closed_

5. After drinking hot or cold fluids, chewing gum, or smoking, an oral temperature should not be taken for _30 min._ (period of time).

6. The clinical glass thermometer with the _short - fat_ bulb is the only one used for rectal temperatures.

7. A thermometer is kept in a patient's mouth for _3 - 5_ minutes minimum.

8. Rectal thermometers are always well-lubricated to prevent _irritation to the rectal area_

9. _rectal_ temperatures are always taken on small children.

10. _femoral_, _temporal_, and _radical_ are three arteries which may be used to take a pulse.

11. _apical_ pulse is the only one recommended to take for children under two years of age.

12. The heart rate has a/an _inverse_ relationship to the blood pressure.

13. _exercise_, _fever_, and _digestion_ may cause an accelerated pulse rate.

14. The correct placement of the stethoscope's earpieces is _tips bent forward_.

15. _thumb_, digit or finger is *never* used to take a pulse.

16. Pressing too hard on a vessel _obliterates_ it.

17. _supine_ position is used to take an apical pulse.

18. _30-50_ per minute is the average respiration rate for infants, and _16-20_ per minute is the average respiration for adults.

19. Cyanosis, confusion, and rapid, thready pulse may be symptoms of low _oxygen_ supply in the blood.

20. The highest point caused by the contraction of the heart is called the _systolic_ pressure.

21. The average blood pressure for an adult is _110-140 / 60-90_.

22. The instruments needed to take a blood pressure are _stethoscope_ and _sphygmomanometer_.

POST-TEST ANNOTATED ANSWER SHEET

A.   1. febrile: feverish, pertaining to fever. (p. 524)

2. bradycardia: slow heart action, rate usually less than 60 per minute in adult, less than 70 per minute in child. (p. 524)

3. tachycardia: abnormally rapid heart action, usually over 100 per minute in adult and over 200 per minute in infant. (p. 524)

4. apnea: absence of respirations. (p. 524)

5. hyperventilation: increase ventilation by excessively rapid breathing. (p. 524)

6. orthopnea: condition in which the patient can only breathe in a sitting or standing position. (p. 524)

7. apical pulse: pulse rate which is taken by means of a stethoscope placed over the apex of the heart. (p. 531)

8. Fahrenheit: a thermometer scale for measuring heat (freezing point is 32° F; boiling point is 212° F). (p. 524)

9. stethoscope: an instrument used to detect, convey, and study the sounds produced by the body, i.e., heart, lung, etc. (p. 532)

10. diastolic pressure: the last sound that is heard as the mercury drops in the blood pressure apparatus. It is the point of greatest cardiac relaxation. (p. 535)

B.   1. vital signs, or cardinal (p. 524)

2. 98.6° F or 37°C (p. 525)

3. time of day, environmental temperature, phase of menstrual cycle or pregnancy, exercise, age, emotions, disease (pp. 525 and 526)

4. mouth breathing due to nasal congestion, nasal surgery, nasal tubes, patients who won't keep mouth closed, small children (p. 525)

5. 30 minutes (p. 525)

6. short, fat (p. 527)

7. 3 to 5 (p. 528)

8. irritation to the rectal mucosa (p. 529)

9. rectal (p. 529)

10. radial, temporal, carotid, femoral (p. 531)

11. apical (p. 531)

12. inverse (p. 531)

13. exercise, fever, digestion (p. 531)

14. with the tips bent forward to the front of ear, or as comfortable as possible with straight ear pieces (p. 534)

15. thumb (p. 533)

16. obliterates (p. 533)

17. supine (p. 533)

18. 30 to 50; 16 to 20 (p. 535)

19. oxygen (p. 535)

20. systolic (p. 535)

21. $\dfrac{110 \text{ to } 146}{60 \text{ to } 90}$ (p. 535)

22. stethoscope; blood pressure apparatus or sphygmomanometer (p. 536)

WORKSHEET

Directions: Refer to the blank graphic sheet (Sample A). The graphic sheet has space for recordings for 7 days. Each space is ruled into A.M. and P.M. columns. The A.M. and P.M. columns are each divided into three hourly columns for recording purposes. They are numbered for:

4 A.M. (0400)   8 A.M. (0800)

4 P.M. (1600)   8 P.M. (2000)   12 midnight (2400)

How to Record Temperature: The top half of the graphic sheet is for recording the temperature. Note that the temperature range of degrees is 96° to 106°F.

1. Record in even tenths or even numbers.

2. Place a dot on the center of the appropriate line; the dot should be at the intersection of the appropriate hour and temperature reading.

3. Using a ruler, connect dots with a straight, accurate line.

4. If temperature is rectal, indicate above dot with Ⓡ.

5. If temperature is axillary, indicate above dot with Ⓐ.

Now refer to the Graphic Sheet (Sample B).

Temperature was 99.8°F. Note that each line stands for two-tenths of a degree. 99° is the line on which it is written and each line above it is two-tenths until the next number is reached. Therefore, the heavy dot is on the last line before 100°.

Directions: Refer to the blank graphic sheet (Sample A).

How to Record Pulse: The bottom third of the graphic sheet is for recording the pulse. Note that the pulse range is from 60 to 160. When the pulse rate to be recorded is one of the numbers indicated on the sheet (such as 90, 110), then place the dot in the center of the appropriate line. Otherwise the dot is centered the correct vertical distance between two lines.

Example: Pulse 92 is recorded as   ——— 100

——— 90

Now refer to Graphic Sheet (Sample B).

1. Pulse is 94; note that 90 appears on the line it represents, and the heavy dot is placed about one-third of the way toward the next number.

Record in even numbers, such as 86, 102. Using a ruler, connect dots with a straight, accurate line.

— — — — — — — — — — — — — — —

Directions: Refer to the blank graphic sheet (Sample A).

How to Record Respiration: The bottom third of the graphic sheet is for recording the respiratory rate. Note that the respiration scale is from 10 to 50. When the respiratory rate to be recorded is one of the numbers indicated on the sheet (such as 20, 40), then place the dot in the center of the appropriate line. Otherwise the dot is centered the correct vertical distance between two lines.

Example: Respiration 48 is recorded as   ——·— 50

——— 40

Record in even numbers such as 22, 46. Using a ruler, connect dots with a straight, accurate line.

Now refer to Graphic Sheet (Sample B).

1. Respiration is 24. Note that 20 appears on the line it represents, and the heavy dot is placed about one-third of the way toward the next number.

— — — — — — — — — — — — — — — — — —

Directions: Refer to Mr. James Danner's Graphic Sheet. Read and record on this sheet the TPR for Mr. Danner from 12/1/70 through 12/7/70.

Dates	Temperature	Pulse	Respiration	Time
12/1/70				

GRAPHIC CHART

Sample "A"

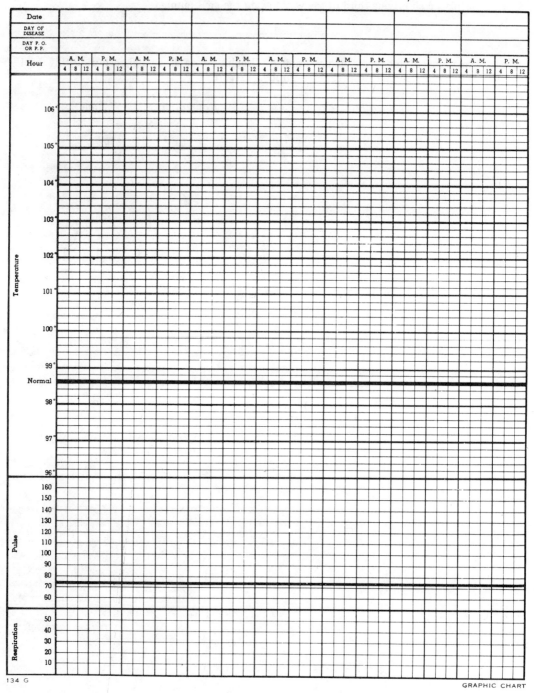

134 G

GRAPHIC CHART

GRAPHIC CHART

Sample "B"

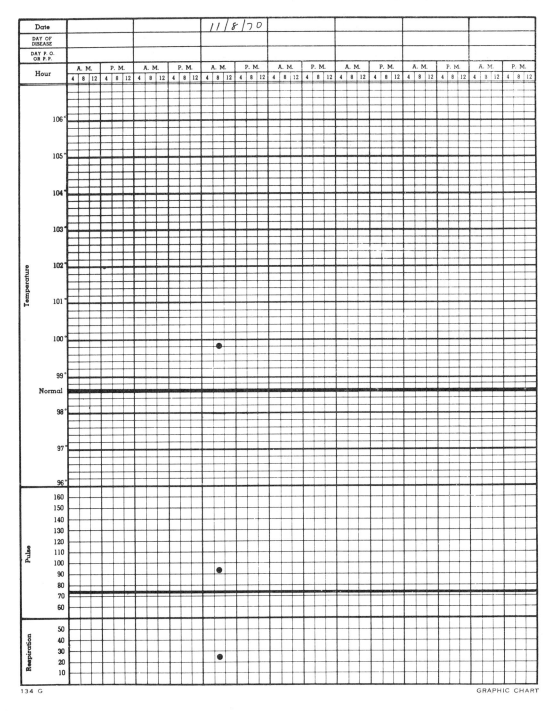

UNIT
26

134 G

GRAPHIC CHART

GRAPHIC CHART

Mr. James Danner

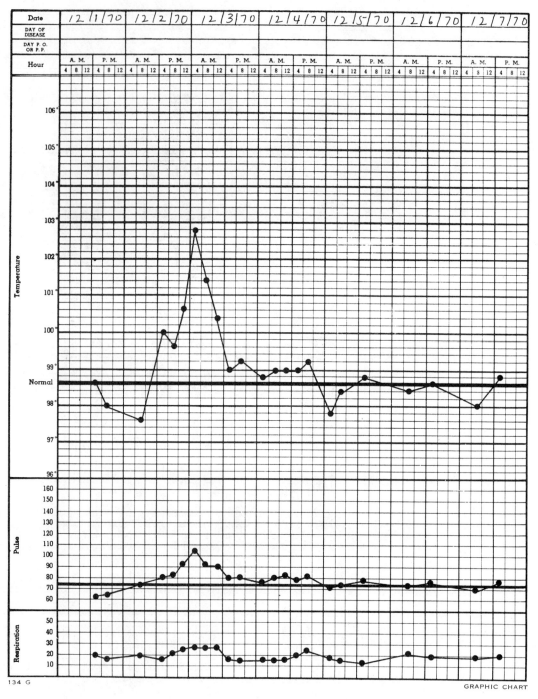

134 G

GRAPHIC CHART

PERFORMANCE TEST

1. In the skill laboratory you will correctly and accurately take the vital signs (T, P, R and B/P) on your partner using the procedures presented in class, e.g., oral, rectal, axillary temperatures; radial, femoral, temporal, carotid, and apical pulse.

2. In addition, you will accurately chart the vital signs you took on your lab partner on a practice nurse's notes and graphic record.

3. Complete the attached Cardinal Signs Worksheets.

PERFORMANCE CHECKLIST

CARDINAL SIGNS

ORAL TEMPERATURE WITH GLASS THERMOMETER

The student will demonstrate correct method of taking an oral temperature with a glass thermometer.

1. Wash hands.

2. Approach patient and explain procedure.

3. Obtain equipment.

4. Prepare equipment for use: clean thermometer according to agency regulations; rinse thermometer in cold water if necessary.

5. Check level of mercury in thermometer; if above 96° Fahrenheit, level must be lowered by shaking.

6. Place thermometer in patient's mouth:

   A. Place under tongue.

   B. Place deep into area.

   C. Request patient to keep mouth closed.

7. Leave thermometer in place from 3 to 5 minutes.

8. Remove thermometer, holding top end between thumb and index finger.

9. Wipe thermometer with tissue, making sure to wipe from top to bottom.

10. Read thermometer.

11. Place thermometer in holder.

12. Record appropriately on chart.

ORAL TEMPERATURE WITH ELECTRIC THERMOMETER

The student will demonstrate the correct way to take an oral temperature with an electric thermometer.

1. Wash hands.

2. Approach patient and explain procedure.

3. Obtain equipment.

4. Prepare electric thermometer for use: place clean cover on probe; warm up machine.

5. Insert probe under patient's tongue.

    A. Ask patient to keep mouth closed.

    B. Make sure to insert probe into rear of oral cavity.

6. Leave thermometer in place from 10 to 20 seconds.

7. Remove thermometer.

    A. Wipe thermometer with tissue from top to bottom.

    B. Remove disposable cover.

8. Read scale.

9. Record temperature on patient's chart or appropriate worksheet.

OBTAINING RECTAL TEMPERATURE WITH A GLASS THERMOMETER

The student will demonstrate the correct procedure for obtaining a rectal temperature with a glass thermometer.

1. Wash hands.

2. Identify and approach patient.

3. Obtain equipment: thermometer; KY jelly.

4. Position patient in Sims' position, being careful to maintain his privacy and warmth.

5. Insert thermometer into rectum: lift upper buttocks slightly; insert lubricated end of thermometer about 1½ inches into rectum.

6. Leave thermometer in cavity from 3 to 5 minutes. Make sure to hold thermometer during entire time because it could slip into rectum.

7. Remove thermometer and wipe it clean with gauze or tissue, wiping from top to bottom.

8. Read temperature.

9. Record temperature on chart.

10. Make sure to indicate temperature as taken rectally ®.

OBTAINING RECTAL TEMPERATURE WITH AN ELECTRIC THERMOMETER

The student will demonstrate the correct method used to obtain a rectal temperature using an electric thermometer.

1. Wash hands.

2. Approach and identify patient, and explain procedure.

3. Obtain equipment.

4. Prepare equipment for use: insert a probe on the thermistor; warm up machine; coat probe with lubricant.

5. Position patient in Sims' position, being careful to maintain his privacy and warmth.

6. Insert thermometer into rectum: lift upper buttocks slightly; insert lubricated end of thermometer about 1½ inches into rectum.

7. Leave thermometer in cavity from 10 to 20 seconds. Make sure to hold thermometer during entire time because it could slip into the rectum.

8. Read temperature on dial indicator.

9. Record temperature on chart.

10. Indicate temperature as taken rectally ®.

TAKING TEMPERATURE BY AXILLARY METHOD

The student will demonstrate the correct method used to obtain axillary temperature.

1. Wash hands.

2. Identify patient and explain procedure.

3. Obtain equipment—glassblown thermometer.

4. Prepare equipment for use: shake down thermometer if necessary; rinse and wipe dry if necessary.

5. Place thermometer in patient's axilla—make sure it is dry.

6. Leave thermometer holding top end between thumb and index finger for 10 minutes.

7. Remove thermometer, holding top end between thumb and index finger.

8. Wipe thermometer with tissue, making sure to wipe from top to bottom.

9. Read thermometer.

10. Place thermometer in holder.

11. Record on chart indicating axillary temperature Ⓐ.

TAKING PULSE (RADIAL, FEMORAL, TEMPORAL) AND OBSERVING RESPIRATORY RATE

Show correct procedure for taking radial, femoral, and temporal pulse and observing respiratory rate.

Taking pulse.

1. Wash hands.

2. Identify and approach patient.

3. Explain procedure to patient.

4. Place three middle fingertips over the appropriate artery.

5. Count the pulsations for specific period of time—usually 60 seconds.

6. Note rate, force, and rhythmicity of beats.

7. Record appropriately.

Observing respiratory rate.

1. Identify patient.

2. *Important that patient is not aware of procedure.*

3. Observe rate, depth, and rhythm of respiration.

4. Record appropriately on chart.

TAKING AN APICAL PULSE RATE

Demonstrate the correct procedure for determining apical pulse rate.

1. Wash hands.

2. Identify patient and explain procedure.

3. Obtain equipment.

4. Position patient and provide for his privacy, warmth, and comfort.

5. Warm stethoscope with hands.

6. Place diaphragm of stethoscope over apex of heart.

7. Insert earpieces in ears; the bend should be forward in the ears.

8. Listen for heart sound, and adjust location of diaphragm if necessary.

9. Record apical pulse rate noting rate, force, and rhythm.

10. Remove stethoscope from ears and chest.

11. Record information on patient's chart.

12. Clean and replace equipment in proper area.

BLOOD PRESSURE

The student will demonstrate the correct procedure for taking a patient's blood pressure.

1. Wash hands.

2. Identify patient and explain procedure.

3. Obtain equipment.

4. Position patient.

5. Attach equipment to patient appropriately: place cuff at approximately heart level, 2 inches above elbow; wrap cuff neatly around arm; secure cuff end with tape or adhesive.

6. Attach tubes from blood pressure cuff to air pump and sphygmomanometer.

7. Adjust stethoscope position: arrange ear pieces; place diaphragm over *brachial* artery.

8. Close valve on air pump.

9. Inflate cuff to a minimum of 180 mm. of mercury and inform patient that this may cause some tingling.

10. Open valve of air bulb—release pressure *slowly.*

11. Observe mercury column and listen to pulse sounds carefully. Record the value when the mercury begins to fluctuate and when the first sound is heard.

12. Continue to decrease pressure slowly.

13. Record value when mercury ceases to fluctuate and when last sound is heard.

14. Repeat process to check recording.

15. Remove equipment from patient's arm.

16. Return materials and equipment to storage.

17. Record readings on patient's chart.

18. Clean stethoscope and return it to storage.

NOTES

Unit 27

ADMISSION, TRANSFER AND DISCHARGE

I. DIRECTIONS TO THE STUDENT

You are to proceed through the lesson using this workbook as your guide. You will need to practice the tasks using the different types of equipment with the mannequin or a student partner in the skill laboratory. After you have completed the lesson and the practice, arrange with your instructor for the post-tests.

II. GENERAL PERFORMANCE OBJECTIVE

When you have completed this lesson, you will be able to admit, transfer, or discharge a patient correctly while demonstrating concern for his physical and emotional well-being as well as for his personal belongings.

III. SPECIFIC PERFORMANCE OBJECTIVES

After finishing this lesson, you will correctly:

1. Take and record your observations of the patient's physical and emotional condition at the time of admission.
2. Explain to the patient about the hospital environment and routine (including the operation of the electric bed controls, the TV controls, and the nurse-call communication system).
3. Take safe care of the patient's personal belongings during his stay in the agency or during transfer to another location.
4. Prepare the patient and his belongings for discharge.
5. Complete the necessary admission, transfer, and discharge forms.

IV. VOCABULARY

Words commonly used in charting the procedures for this unit can be found in the unit on Charting. You will practice charting these procedures using the terms listed. When you are able to use these words effectively and correctly, you will have increased your vocabulary greatly.

V. INTRODUCTION

The admission of a patient to a health care facility is usually a difficult time for the patient and his family. The patient is frightened and may be having pain or discomfort. Kindness, courtesy, concern, patience, and confidence in what you are doing are vitally important. You must also convey the assurance that everything in his records will be kept strictly confidential—by you and other health personnel.

The preliminary routine admission procedures (obtaining personal facts for the admission record, getting a signed general consent for care, assigning the patient to a bed, applying the patient's identification bracelet) are usually handled by the Admitting Office staff. They may be a part of the Business Office section or the Nursing Service, depending on the agency. (Emergency admission procedures may vary from the routine admission procedure.) Although each agency has its own policies, the general procedure is similar.

After completing the initial (first) admitting procedures, the admitting office will notify the nursing unit by telephone that the patient will be arriving shortly to occupy a specific bed. Other information is included in this call: the patient's full name, the physician's name, the diagnosis, and any other information which the admitting clerk determines is needed.

The patient will be sent to the unit on foot, in a wheelchair, or on a stretcher, depending on his condition. He will be accompanied to the nursing unit by a volunteer, a member of the escort service, or someone from the admitting office or the nursing unit to which he is going, depending on agency procedure.

The patient's admission chart will also accompany him. Usually it is carried by the health worker. The chart will include the admission record, consent for care, and sometimes the doctor's order. Sometimes preadmission laboratory work has been completed and the reports will be on the chart.

The first contact that the patient and his family have with the health personnel is crucial. You should therefore take this opportunity to greet the patient warmly by name, and introduce yourself. Be helpful in any way you can—answer questions which the patient or his family may ask. This should be done by every health worker who meets the patient and his family, regardless of responsibility to the particular patient.

ITEM 1. PREPARATION OF ROOM FOR NEW ADMITTANCE

Upon notification that a patient will be admitted, you will prepare the patient's room for his arrival.

Important Steps	Key Points
1. Lower the bed.	This makes it easier for the patient to get in. (However, if he is coming by stretcher, the bed should be placed in the high position.)
2. Open the bed.	Turn back the covers, fluff the pillow, and adjust lights, temperature, and ventilation.
3. Place gown on top of bedding.	A patient usually changes into the hospital gown immediately. However, if he is not too ill (e.g., if he is to have diagnostic studies or to undergo surgery the following morning), he may prefer his own sleeping garments, and he may wear them.
4. Assemble admitting equipment.	Obtain urine specimen container, sphygmomanometer and stethoscope, thermometer, admission checklist (if used), and any other special equipment your team leader suggests, such as oxygen equipment or IV standard. Await the arrival of the patient.

ITEM 2. PATIENT'S ARRIVAL AT ROOM

Upon arrival of the patient to the unit:

Important Steps	Key Points
1. Greet the patient.	Call him by name, check his identification band. Give his chart to the ward clerk or nurse.
2. Introduce yourself.	Tell the patient and his family, "I'm Miss Jones, the nurse's aide (or nursing student) assigned to take care of you." Be warm, friendly, and courteous. First impressions are often lasting. Endeavor to make the patient feel that he has been expected (sometimes patients arrive on the nursing unit before, or at the same time as, the notification of the admission comes from the admitting office; or the patient formerly occupying the bed has not yet left the room). These two situations occur frequently. Still you must make every effort to welcome the patient in a warm, kind, and unhurried manner. Tell him the cause for delay if he has to wait and, if his condition permits, ask him to be seated in a nearby chair or in the waiting room in case the room is still occupied. If his condition is serious, your charge nurse may need to help you arrange an alternative solution, such as putting the patient to bed in another room (after confirmation with the Admitting Office).

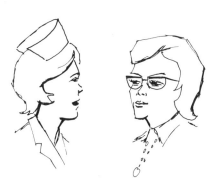

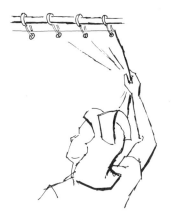

3. Take the patient to his room.	Wash your hands. Assist him to get ready for bed. Carry on a friendly conversation, explaining each step as you go along. Gain his cooperation. Introduce him to his roommate if there is one.
4. Screen the patient.	Pull the curtains to give him privacy as he changes into either the hospital gown or his own sleeping garments. Be sure the room is warm and free of drafts. If you do not have a screen available (as in a private room) or curtains, be sure to close the corridor door securely.

Important Steps	Key Points

5. Obtain a urine specimen.

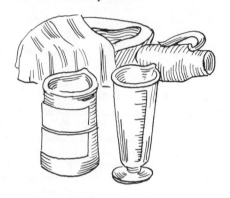

If the patient is ambulatory, ask him to give you a urine specimen (if possible) before going to bed. If he is on bedrest, give him a clean bedpan/urinal and ask him to give you a specimen. (Follow procedure used in the unit on Urine Elimination.) If he is unable to give you a urine specimen at this time, leave the container in the room and tell him you need the specimen as soon as possible.

6. Take care of patient's belongings.

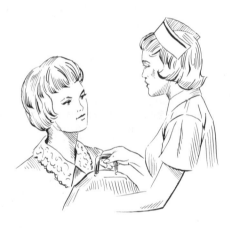

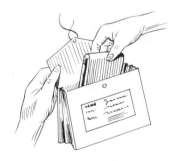

While he is getting the urine specimen, hang his clothes neatly in the clothes closet, and unpack his personal belongings, e.g., tooth brush, tooth paste, comb, deodorant, and place them conveniently in the bedside cabinet. Store the suitcase in the clothes closet.

Note: When you hang the clothes in the closet, inspect the clothing for pediculi (lice) or bedbugs. If found, report immediately to the nurse so the doctor can prescribe treatment for the patient. In some instances the clothes must be burned or sterilized. Check your agency procedure.

Ask patient if he has any *valuables* or money over $2.00; if so, they should either be taken home by a family member or placed in a special "Valuables Envelope" and taken to the safe in the Business Office for storage until he is discharged. When you use a Valuables Envelope, follow your agency procedure. Be sure to record the envelope number and where you stored the envelope on the nurse's notes. Also ask if he has any *medications* with him. If so, these should either be sent home with the relatives or taken to the drug room for safekeeping while he is in the hospital. (They are returned to him on discharge.) If the patient has money or valuables but will not give them to you, report this to your team leader. You are not to search the patient's wallet, handbag or suitcase for such articles. See your agency regulations for handling this type of problem.

7. Take the patient's physical inventory.

Record the information on your admitting record as you proceed. Later it will be transferred to the patient's chart.

A. Take the T, P, R and B/P.

B. Weigh the patient (use either the portable scales or the health scales in the treatment unit).

Important Steps	Key Points

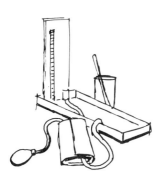

C. Observe the patient carefully during the entire procedure for:
—his general condition (good, alert, drowsy, emaciated or thin, etc.)
—the condition of his skin (clean, dirty, birthmarks, dry, bruised, cut, etc.)
—difficulty in breathing (dyspnea)
—coughing: what kind, i.e., dry, wet, hacking, productive (amount, color, odor, etc.)
—breath (odor)
—level of consciousness (alert, partly conscious, comatose)
—pain (location and type)
—speech (fluent, articulate, incoherent, and what language)
—his complaints, e.g., "I have a headache."
—ability to move easily
—ability to hear (deafness)
—ability to see (blindness)
—prostheses (wigs, dentures, bridges, glass eye, contact lenses or eyeglasses, artificial leg, etc.)

All of these must be recorded on the patient's chart. A list of descriptive terms useful when charting your admission notes can be found in the unit on Charting.

UNIT 27

8. Explain the use of hospital equipment.

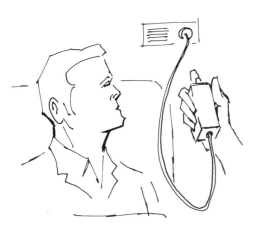

Demonstrate how to use the *call-button* and intercom (communication system) for calling the nurse. Attach call light conveniently within the patient's reach; also demonstrate use of the bathroom *emergency call button.* Explain how to operate the *bed controls* for the bed; demonstrate operation of the *TV controls;* and explain how to use the telephone for outside calls. Be sure that the telephone is easy to reach.

Since each of these items may vary from agency to agency, follow your agency procedure.

9. Explain hospital routine.

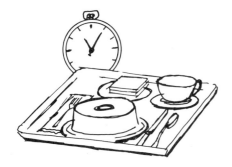

Tell him when *meals* will be served, e.g., 8 A.M., 12 noon and 4:30 P.M. Explain the *visiting hour* regulations: afternoon 2 to 4 P.M., evening 7 to 8:30 P.M. These vary among agencies, so tell him your agency's visiting hours.

There are Public Health Regulations which prohibit children under 14 years of age from visiting (exceptions can be made in critical cases, however, so check with your team leader). This is done to minimize the possibility of children bringing infectious diseases to already sick patients and to prevent the chil-

Important Steps	Key Points

dren from contact with patients who have infectious disease.

Special Care units (obstetrics, pediatrics, CCU, ICU, etc.) have special visiting hours. Check your agency regulations. Exceptions are also made for critically ill or pre-operative patients.

Visitors are usually limited to two at a time per patient. This is done for several reasons:

(1) To avoid overtiring the patient, who usually makes an effort to entertain visitors; this is *very* tiring.

(2) Because of limited space and chairs available for visitors in the patient's room.

(3) To keep the noise level at a minimum. Many people crowded into a small area tend to talk loudly.

Explain that laboratory and X-ray procedures may be done on admission, or they may be taken care of later, after the patient arrives on the floor. If the patient is pre-operative, explain that surgical preps (shaves) are usually done on the evening of admission by someone from the operating room. Inform him about the *volunteer service* to obtain newspapers, toilet articles, reading materials, etc.

Describe the uniforms and duties of various personnel the patient will have contact with, e.g., nurse's aide, orderly, LVN (LPN), RN, student nurses of several types from various programs, and personnel from other departments: housekeeping, dietary, maintenance, etc.

10. Provide for patient's safety.

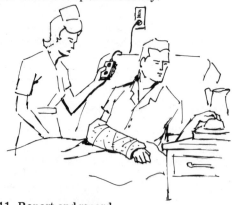

Lower bed to lowest position. Raise siderails if indicated (observe your agency rules). Place call light within easy reach, also the TV and bed controls. Have bedside stand near the bed so the patient will not have to reach (possibly fall out of bed). Arrange bedding and patient for comfort and proper body alignment.

11. Report and record.

Transfer information from your admission form to the nurse's notes. Report any unusual findings to your team leader. Take urine specimen (properly labeled) immediately to the laboratory. Charting example:

5:40 P.M. White male admitted ambulatory. To bed in 602, appears alert and in good condition. States he is in for general cardiac workup. Valuables sent home with wife. Urine specimen obtained, sent with requisition and charge voucher to the laboratory. Oriented to equip-

Important Steps	Key Points

ment in room and general hospital routine.

J. Jones, SN

TPR/BP/weight will be recorded on graphic sheet. May also be recorded in nurse's notes depending on agency procedures.

ITEM 3. TRANSFER PROCEDURE

Transfers, moving a patient from one bed to another, or to another room or unit, are common occurrences in health agencies. They are necessary for a variety of reasons:

A. The patient requests a private or semi-private room on admission. If none is available, he must wait and stay in a multi-bed room until a private one is vacated.

B. The patient's condition changes and he must be moved to a special care unit, e.g., ICU, CCU, or an isolation room. Certain persons in a room may not get along; one must be moved so that both can rest.

C. The patient may request a bed by the window when it becomes available.

A patient may be apprehensive about a transfer requested by the doctor. You must reassure him and explain why he is being transferred. Be sure that the room to which he is going is ready for his occupancy.

Important Steps	Key Points

1. Wash your hands, identify the patient, and collect his personal items.

Explain to patient that he is being transferred. It helps to use a utility cart or a wheelchair in transporting his personal items and supplies. Be sure to take *all* of his *clothes* (check bedside stand and clothes closets), luggage, personal items, and *dentures*. (These are frequently lost during a transfer; if so, *you* may have to pay to have them replaced. Some agencies have an emergency fund to cover this expense. However, it is not only the cost of $200 to $500 but the embarrassment and inconvenience for the patient.) Collect all his equipment (bedpan, wash basin, emesis basin, etc.). In some agencies you may order clean equipment on transfer. Whichever is the case take them to the patient's room.

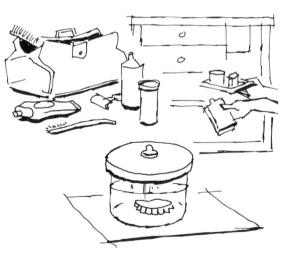

2. Transfer patient.

Move the patient by wheelchair or stretcher, depending on his condition, to his new room. Remember to use good body movement both for yourself and your patient during this procedure. Take necessary safety precautions (use safety belts if available; use equipment which is

Important Steps	Key Points

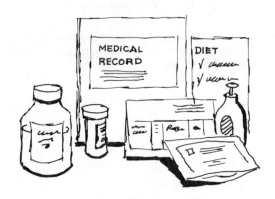

in good working order). Push wheelchair or stretcher in correct manner.

Note: Patient may be moved in his own bed if his condition warrants it. You will need assistance in moving the bed.

Take the patient's *chart* and *medications* with you when you are transferring him to another unit.

3. Secure patient in new bed.

Assist him into bed. Position the patient for comfort and safety. Adjust siderails if indicated. Place call button, bed and TV controls conveniently. Put bedside stand near head of bed in easy reach of the patient. Store patient's supplies and equipment in bedside table. Get fresh water and a pitcher of ice for patient (if permitted).

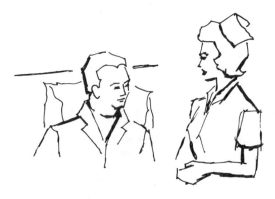

4. Introduce patient to new roommate.

It is also helpful to introduce him to new ward personnel. Leave patient neat and comfortable.

5. Return wheelchair/stretcher to storage area.

Remove soiled linen from stretcher and replace with clean linen ready for next usage.

6. Go back to patient's former unit.

Strip room of used linens and supplies. Make ready for terminal cleaning by housekeeping personnel (or nursing personnel, according to your agency procedure). After cleaning, a closed bed is made for new admission. Be sure that room is neat and restocked with admission equipment (bedpan/urinal, emesis basin, wash basin, gown, etc.).

7. Report and record.

Note transfer on the patient's chart (time, from room number and bed, to room number and bed via wheelchair or stretcher). Chart any unusual occurrences. Give chart and medications to charge nurse. Give an oral report on patient's condition. Charting example.

10:45 A.M. Transferred to room 407 via wheelchair. All personal items including dentures with patient. Settled into new surroundings. Is looking forward to the new experience.

          J. Jones SN

Important Steps	Key Points
8. Receiving the transfer patient.	The assigned personnel will assist in getting the patient to bed and settled. The charge nurse will take the patient's chart, his medications, and a verbal report from nursing personnel bringing the patient to the unit (specimens required, special care needed, procedures which must be completed). Be sure to introduce patient to new staff. Make him feel welcome. Be courteous and friendly.
9. Explain routines.	If routines in new area are different (meals, visiting, etc.), they should be thoroughly explained to the patient and his family.
10. Record on patient's chart.	Make a note of the time, method of transportation, and general condition of patient at time of transfer. Charting example:
	10:55 A.M. Received on unit via wheelchair from room 602, in good condition. To bed after orientation to unit routines and introductions. J. Jones, SN

UNIT 27

ITEM 4. DISCHARGE PROCEDURE

The physician usually writes an order for the patient's discharge; however, a patient may leave Against Medical Advice (termed "AMA"—in this instance he must sign a special release), or he may have expired. (In that case follow the procedure for postmortem care.) Patients are normally happy to go home, but they are often weak and need your careful, considerate assistance. Before the patient can be released from a nursing unit, certain financial arrangements must be made with the Business Office. These arrangements can be handled by the patient or his relatives. The Business Office will notify the nursing unit when these arrangements have been made.

If the doctor wrote orders for medications to be sent home with the patient, be sure they are available on the nursing unit. Occasionally, the patient will have a special diet to follow. Be sure that the dietitian has conferred with the patient or relatives before he is discharged.

Patients may be discharged by ambulance service. In this case, a time is usually scheduled for the departure. Make sure that the patient is completely ready for discharge when the ambulance personnel arrive. Again, be courteous and helpful as you assist the patient in packing his personal belongings and leaving.

Important Steps	Key Points
1. Obtain discharge order.	The order usually will be written by the physician, and you will be given the assignment by your team leader.
2. Wash your hands, identify the patient and explain procedure to him and his family.	Ask for their cooperation. Determine the expected time of discharge and the time when family, friends, or ambulance can arrive to take him home.

Important Steps	Key Points
3. Obtain valuables from safe. 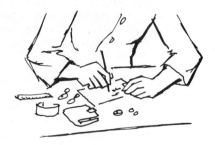	If he has valuables stored in the safe, the patient must sign the release tab on the Valuables Envelope indicating that he has received the items. The signed receipt will either be attached to the patient's chart or returned to the Business Office for filing. (Follow your agency procedure.)
4. Check special instructions for the patient to be sure they have been carried out.	Be sure that take-home medications are received by the patient or his family and that instructions for taking them are given. (This is usually taken care of by the Registered Nurse.) If the patient is to follow a special diet after discharge, be sure the dietitian has discussed it with the patient or his family. If the patient is to return to the clinic for follow-up appointments, be sure he has the appropriate forms and directions.
5. Check dressings and/or bandages.	If they need changing, be sure this is done before the patient leaves. Your team leader will determine if they should be changed; see that it is done if indicated. Usually the entry-level nurse does not do the actual dressing change; the LVN or RN will complete the procedure.
6. Assist patient to dress and pack. 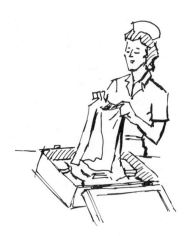	Offer to help the patient pack. Be sure you check the bedside stand and clothes closets for all his belongings. Assist him to dress as needed. If the patient asks questions you cannot answer about his condition or what he is to do at home, immediately ask your team leader to come and clarify them.
7. Check to see if Business Office procedure has been completed.	Most agencies require a special release form which must be completed for the Business Office before the patient can leave. Usually the patient or a member of the family will have to go to the Business Office to take care of the financial arrangements. (Follow your agency procedure.)

Important Steps	Key Points
8. Obtain a wheelchair and utility cart to transport belongings.	Although many patients claim that they feel well enough to walk out, be sure they take a wheelchair. They are not as strong as they think they are, and an unnecessary delay (e.g., waiting for an elevator) may lead to weakness and possible fainting. If there are safety belts on the wheelchair, make sure they are secured. The utility cart is helpful to transport the luggage.
9. Transport patient and belongings to waiting vehicle.	Most agencies provide a discharge area where the patient is protected from the weather when getting into the car. Assist patient into the car. Install belongings in car.
10. Return wheelchair and utility cart to storage area.	Some agencies have a special area for returning supplies so they can be thoroughly cleaned before use. In any event, when you return the equipment, be sure it is clean (you may need to wipe it with a cleaning solution) and in good working order. If it needs repair, place a repair notice on the article and notify the maintenance department, by phone or requisition, of the necessary repair work.
11. Return to patient's room, strip bed, and prepare for terminal cleaning.	In most agencies, nursing personnel are responsible for this activity, but the actual cleaning is the responsibility of the housekeeping department.
12. Report and record.	Report to team leader and ward clerk that patient is gone. Chart the discharge on the nurse's notes. Information should include time, whether by stretcher or wheelchair, a statement about the general condition, destination (home or another health facility), and any other appropriate comments. It is helpful to note the name and location of the other health agency for future reference. Sign your name and title. Remove chart from chart holder and place in area designated for discharge charts. Charting example:

2:30 P.M. Discharged via wheelchair to home in good condition. Dietary instructions and medication were explained. Patient stated all personnel were most kind, thorough and conscientious.   J. Jones, SN

U
N
I
T
27

POST-TEST

True or False: Circle "T" if the statement is true or circle "F" if the statement is false.

(T) F   1. Introducing yourself to a patient is one of the most important steps in the admitting procedure.

(T) F   2. Checking the patient's skin is part of the admitting procedure.

T (F)   3. On admission, the patient must put on a hospital gown.

(T) F   4. Chart valuables envelope number in nurse's notes.

T (F)   5. All patients should be provided with a full water pitcher and glass on admission.

T (F)   6. When patient is transferred, oral reports are not necessary since information is all on the nurse's notes or nursing care plan.

(T) F   7. Patients should know that they are being transferred to another room or unit.

(T) F   8. Patients may be discharged without a physician's order.

(T) F   9. Patients must sign for clothes and valuables prior to discharge.

10. List at least 10 items that should be observed about a patient upon admission.

A. _attitude_

B. _skin_

C. _dyspnea_

D. _cough_

E. _odor of breath_

F. _level of consciousness_

G. _pain_

H. _speech_

I. _any complaints_

J. _ability to move_

POST-TEST ANNOTATED ANSWER SHEET

1. T (p. 556)

2. T (p. 559)

3. F (p. 556)

4. T (p. 558)

5. F (pp. 560 and 562)

6. F (p. 562)

7. T (p. 561)

8. T (p. 563)

9. T (p. 564)

10. A — general condition

    B — condition of skin

    C — dyspnea

    D — cough

    E — odor of breath

    F — level of consciousness

    G — pain (p. 559)

    H — speech

    I — patient's complaints

    J — ability to move

       — hearing deficit

       — sight deficit

       — protheses

(In any order)

PERFORMANCE TEST

1. Read the following situation through. Record the appropriate information on nurse's notes.

On December 22, 1970 at 2:15 P.M. a Caucasian male age 63 was admitted via wheelchair to room 466. He undressed and was assisted to bed. Vital signs 98.2–82–22, BP 122/82, Wt. 152 lbs., Ht. 6 ft. He was alert but appeared to have difficulty moving his right arm and leg. He complained of nausea and vomiting and stated his stomach hurt. While assisting him to bed, you noticed a small bruise on his right ankle and a large reddened area on his sacrum. A urine specimen was obtained and sent to the lab. His doctor was notified.

2. Given a partner in the skill laboratory, you will prepare the "patient" and carry out the procedure for: Admission, transfer, or discharge. You will assemble the necessary equipment, supplies, and records, explain to the patient what you are going to do, follow the procedure established in the lesson, and practice the charting of your activity on the nurse's notes. Explain *what* you are doing and *why* so that both the "patient" and your instructor will be able to follow your line of reasoning.

PERFORMANCE CHECKLIST

ADMISSION, TRANSFER, AND DISCHARGE

ADMISSION

Demonstrate procedure followed for admission of a patient.

1. Adjust height of bed—on notification patient is to be admitted (low, if patient is ambulatory; high, if on stretcher).

2. Prepare environment: open bed, adjust lights, temperature, and ventilation.

3. Place gown on top of bed.

4. Assemble admitting equipment: urine specimen container, sphygmomanometer, stethoscope, thermometer, and admission checklist.

5. Await patient's arrival.

6. Greet patient and check his identification band.

7. Give chart to nurse.

8. Introduce self.

9. Take patient to room.

10. Wash hands.

11. Pull screen.

12. Assist patient into gown (own or hospital).

13. Obtain urine specimen.

14. Hang clothes neatly in closet.

15. Inspect for pediculi.

16. Inquire about valuables and medications, take necessary steps.

17. Do patient physical inventory: temperature, blood pressure, weight; observe objective symptoms and elicit subjective symptoms from patient.

18. Explain hospital procedures: call signal and emergency call system, and the television and bed controls.

19. Explain agency schedules and procedures: meals, visiting, laboratory and X-ray exams, prep, volunteer service, uniforms, and types of personnel.

20. Provide for safety: lower bed; position siderails; check controls; and make sure there is a bedside stand nearby.

21. Leave patient comfortable and in good body alignment.

U
N
I
T
27

TRANSFER

Demonstrate the correct procedure for transferring a patient.

1. Wash hands, identify patient and explain procedure.

2. Collect patient's personal items.

3. Obtain stretcher or wheelchair to transport patient.

    A. Obtain utility cart to transfer patient's personal items, if needed.

    B. Check equipment for safety.

4. Transfer patient to new location.

    A. Use good body movement for self and patient.

    B. Use safety precaution with mechanical aid, i.e., safety belt.

5. Take chart and medications with patient.

6. Install patient in new unit and leave patient neat and comfortable.

7. Introduce new roommate and staff.

8. Return stretcher or wheelchair to storage area.

9. Return to former patient unit and strip room for terminal cleaning.

10. After room is cleaned, restock supplies, and make ready for new admission.

11. Chart procedure on nurse's notes.

DISCHARGE

The student will demonstrate the procedure for discharge of a patient.

1. Obtain discharge order.

2. Wash hands, identify patient, and explain procedure to patient.

3. Obtain valuables.

4. Check to see if special instructions have been carried out, e.g., take-home medications available, special diet instructions given.

5. Check dressings or bandages, and change them if necessary.

6. Assist patient to pack and dress (make sure all personal items are packed).

7. Verify final Business Office clearance.

8. Obtain wheelchair and utility cart for transportation, and check safety features, i.e., safety belts.

9. Transport patient and belongings to discharge area.

10. Assist patient into car:

    A. Use good body movement for patient and self.

    B. Use safety principles, i.e., lock wheels of chair.

11. Return wheelchair to storage area.

    A. Clean and check wheelchair for needed repairs.

    B. Prepare work requisition if repairs are needed.

12. Return to patient's room, strip and make ready for terminal cleaning.

13. Make room ready for new patient after cleaning is completed.

14. Record activity on nurse's notes.

Unit 28

CARE OF THE DYING PATIENT AND POSTMORTEM CARE

I. DIRECTIONS TO THE STUDENT

Proceed through this lesson. When you have finished, practice the preparation of the body on a mannequin in the presence of your instructor. Complete the post-test.

II. GENERAL PERFORMANCE OBJECTIVES

Following this lesson, you will be able to prepare a body after death, including the care of skin, body orifices, tubings, and valuables.

III. SPECIFIC PERFORMANCE OBJECTIVES

When you have completed this lesson, you will be able to:

1. Name and describe the five stages of dying.

2. Demonstrate concern and respect for the patient's body by moving it gently and carefully and without injury.

3. Protect the patient's valuables no matter how small and seemingly insignificant.

4. Demonstrate the correct care of drainage tube.

IV. VOCABULARY

autopsy—postmortem examination of the organs of a dead body to determine cause of death, or pathological conditions.

coroner—pathologist employed by the city, county, or state (may or may not be a physician) who examines a dead body to determine the cause of death in unusual circumstances, e.g., drowning, shooting, suicide, murder, auto accident.

coroner's case*—coroner has legal authority to perform an autopsy without family consent in certain cases; examples of coroner's cases include:

(1) A person dies within 24 hours after admission to the hospital.

(2) Possibility of death resulting from injury or accident.

(3) A person dies without having seen a physician within 72 hours prior to death.

deceased—dead or expired.

morgue—a place where dead bodies are kept before they are released to the mortuary.

next of kin—person related to the deceased with legal authority to sign documents. See your agency consent manual for more details.

pathologist—a specialist in diagnosing the morbid (death-related) changes in tissues removed during operations and postmortem examinations.

---

*Coroner's cases vary from state to state; check with your particular agency for a list of coroner's cases in your area.

pathology—study of the nature and cause of disease which involves changes in structure and function.

postmortem—after death.

rigor mortis—temporary rigidity of muscles occurring after death.

shroud—a large sheet, usually muslin or plastic, used to wrap dead bodies.

supine position—lying on the back with the face upward.

V. INTRODUCTION

Death and dying are fearful concerns for all of us. It is difficult for many of us to accept the fact that we are not immortal. At the same time, we know that death is a certainty for each of us. Our attitude toward the dying patient is usually uneasy and fearful. Frequently the patient is abandoned by all, even by the very people who care most about the patient. Health workers may avoid visiting these patients because they feel that they are beyond help.

It is actually very important for you to be with the patient as often as possible during the terminal stages of his illness. Continue to display concern, support, and comforting nursing attitudes toward him. Often you will find that the patient is longing just to have someone near. Sometimes, he wants to talk about his feelings toward death and dying. It will be hard for you to talk with him because of your own feelings, apprehensions, and lack of understanding about the process of dying. However, more information is becoming available each day which will help you to meet this important opportunity for service to the patient.

There are researchers working currently with terminally ill patients to find ways to help them cope with the last crisis of life. Five stages have been identified as characteristic of the process of dying. They are:

1. *Denial*—when the patient cannot believe the fact. He may respond, "No, not me!"

2. *Anger*—when he lashes out all around him, frequently saying "Why me?"

3. *Bargaining*—when he tries to find a way out of the situation by saving himself. He may respond, "If you give me six months more so I can see my son graduate, I'll donate my body or my heart to science."

4. *Preparatory grief*—this is the time when the patient begins to deal personally with the fact of dying. He is quiet, noncommunicative, and depressed. This may be the most difficult time for you. Sometimes just sitting quietly by the patient while he works the problem through will be of assistance to him. Your presence is his greatest need at this time.

5. *Acceptance*—This stage is not resignation, but one of peace and understanding that he has fulfilled his task; he is ready to go. In other words, he has resolved his own feelings.

It is helpful to know that most persons will move through the various stages of the process as they approach the final acceptance of death. Sometimes the stages overlap and are of very brief duration. In other instances, a patient may never move beyond the denial stage. In all cases, your continued understanding of their struggle, and your support (physical, emotional, spiritual) will help the patients and their families. As you continue your nursing career, you will begin to see the pattern of the dying process evolve in your patients. With each experience, your increasing awareness and understanding of the patient will make it easier for you to help him.

When the patient expires (dies, is deceased), you will be expected to perform the final postmortem procedure. Usually you will have another coworker to help you with the procedure. It will be helpful to you to have some background information before you proceed.

VI. BASIC INFORMATION

The patient is not considered legally dead until the physician has certified his death, and you should avoid doing anything that would interfere with life, because there is always a possibility of life remaining in the body. The undertaker cannot accept the body or prepare it for burial before the official pronouncement has been made.

Bodies are usually embalmed (chemically preserved) in this country and made to look as natural as possible. Embalming is not carried out in all countries of the world, however. Distortion, discoloration and scarring of the body are distressing to the family and friends, and therefore should be avoided by moving the body gently and carefully. The body itself should be clean and wrapped in a clean covering when sent to the hospital morgue or to the undertaking establishment, and should be plainly marked to avoid mistakes in identity.

The death certificate, which is sent to the local or state health department, is made out by the physician, the undertaker, and/or the pathologist if an autopsy is performed. State laws regulate the disposition of unidentified as well as identified bodies. In obtaining permission for autopsies when an unidentified person dies in a hospital, a local agency (police, health or coroner) is notified, and this agency assumes responsibility for trying to determine the identity of the body and for burial arrangements.

When a person has a family or is in the custody of friends, most state laws require that permission of the next of kin or the custodial friend be obtained before an autopsy is performed. If circumstances of death necessitate a coroner's inquest, the state is permitted to conduct an autopsy without the consent of relatives of the deceased.

Because ideas about death and the hereafter differ among people of various backgrounds, it is important for you to be familiar with certain religious beliefs:

The Catholic patient should be baptized if he had not already been baptized. Prayers for the Dying should be offered for him at this point. (Review unit Assisting with Spiritual Care.)

If the patient is an Orthodox Jew, do not touch the body until the rabbi has arrived to perform the final rites.

You should not inflict your religious beliefs on the patient or family, but stand ready to assist them in any way you can. However, dying is a lonely and frightening experience for the patient (if he is conscious) and a traumatic one for his family. Remain nearby to comfort patient and family in any way you can, such as offering to assist them with telephone calls, summoning a clergyman, obtaining coffee, or offering other services.

There are certain signs of approaching death which may appear:

1. The reflexes gradually disappear and the patient may be unable to move; the sphincter muscles (rectal and urinary) relax, causing incontinence. Be sure to keep the patient clean and dry during his last hours.

2. The typical respiration of the dying is called Cheyne-Stokes; it begins with slow, shallow breathing, gradually increasing in depth and rapidity, followed by a short period of apnea (no respiration), then repeating the cycle, until there is no recovery from the periods of apnea.

3. The circulation slows and the extremities (feet and hands) become cold and mottled blue in color (cyanotic). The pulse becomes rapid and weak; the blood pressure is lowered.

4. The eyes stare (become fixed); they do not respond to light.

5. The hearing is the last sense to fail. Even though the patient appears unconscious, he can usually still hear very well. Therefore, you must be extremely cautious about what you say in his room. Caution the family about saying anything which may adversely affect the patient while they are in his room.

6. When both the breathing and the pulse stop, notify the RN in charge immediately.

UNIT 28

The family may need a quiet room in which to discuss matters concerning the choice of the mortuary to handle the funeral services. Because this is a highly emotional ordeal, it is important to have a quiet, secluded room (often near the chapel) where they can have privacy to release their feelings. Provide coffee or tea for them if indicated. Stay nearby to help if the need arises.

When a patient dies in the hospital, the RN in charge is responsible for obtaining a form called "Release of the Body to the Mortuary" and having it properly filled out and signed. There is another form, an autopsy release, which she must also have prepared and signed when circumstances require it.

Upon the pronouncement of death you will be expected to carry out the following procedure:

Important Steps	Key Points
1. Gather equipment and take it into room.	Obtain the "death care kit" of two large shipping tags, clean gown, rubber bands, envelopes or containers for valuables, shroud, gauze 4 X 4's, cotton balls, paper bags, and valuables list.
2. Draw curtains 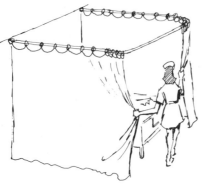	When death occurs in a multi-bed unit, provide others with privacy; close the door to the corridor. Wash your hands.
3. Elevate the bed to working height and flatten.	Use proper body alignment, balance and movement while you work. Review lesson if necessary.
4. Place the body in supine position as if sleeping. 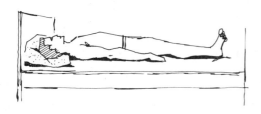	Close the eyes; you may use cotton gently applied over eyelids and held in place by tape if the eyes will not stay closed. Straighten the body, with the arms laid to each side, palms down. Some agencies may prefer to have the arms gently crossed over the body at the waist or across the abdomen. Replace dentures and close the mouth. If the mouth will not remain closed, place a towel rolled as a cylinder under the chin to keep the mouth closed. Place a pillow under the head. Move the body gently to avoid bruises and breaks. In general, the body should be put in a sleeping position as soon as possible, so that when stiffness (rigor mortis) occurs, the body will be positioned for an open casket, which many families request during funerals. After rigor mortis sets in, it is difficult to change the position of the body.
5. Remove jewelry and list all personal articles.	In general, all rings, earrings, bracelets, beads, hairpins, etc., should be removed and placed in a container provided for valuables. Include eyeglasses, cards, letters, keys, religious articles.

Important Steps	Key Points

Nothing is too small to be listed on the valuables list, for these articles are valuable to the family. Review agency policy regarding the disposition of these articles. If wedding or other rings worn are too tight to remove, it is advisable to place cotton over stones, then tape the ring to the finger. Note this on the valuables list as well as on your nursing notes, or wherever your agency requires this to be noted. If the family is present, all personal articles, including the above, should be given to the next of kin. In the nurse's notes, list the items and the name of the person who takes the belongings.

6. Clean the body.

Using plain water, wash the areas of the body that may be soiled with blood, feces, or vomitus. Especially make sure that all body orifices (openings) are cleansed and dried. If leakage occurs around the rectum, urethra or vagina, place a gauze 4 X 4 over each opening and secure it with tape to prevent further soiling. Following death, sphincter muscles relax, often causing incontinence of feces and urine.

7. Arrange the hair.

Brush and comb the hair neatly, so that if the family wishes to see the body before it is moved, grooming will be in order. (Review lesson on hair care if necessary.)

If the family wishes to view the body, place it in sleeping position, supine, eyes closed, arms gently crossed on lower abdomen. Straighten bedding (sheet and spread) as though you had completed a bath and prepared the patient for a nap. Remain with the family during the visit.

8. Care for tubes.

If there *is* to be an *autopsy*, the tubes are generally left in the body; remove the drainage bottles or bags from the tube and fold tube over twice; secure the end with a rubber band to avoid leakage. If there is no autopsy, tubes usually may be removed. Make sure you deflate balloon tips so that you do not injure the body tissues upon removal. Review your agency policy about tubes after death.

9. Change dressings.

Soiled dressings should be replaced with fresh ones. Old adhesive tape marks may be removed with benzene or a similar solution used by your agency.

10. Dress the body. (Follow agency policy; some do not dress body in a clean gown.)

If it is your agency's policy, dress the body in a clean gown. Gowning the body is usually done for the family's viewing of the body.

11. Identify the body.

Label the tag(s) with the patient's name, age, sex, date, hospital number, room number and physician's name. Tie the tag to the wrist or ankle according to hospital policy. Tie the tag tight enough so it will not slip off, yet loose enough that it will not cause bruises. Some agencies tape the label to the patient's anterior chest.

UNIT 28

Important Steps	Key Points
12. Place the body on a shroud if this is your agency's policy. 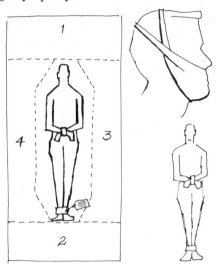	Place the body on the shroud (large square piece of muslin or plastic). As shown in the sketch, wrap side 1 down around the head, followed by side 2 up over the feet. Wrap sides 3 and 4. You may need to tie a bandage lightly under the jaw and up around the head to keep the jaw closed. Also, some agencies lightly bandage the wrists together criss-crossed over the abdomen to prevent the arms from falling off the stretcher when moving the body to the morgue. A large safety-pin or masking tape may be used to keep the shroud in place. (If your agency provides instructions for wrapping a body in a shroud, follow those directions.)
13. Apply outside label. 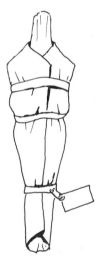	Tag the outside of the shroud with the patient's name, age, sex, hospital number, room number, physician's name, and the date. Safety-pin this tag to the outside of the shroud.
14. Transport the body to the morgue. (Some agencies leave the body in the room until a mortician or coroner's officer removes it. Check your agency's policy.) 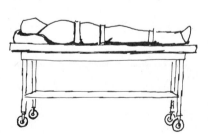	Using proper body alignment and movement, slide the body gently onto a cart or stretcher. Cover the body with a sheet. In some agencies, the face remains uncovered; others cover the face, particularly when the shroud is used. Follow your agency policy. Secure the body with stretcher straps at the chest and knees. Apply the straps tight enough to prevent the body from slipping off, but loose enough so as not to cause bruising. When transporting the body, try to use non-public elevators and corridors to avoid disturbing visitors. If an elevator is used, secure an elevator key and ask visitors to step off to avoid distress and to make the transfer as fast as possible.

Important Steps	Key Points
	When the assigned personnel have left the body in the morgue, take the stretcher back to the unit, remove the linen and place it in the hamper, wash (or take it to the central processing area for cleaning), and make it up with clean linen.
15. Strip the patient's room.	Return to the patient's room. Remove the soiled linen, bottles, pitchers, etc., and put them in the place provided for their processing. Call department for room cleaning, or proceed to clean, whichever is your agency's policy.
16. Provide security for valuables.	This step may be completed whenever it is possible. Follow your agency's policy for the disposition of valuables. *Never* leave valuables unattended. Place them in the Nursing Station until they can be stored in a secure place or given to the family.
17. Record.	In your nursing notes, record the time and date the body was taken to the morgue or by the undertaker. If valuables were placed in safekeeping, indicate this in writing. If valuables were given to the family or friends, record the name of the persons to whom they were given, the relationship to the deceased, time and date. Have a co-worker who witnessed this action cosign with you in the notes. Charting example: 2:10 A.M. Transferred to morgue. Valuables (watch, wedding ring, and 2 nightgowns) sent home with son, John. J. Jones, SN M. Maye, SN

U
N
I
T
28

VII. ADDITIONAL INFORMATION FOR ENRICHMENT

For those who are interested, the instructor will be able to give some additional reading assignments which will be helpful to you as you learn about the dying process. In some agencies, a staff psychiatrist confers with the personnel to help them work through their personal feelings about death. If you have the opportunity to participate in such discussion groups, you might find it interesting and helpful.

POST-TEST

1. A person is considered legally dead only after a _____ has certified the death.

2. List two kinds of cases that are considered to be coroner's cases:

   a. _____

   b. _____

3. If an autopsy is to be done, all body tubes are usually _____ in the body.

4. In caring for the body after death, place the body in a _____ position, with eyes _____ and dentures _____

5. An autopsy is performed for the purpose of _____ and/or _____

6. Circle "T" or "F" if the following statements are true or false:

   T   F   a.   Dentures are removed from the body at death.

   T   F   b.   Jewelry may be left on the body at death.

   T   F   c.   Soiled dressings are changed before the body goes to the morgue.

   T   F   d.   Stretcher straps are not necessary when transporting the deceased.

   T   F   e.   Identification tags are placed on the body and the shroud.

   T   F   f.   Letters and greeting cards of the deceased may be thrown away.

POST-TEST ANNOTATED ANSWER SHEET

1. physician (p. 573)

2. unidentified bodies; questionable circumstances surrounding the death (p. 573)

3. left (p. 575)

4. supine; closed; in place (p. 574)

5. determining cause of death; determining pathological conditions (p. 571)

6. a.   F   (p. 574)

   b.   T   (p. 574)

   c.   T   (p. 575)

   d.   F   (p. 576)

   e.   T   (p. 576)

   f.   F   (p. 574)

PERFORMANCE TEST

Discuss the five stages of dying with your instructor.

In the skill laboratory you will prepare the mannequin (Mrs. Chase) as though she were a dead body. You will cleanse her, pack her body orifices, label the body, wrap her in a shroud, label the outside of the shroud, and prepare to transport her to the morgue.

Practice charting the activity on the nurse's notes. Your instructor will give you a set of comments which you will appropriately record on the nurse's notes.

PERFORMANCE CHECKLIST

POSTMORTEM CARE

Demonstrate correct postmortem care procedure

1. Assemble equipment in room.

2. Screen patient (draw curtains and close door).

3. Adjust bed to working height, flatten bed.

4. Place body in supine position, eyes closed, dentures in place, arms at side or across chest, and pillow under head.

5. Remove jewelry and list personal articles.

6. Clean body and pack orifices.

7. Arrange hair.

8. Remove tubes (if no autopsy). Tubes remain in if an autopsy is to be performed.

9. Change dressings.

10. Change patient's clothing according to agency procedure.

11. Identify body with labeled tag on toe, wrist, chest (follow agency procedure).

12. Wrap body in shroud and attach label.

13. Move body to stretcher using correct body movement and alignment.

14. Secure safety belts at knees and chest.

15. Transport body to morgue.

16. Return to room for stripping and final cleaning.

17. Dispose of valuables according to agency procedure.

18. Record activities on chart.

Unit 29

CARE OF PATIENTS RECEIVING OXYGEN THERAPY

I. DIRECTIONS TO THE STUDENT

Read the introduction and procedures in this lesson carefully. They will tell you what you need to know regarding the nursing care of patients receiving oxygen therapy. Arrange with your instructor to practice using the various types of oxygen apparatus in your skill laboratory.

II. GENERAL PERFORMANCE OBJECTIVE

You will demonstrate your knowledge of the various oxygen therapies as well as the nursing care indicated when caring for patients receiving oxygen therapy.

III. SPECIFIC PERFORMANCE OBJECTIVES

Upon completion of this lesson and your laboratory practice, you will be able to correctly:

1. Describe and identify the methods of oxygen therapy administered to patients.

2. Demonstrate how to regulate oxygen flow and how to care for a patient with an oxygen tent, nasal cannula, nasal catheter, oxygen mask, or IPPB (intermittent positive pressure breathing apparatus), and properly record your activities.

3. Demonstrate and discuss safety precautions which must be observed when patients are receiving oxygen therapies.

IV. VOCABULARY

anoxia—deficiency of oxygen.
atelectasis—lack of air in the lungs due to blocking of small bronchial tubes.
bronchioles—terminal ends of the bronchi.
bronchus—one of two branches of the trachea (plural, bronchi).
complication—an added difficulty, e.g., post-operative appendectomy patient gets pneumonia.
cough—violent expiratory effort to rid the respiratory track of an obstruction; mouth is open.
diaphragm—the musculomembranous wall separating the abdominal and thoracic cavities.
diffusion—chemical process whereby a liquid or gas mixes its chemical components.
dyspnea—difficult or labored respiration.
epiglottis—small pedicle over the larynx (voice box) which closes when swallowing to permit food to go down the esophagus and to shunt air to the trachea.
expiration—breathing air from the lungs.
hiccough (singultus)—spasmodic contraction of the diaphragm due to an irritation of the stomach.
humidifier—an apparatus to increase the moisture content of the air.
hypoxemia—low oxygen content in the blood.
hypoxia—low oxygen content in the tissues.

inspiration—breathing air into the lungs.

medulla—enlarged portion of the spinal cord just inside the cranium.

nasal catheter—a tube, rubber or plastic, used to give oxygen through the nose.

nebulizer—atomizer or sprayer.

pharynx—throat, common passageway for food and air.

pleura—covering of the lung.

respiration—the act of breathing (inspiration and expiration).

sneeze—similar to a cough except that the violent expiratory effort is through the nose.

spirometer—an apparatus used to measure lung volumes of inspired and expired air.

syncope—fainting.

therapeutic—treatment given for the purpose of healing.

trachea—windpipe, 4½-inch-long tube from the larynx to the bronchial tree.

trauma—injury.

vertigo—dizziness

yawning—deep, long inspiration usually due to mental or physical fatigue.

V. INTRODUCTION

Breathing (respiration) is essential to life. Breathing is regulated by the respiratory centers located in the medulla and pons of the brain as well as some peripheral centers which are composed of clusters of chemosensitive cells known as carotid bodies and aortic bodies. Through the act of breathing in (inspiration), we take in air which has 20.93 per cent oxygen (O_2) and .04 per cent carbon dioxide (CO_2) and carry it to the respiratory system (nose, pharynx, larynx, trachea, bronchi, and lungs). The oxygen is absorbed into the circulatory system, which in turn carries it to all parts of the body. The oxygen content in the blood is a necessary chemical component upon which all tissues and living cells exist. Without oxygen some cells begin to die in 30 seconds.

When oxygen is prevented from entering the blood stream in the proper concentration, steps must be taken to assist the patient in getting more oxygen into his system. Disease or obstruction in some part of the respiratory tract may prevent the proper intake of oxygen.

Oxygen is carried by the hemoglobin in the red blood cells. It is a clear, odorless, tasteless gas that is heavier than air. It is a component of all living tissue and it supports combustion (the act of burning or fire). Because of this combustive characteristic, special precautions must be taken by the patient, staff, and visitors to prevent fire or an explosion during oxygen treatments. Cautionary NO SMOKING signs are placed in strategic places around the patient (on the oxygen equipment, at the head of the bed, and on the door to the patient's room). Most fires and explosions connected with oxygen therapy are caused by lighting a match in the immediate vicinity of the oxygen. Sparks from improperly working electrical equipment (electrical connections, electric shavers, radios, and TV's), or from static electricity, which can be generated by wool blankets and synthetic clothing, may produce a fire or explosion when in the presence of a high oxygen concentration. Most health agencies therefore use cotton blankets and request personnel to wear cotton clothing.

In the Additional Information for Enrichment segment of this unit you will learn more about the anatomy and physiology of the respiratory system. Some signs and symptoms you may observe in your patient who is not getting enough oxygen are as follows:

1. He may comment that he "can't breathe" or he "feels as though he is suffocating."

2. He will appear restless and irritable, anxious or frightened (he won't know why).

3. He will have decreased muscle coordination and slowed mental capacities. (Remember, all living tissue must have oxygen in order to continue proper functioning.)

4. He may become dyspneic (have difficulty breathing).

5. He may become cyanotic (bluish in color), because of diminished oxygen content in the blood.

6. He may increase the rate and depth of respirations to try to get enough oxygen from the air to supply the needs of the body.

7. He may faint (syncope) or complain of vertigo (dizziness) which is caused by a lack of oxygen in the brain.

Treatment of patients with respiratory diseases can take one of several forms:

1. Maintenance of an open breathing passage:

   a. The nurse may suction (a method of sucking up obstructing material by changing air pressure), if the patient can't cough up mucus and obstructions.

   b. You can also insert an airway for easier breathing. The airway keeps the tongue from falling into the back of the throat and obstructing the passage of air. You will recall the procedure from the unit on post-operative care.

   c. Another method of keeping an open air passage is to thin out the mucus secretions so that they can easily be removed by coughing or suction. This can be done by giving the patient steam inhalation treatments, nebulizers with or without medication, and intermittent positive pressure breathing (IPPB) with aerosol attachment.

2. Increasing the oxygen content by giving oxygen directly to the patient via one of several methods, e.g., nasal catheter, nasal cannula or naso-inhaler, nasal mask, or hyperbaric oxygen chamber.

U
N
I
T
29

ITEM 1.   ADMINISTRATION OF OXYGEN BY NASAL CATHETER

Oxygen is given by nasal catheter when high concentrations of oxygen are required (up to 35 per cent). This method is the most frequently used because it is efficient, it is not frightening to most patients, it permits easy observation of the patient by nursing personnel, and it gives the patient freedom to move about in bed. The catheter may cause some irritation to the nasal passages if it is left in for a long period of time; therefore, a humidifier is always used with this type of administration to keep the passageways moist. Although, as a beginning nurse practitioner, you will not initiate the use of the various nasal oxygen techniques, you may be responsible for starting and stopping the oxygen flow per doctor's or patient's orders. Oxygen therapy is given only on a doctor's order except in certain emergency situations established by the agency, e.g., in Coronary Care Units, Intensive Care Units, Recovery Room or Emergency Room, or other special care units within the agency.

You should be aware of the techniques for beginning administration so that you can assist the nurse or doctor and the patient. You must know how to regulate the oxygen flowmeters.

In the skill laboratory, given an emergency patient who is having severe breathing problems, you will assist in obtaining, assembling, and initiating oxygen by using a nasal catheter.

Important Steps	Key Points
1. Wash your hands, approach and identify the patient, and explain what is to be done.	Check his identification band. In this way it will be easier to obtain his cooperation. The patient may be frightened, anxious, irritable, and somewhat slow to comprehend (understand) your explanations. Refer to the signs and symptoms of insufficient oxygen intake on the previous page. Speak slowly, kindly, and with patience. Gain his confidence and cooperation. Instruct him on safety precautions, e.g., no smoking, restricted use of electrical appliances.

Important Steps	Key Points
2. Assemble equipment.	You will need an oxygen flowmeter and humidifier with connecting tubing and nasal catheter, glass of water, lubricant, piece of gauze, and NO SMOKING signs. (Equipment can be obtained from storage, from the supply department, or the inhalation therapy department.) The nasal catheter may be rubber or plastic. It is about 16 inches long, with several small holes in the tip of the catheter so that the oxygen can come out of the tube in several places. The type and size of the catheter for an adult is usually a #14 French. Always check equipment to see that it is in good working order.

3. Connect apparatus.

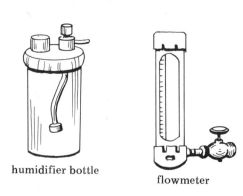

humidifier bottle   flowmeter

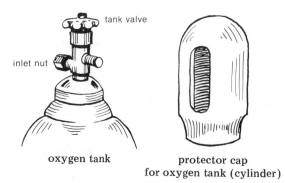

tank valve

inlet nut

oxygen tank   protector cap for oxygen tank (cylinder)

a. First fill the *humidifier bottle* (usually the bottle will come to you with distilled water in it, filled to the level marked on the outside of the bottle—about 2/3 full). If the water is not in the humidifier, you must fill it from your stock supply to the level marked on the bottle. To do this you unscrew and remove the bottle cap (counterclockwise). Fill with distilled water, (Tap water may be used with some equipment). Follow your agency procedure. Replace bottle cap (screw in clockwise motion).

b. Attach top of humidifier to oxygen regulator (or *flowmeter*). Attach flowmeter to oxygen outlet on the wall for piped-in oxygen by pressing it firmly into the outlet. To attach it to an oxygen tank: open the tank valve slightly to clear oxygen passageway of dust particles (this is known as "cracking the tank or valve").

Close immediately (turning counterclockwise). Connect the flowmeter to tank by inserting it into the cylinder outlet valve. Tighten inlet nut with a wrench (raise wrench upward) until nut is tight and holds regulator firmly.

c. Attach *connector tubing* from apparatus to nasal catheter.

d. Attach *nasal catheter* to connector tubing.

Important Steps   **Key Points**

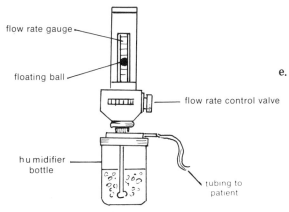

flow rate gauge

floating ball

flow rate control valve

humidifier bottle

tubing to patient

One style of oxygen setup.

e. Turn on wall-mounted oxygen supply. This is done by turning the flow adjustment valve upward toward the "on" position. (See accompanying diagram.) Continue turning valve upward until the desired flow level is reached; this level is recorded on the gauge just above the flow adjustment valve. The flow is recorded in liters of oxygen per minute. The doctor will usually prescribe the rate of flow, usually 3 to 4 liters. To turn on cylinder regulators: open the valve slowly and regulate flow-meter gauge.

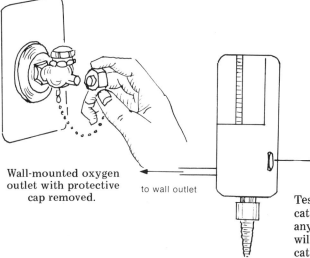

Wall-mounted oxygen outlet with protective cap removed.

to wall outlet

flow adjustment valve

Test oxygen flow by inserting tip of nasal catheter into a glass of water. You can see if any of the holes are plugged. The oxygen will bubble out through the holes in the catheter.

Wall-mounted oxygen gauge.

4. Pick up catheter and measure nasal catheter length for insertion.

The depth to which the catheter is to be inserted is determined by holding the catheter near the patient's face, measuring the distance from the tip of his nose to his ear lobe. Mark the length with the thumb of your left hand (you can use a piece of tape, if you prefer). (Reverse hand positions if you are left-handed.)

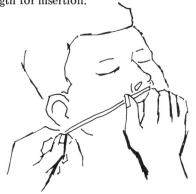

Important Steps	Key Points
5. Squeeze some lubricant onto a gauze square.	The nasal catheter needs to be well lubricated for ease of insertion. The easier the insertion, the less trauma (or injury) to the delicate mucous membrane lining in the nasal cavity. (Mineral oil and vaseline are not used because they are irritating to nasal lining.) Lubricate the tip end of nasal catheter in the agency prescribed jelly (a *water* soluble lubricant).
6. Insert nasal catheter. 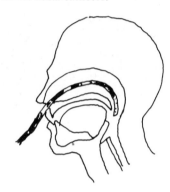	In your right hand, holding the catheter at the level marked on it for insertion, gently introduce catheter into one side of the nasal passageway. This is easier to do if with your left hand you pull the external nares back and up so you can see the nares very clearly. (Reverse hand positions if you are left-handed.) Do not use force to get catheter in. If you hit an obstruction, remove catheter and insert it into the other nostril.
7. Check level of catheter in back of throat. 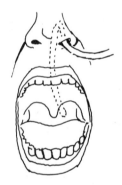	Have patient open his mouth wide. (You may need a tongue blade to hold his tongue flat so you can see the back of his mouth.) The tip of the catheter should be seen slightly to one side of the uvula (small pedicle of tissue hanging down from roof of mouth at the back).
8. Adjust oxygen flow.	Set it at the rate prescribed by the physician. (You may have done this under Step 3.)
9. Secure nasal catheter to patient's face with tape. 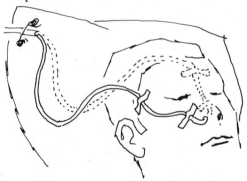	Split a 2-inch piece of adhesive tape in half to about the center of the strip. Wrap one split end around the catheter and attach the other to the patient's face. The catheter can be placed in one of two positions: (1) bring to side of nose (used for insertion) and fasten to face, or (2) bring back up over bridge of nose and fasten to forehead. Make patient comfortable in good body alignment, with call light and bedside stand conveniently located, fresh water at hand.

Important Steps	Key Points
10. Place "No Smoking" sign strategically.	Put signs on head of bed, on oxygen equipment, and on patient's door. Restate no smoking precautions. Although oxygen does not burn, it provides the climate for fires to start. Fire, like living tissue, needs oxygen to burn.
11. Record	Record initiation of oxygen. Note the method, time, flow rate, and any observations about the patient's condition, e.g., color pinked-up, breathing less labored. (Remember the *initiation* of the oxygen treatment is usually done by the nurse.) However the oxygen may be ordered PRN and you may be responsible for turning the flowmeter on or off as the patient requests. Be sure to record each administration. Charting example:

Nasal oxygen started at 3 L per minute. Respirations seem less labored, color pinked up. Seems less apprehensive.   C. Wyno, RN

UNIT 29

ITEM 2. SPECIAL CARE FOR PATIENTS RECEIVING NASAL OXYGEN

In caring for the patient who is receiving nasal oxygen, you will need to pay special attention to a number of details:

A. The nasal catheter will probably be exchanged for a clean one q̄ (every) 8 hours (or follow your agency procedure). Fresh lubrication will help to keep the nasal passageway moist and will be less irritating for the patient.

B. Observe the water level in the humidifier bottle several times during your tour of duty. Keep the water at the prescribed level (2/3 full). Turn off the oxygen supply while you unscrew the top of the water bottle for refilling. Fill bottle to prescribed level with distilled water, replace cap, reattach to flowmeter. Turn on oxygen and adjust flow rate. Remember, oxygen is extremely drying to tissue when given in this manner, and moisturization is very important for the comfort of the patient.

C. Be sure the tubing is not kinked (this will stop the oxygen flow to the patient). Be sure that there is enough slack in the tubing to permit him to move about freely.

D. Check the oxygen flow level—be sure it is maintained at the designated level. Become accustomed to checking the oxygen level each time you enter the patient's room.

If you are using an oxygen tank to give the oxygen treatment, you will need to watch the content in the tank so that it can be changed immediately when the tank registers empty. Occasionally the oxygen level gets low in the central oxygen system with piped-in oxygen. It is always necessary, therefore, to check the oxygen level frequently when your patient is receiving the treatment.

E. Observe the skin where the tape is attached to the patient's face. Watch for any marked irritation. Some patients may be allergic to the tape and you will have to fasten the catheter in some other way, e.g., tie gauze around the catheter and attach it with a pin to the sheet. (Care must be taken not to puncture the catheter with the pin.)

F. Give frequent oral hygiene to these patients. Since the oxygen is drying to tissue, the mouth becomes dry and stale-tasting. It must be refreshed frequently throughout the 24-hour period.

ITEM 3. SPECIAL CARE FOR PATIENTS RECEIVING OXYGEN BY NASAL CANNULA

The nasal cannula (or naso-inhaler) is used when the required concentration of oxygen is less than 35 per cent. The cannula consists of a rubber or plastic tube that splits into a V-shape at the tip. Each tip end of the V is inserted into one nostril about ¼ to ½ inch. The cannula is held in place with an elastic retainer which fits snugly around the head and attaches to the cannula, and can be easily adjusted for the patient's comfort. There is no need to fasten the cannula to the patient's face with tape; therefore, with this method of oxygen therapy the skin will not become irritated. This is an inefficient method since the patient frequently has his mouth open and the oxygen escapes around the external nares (nostrils) as well as through the mouth.

Follow same precautions in caring for the patient receiving oxygen by nasal cannula as those learned in the previous section.

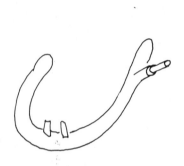

Nasal cannula.

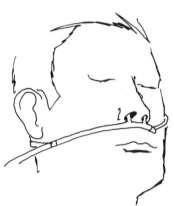

Cannula in place.

ITEM 4. ADMINISTRATION OF OXYGEN BY FACE MASK

Face masks are used when the concentration of oxygen must be very high—near 100 per cent: this method is often used as an emergency measure. Patients who must receive oxygen therapy over a long period of time dislike this method because they feel as though they are "going to suffocate" and they "can't breathe."

The face mask may cover the nose, or the nose and mouth, depending on the kind of mask you are using. Masks are adjusted over the nose and/or mouth and held in place by an elastic, adjustable head strap which fits snugly around the head.

In the skill laboratory, given a middle aged lady who is having an asthma attack, you will obtain and assemble equipment, and assist in the initiation of oxygen via a face mask.

Important Steps	Key Points
1. Wash your hands, approach and identify the patient, and explain what you will be doing.	Check the identification of the patient. Explain in detail what you are going to do. Answer all the patient's questions thoughtfully and correctly. If you are unable to answer the questions, refer them to the nurse or doctor. All of the patient's questions should be answered if possible.

Important Steps	Key Points

2. Assemble equipment and demonstrate its use.

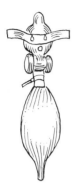

Obtain designated mask and oxygen flow meter. Select mask size to fit patient's face (small, medium, large, or infant). Show patient the correct placement of the mask by holding mask near your face. Demonstrate how the retaining strap will fit around his head to hold the mask securely in place. (It can be adjusted by the patient for his comfort.) If the patient has flown on an airplane, he may recall the stewardess's demonstration and explanation of the oxygen mask.

3. Attach mask tubing to oxygen flow.

Start oxygen flow at about 14 liters per minute. Most patients become apprehensive when the mask is placed over the nose and they breathe quite deeply. To prevent fright, they must be able to feel the oxygen coming in to the mask. (Flow will be decreased after the patient becomes accustomed to the mask.)

U
N
I
T
29

4. Place mask on patient's face.

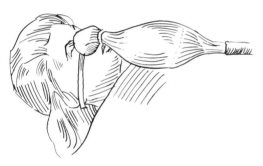

Adjust mask so that it fits comfortably on the face. Be sure there are no leaks of oxygen around the edges of the mask. The mask will fit over the patient's nose and/or his mouth, depending on the type of mask being used. You may need to pad the leaking areas with gauze or cotton if the mask does not fit the face tightly. Ask the patient to breathe naturally as you apply the mask. Talk quietly to him during the application of the mask. Help him to relax and breathe normally. Stay by his side until he has adjusted his breathing into the mask.

5. Secure the head retainer.

Adjust it so that it is comfortable for the patient and holds the mask securely in place.

6. Adjust oxygen flow rate.

Set it according to doctor's order. The flow may require adjusting from time to time as the patient's needs change. A humidifier can be used in the room if needed while the patient is wearing the nasal mask.

Important Steps	Key Points

7. Leave the patient comfortable.

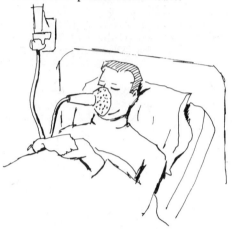

Usually most patients receiving oxygen therapy do best when in the semi-Fowler's or high-Fowler's position.

Tell your patient when you will be returning (e.g., in 15 to 30 minutes); this will help decrease his apprehension. Be sure that you return when you promised you would. Keep close check on these patients (at least hourly). Leave call light and bedside stand within easy reach.

Note: Remove face mask for cleaning PRN when it becomes excessively moist inside. Replace mask immediately.

8. Record.

The initiation of the treatment, e.g., time, method, rate of flow and patient's response. Charting example:

10 A.M. O_2 mask initiated at 8 L. Very apprehensive at onset. Quieted quickly after initiation of treatment. Pulse and respirations became slower. Color good.   A. Turno, RN

Note: Sometimes oxygen is ordered PRN. The oxygen will therefore be turned off and on at the patient's request. You may be responsible for regulating the flow meter on these occasions. Again, the initiation of the treatment is done by the nurse.

ITEM 5. ADMINISTRATION OF OXYGEN BY TENT

Oxygen tents are used less frequently than they were some twenty years ago. They supply a relatively high concentration of oxygen (50 to 60 per cent) and provide a means of circulating the moist air around the patient. The temperature of the air can be somewhat controlled and it provides comfortable air-conditioning for the patient. The oxygen tent is not economically efficient because of the high volume of oxygen needed to maintain the designated concentration, as well as loss of concentration when the oxygen tent is raised to permit working with the patient. Also, the equipment is hard to maintain and clean.

The concentration of oxygen is lost each time a part of the oxygen tent is raised. There should therefore be a minimal amount of disturbance to the patient. You must plan your work so that you loosen the oxygen tent infrequently, but on those occasions you will do several things for the patient.

While many patients like the oxygen tent because they can move about freely, they sometimes have a feeling of isolation. You must therefore talk with these patients frequently. If you speak loudly and clearly, they can hear you without your disturbing the tent.

Most oxygen tents now in use are electrically cooled models. When taking care of children in pediatrics, an apparatus is used similar to the oxygen tent. Called a mistogen tent (or Croupette), it provides both oxygen and very high humidity (moisture content). The Croupettes are commonly used for children who have pneumonia or tracheobronchitis.

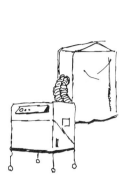

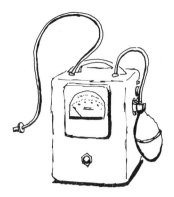

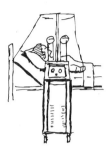

One type of
oxygen tent.

Oxygen analyzer
(records oxygen
concentration).

Oxygen tent
in operation.

In the skill laboratory, given a young male patient who has pneumonia, you will assist in setting up and regulating the oxygen tent.

Important Steps	Key Points
1. Wash your hands, approach and identify the patient, and explain what you are going to do.	Identify the patient. Answer all his questions. Speak audibly, clearly, kindly, and knowledgeably. (If you are unable to answer a question, get the answer from your team leader immediately.)
2. Obtain the equipment.	Get the oxygen tent. (The tent may be set up by someone from the Central Service Department, the Inhalation Therapy Department, or someone in nursing.)
3. Assemble the oxygen tent.	a. Move the tent to the head of the bed. Place it along one side of the bed with the regulating dials facing away from the patient. Extend the canopy arm to a horizontal position.

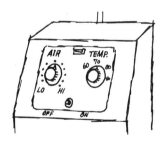

Oxygen tent control panel.

b. Plug the cord into the electrical outlet. Check the cord to be sure it is not frayed. (If frayed, it could be a fire hazard. Replace it with a new cord.)

c. Turn the motor on and set the control knobs on the control panel.

d. The temperature is usually set at 70° F.

e. The circulation dial is set halfway between low and high.

f. Connect the oxygen outlet to the oxygen flowmeter and start oxygen at 15 liters per minute.

g. The water tray at the back of the machine must be checked often and emptied of accumulated water. (Not all units have a water tray.)

h. Arrange canopy over the patient. (Do not drag it over the patient's face.)

Important Steps	Key Points
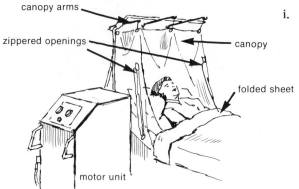 canopy arms, zippered openings, canopy, folded sheet, motor unit	i. Secure the edges in place by folding a drawsheet in half lengthwise and laying it across the patient's abdomen, then placing the bottom edge of the tent canopy edges securely under the mattress at both sides of the bed and at the head of the mattress. *Note:* Be sure zippered openings in sides of canopy are tightly closed.
4. Leave patient comfortable.	Place patient in good body alignment. Put a *manual call bell* within his reach. (The conventional electric call bell is not used because it could provide an electric spark when activated in the high oxygen concentration and start a fire or explosion.) Raise siderails, if appropriate.
5. Check patient frequently.	This will provide reassurance to the frightened patient and will also give you an opportunity to check the patient's condition and the functioning of the equipment. Empty water trays as needed (if there are any); check oxygen level.
6. Record procedure.	Make a note of the initiation of the treatment, e.g., time, method, level of oxygen flow, response of the patient. Charting example:

8:30 P.M. Oxygen tent initiated at 8 L. Quickly quieted. Vital signs stable, color good.

M. Mann, RN

9 P.M. Sleeping quietly, no coughing.

M. Mann, RN

ITEM 6. USE OF HYPERBARIC OXYGEN CHAMBERS

Hyperbaric oxygen chambers (rooms) are a recent innovation. They are especially constructed rooms which provide for very high oxygen concentration, used to treat patients who have anaerobic (without oxygen) infections, or in patients whose hemoglobin is not carrying enough oxygen to the tissues. Inasmuch as these units are installed in few health agencies at this time, we will not describe their operation. If you are assigned to this type of patient, you will undoubtedly receive some training in working with a hyperbaric chamber prior to your assignment.

ITEM 7. CARE OF PATIENTS RECEIVING OXYGEN WITH AN INTERMITTENT POSITIVE PRESSURE (IPPB) APPARATUS

IPPB is an inflation of the lungs with air or oxygen given under pressure on an intermittent basis. The IPPB machines permit control of:

A. The inspiration flow rate.

B. Oxygen concentration.

C. Length of the inspiration flow rate.

D. The regulation of the expiration phase of breathing.

E. A sensitive mechanism which triggers inspiration.

F. Nebulization.

The best machines can be adjusted to requirements of the individual patient. Common IPPB machines which are in use are the Bennett PR I, Bennett AP 5, Bird Mark 5 and Mark 7. IPPB treatments are utilized for:

A. Treating or preventing atelectasis and pulmonary edema.

B. Producing mechanical dilatation of the bronchi and lungs and regulating the inspiratory and expiratory rates in patients who do not breathe deeply.

C. Promoting the clearing of bronchial secretions in pneumonia, bronchitis, emphysema, or asthma with the use of aerosol medications.

D. Lessening the effort of breathing for the patient in certain respiratory diseases, operations, and injuries.

IPPB treatment can be given on a PRN (as needed) basis or continuously, depending on the needs of the patient. It is commonly needed on a continuous basis for patients who have had severe head injuries, or whose respirations are critically reduced by drugs, disease, or surgery. In these cases, an interruption of the regular respiratory rate for more than two minutes can lead to the death of the patient. Constant supervision of these patients is mandatory.

Problems which often arise when a patient is using the intermittent positive pressure machines are:

1. Gastric dilatation because air is swallowed. This leads to gastric discomfort and if it goes undetected can lead ultimately to rupture of the stomach. Stop the treatment at once. Explain the proper breathing procedure again to the patient and restart the equipment when he understands what is expected of him.

2. Leaks in the system caused by breaks or cracks in the tubing. This, of course, will lead to minimal mechanical performance. Your action should be to see that the equipment is repaired at once.

3. Pneumothorax, the collection of air or gas in the pleural (lung) cavity. It can be due to the rupture of an emphysematous bleb or a lung abscess in those patients receiving IPPB. It causes abrupt severe chest pain and dyspnea. Stop the treatment at once and have the physician called.

4. Increased pressure within the chest cavity. This causes compression of the blood vessels returning the blood to the heart and results in a reduction of the heart output. Notify the doctor immediately.

5. Contamination of lungs and equipment through improper cleaning and sterilizing methods. You must use meticulous cleaning techniques to prevent your patient from getting a lung infection because of contaminated inhalation equipment.

6. Rapid changes in vital signs, particularly the pulse and blood pressure. These may occur when using certain medications such as aerosols. Treatment should be stopped immediately and reported to the nurse and doctor. Wait for further instructions.

Generally you will not be giving these treatments; they will be given by the nurse or by someone from the Inhalation Therapy Department. You will, however, be required to observe these patients carefully, as you would any patient receiving oxygen therapy. Give frequent oral hygiene and maintain the previously stated safety precautions. If you should give IPPB treatments in your agency you will undoubtedly be given a special training

UNIT
29

program. (Insist on it, since this procedure can be injurious to the patient if not properly given.)

The procedure for setting up and giving the IPPB treatments will be covered in a later publication covering Level II Instructional Materials.

ITEM 8.   GENERAL NURSING CARE FOR PATIENTS RECEIVING OXYGEN

General Nursing Care for these patients is part of your nursing routine and will not be ordered by the doctor (in most instances).

A. The main consideration is to keep the breathing passageways open. The conscious patient can tell you if he is having difficulty; if mucus accumulates in the passageways, he can usually cough it up. If he is unconscious, however, you must be alert to his wet, gurgling respirations. When this occurs, you must see that he is suctioned immediately (either by doing it yourself, if possible, or obtaining assistance at once). If the patient is unconscious, place him in the Sims position so that the secretions can run out of his mouth.

B. For the unconscious patient the Sims position keeps the tongue from falling back into the throat (remember that the head is held high and straight in this position). Also, throat secretions (mucus) can easily drain out of his mouth. The Fowler position for the conscious patient permits fullest lung expansion. Change your patient's position frequently to prevent decubitus ulcers from occurring, and also to expand the lungs fully (the exertion of moving will make him breathe more deeply).

C. Be familiar with the operation of the various oxygen equipment. This will tend to give the patient confidence in what you are doing and will tend to decrease his fright and apprehension. Replace defective working equipment at once.

D. Give good general nursing care to your patient. Keep him clean, dry, and warm. Change his position frequently. Give frequent oral fluids to keep his breathing passages moist; give frequent oral hygiene throughout the day and night.

E. Observe safety precautions and notify patient and family to observe them also.

   1. No smoking—because of danger of fire or explosion.
   2. No wool blankets—sparks from static electricity may start a fire or explosion in the highly concentrated oxygen environment.
   3. Do not give oil or alcohol backrubs to patients in oxygen tents. If this must be done, turn off oxygen flow.
   4. Do not use electrical equipment inside oxygen tent—electrical sparks may be initiated when you turn the equipment on which could ignite the high oxygen concentration and set off an explosion (e.g., call bells, electric razors, radios, hearing aids, suction equipment).
   5. Secure oxygen tank to bed or cart with restraining strap to prevent cylinder from falling.
   6. Use no lighted candles in any religious activity. (This is an extreme explosion hazard.)

F. Take the temperature rectally.

G. You may have to wrap a lightweight cotton blanket around the patient's shoulders while he is in an oxygen tent if he gets too cold. This is particularly necessary for elderly patients.

VI. ENRICHMENT

Attend any additional classes that your employing agency may have on the care of the patient receiving oxygen therapy.

Take a few minutes to review the components of the respiratory tract.

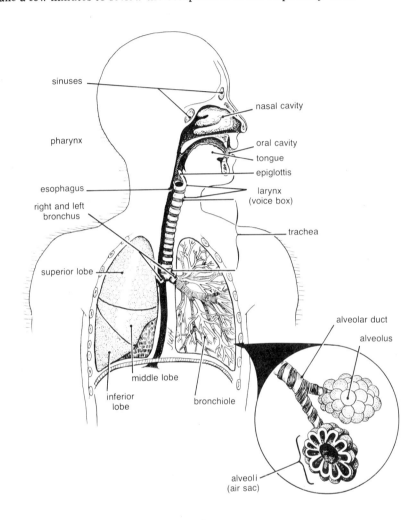

The first organ of respiration is the nose. As air is brought into the respiratory system through the nose, the air is warmed, moistened (by flow over the mucous membranes), and filtered or cleaned by the action of the fine hairs (cilia) in the nasal cavity. Thus, as air passes down the throat and trachea to the lungs, it is warmed, moistened, and cleaned.

The air then goes down to the throat (pharynx) which is a common passageway for both food and oxygen, and then to the larynx or voice box. At this juncture a small pedicle (epiglottis) protects the opening of the larynx when swallowing: food is shunted into the esophagus and air into the trachea. (An inflammation of the larynx is called laryngitis.)

The trachea (windpipe) is a 4½ inch tube extending from the larynx to the bronchial tubes. It, too, is lined with a mucous membrane and cilia, for continuing moistening and cleaning of the air. (An inflammation of the trachea is called tracheitis.)

From here the air goes into the bronchus, which leads directly into the lungs. The right bronchus is short and vertical. (For this reason when foreign objects [peanuts, bones] get into the respiratory tract they go into the right branches and lung.) The left bronchus is double branched and is more horizontal in direction. The bronchi (plural for bronchus) branch into many small tubes called the bronchioles. This part of the respiratory tract is commonly called the bronchial tree because it looks like the trunk of a tree with two limbs and many small branches. (Inflammation of the bronchus is called bronchitis.)

These tiny bronchioles lead to atria (airspaces). The atria join with air sacs in the lung tissue. The walls of the sacs pouch out to form the pulmonary (referring to lung) alveoli. The alveoli are surrounded by a network of tiny blood capillaries. Because of the closeness of these tissues (alveoli and capillaries) gas (O_2) passes into the circulatory system by a process called diffusion. (CO_2 from the blood passes back into the pulmonary alveoli to be exhaled into the air.)

Diffusion is a chemical process whereby a liquid or gas mixes its chemical components. The O_2 and CO_2 from the air mix with the components of the blood; the O_2 and CO_2 tend to distribute themselves equally between the alveoli and the capillaries.

The bronchi, bronchioles, and alveoli are imbedded in tissue called lung (pulmonary). There are two lungs (right and left) located in the chest cavity (thorax). The lungs are encased in a covering called pleura, which is separated from the lungs by a small amount of liquid. (An inflammation of the pleura is called pleurisy or pleuritis.)

The process of the O2 going into the blood through the pulmonary capillaries is called oxygenation of the blood.

The lungs work with several muscles to bring air into the body. The diaphragm is a large, flat muscle separating the chest and abdominal cavities. During inspiration, the diaphragm is contracted and the thoracic cavity is lengthened from top to bottom. The intercostal muscles (between the ribs) contract and enlarge the chest cavity from front to back and side to side. During expiration, the diaphragm and the intercostal muscles relax. Expiration is usually passive, while inspiration is active.

The volume of air in the lung is measured by the use of an instrument called a spirometer. Patients with pulmonary diseases may have a spirometry examination to determine how the lungs are functioning. When a newborn infant takes his first breath, there is already some air in the lungs.

The respiratory regulating center is located in the part of the brain called the medulla and is activated by nerve impulses which respond to the chemical composition of the blood. The cells in the respiratory center are particularly sensitive to CO_2 (carbon dioxide). If there is excess CO_2 in the blood, the respirations become more rapid and deep in order to increase the oxygen (O_2) content of the blood.

Normal respiratory rates are: newborn, 40 respirations per minute; infant—30 respirations per minute; adult, 14 to 18 respirations per minute. The rate is influenced by disease, drugs, and activity.

The cough is nature's mechanism for ridding ourselves of a respiratory tract obstruction or blocking. It is an abrupt expiration with the mouth open. A sneeze is a similar action to relieve the respiratory tract of a foreign object; however, the expiration of air is through the nose. Hiccough (singultus) is a spasmodic contraction of the diaphragm due to irritation of the stomach. Yawning is a deep, long inspiration usually due to mental or physical fatigue (tiredness). A sigh is a prolonged inspiration followed by a long expiration.

All these mechanisms may be observed as you care for patients with respiratory diseases or conditions. The symptoms may be significant clues in the progress of disease and should be observed and recorded.

POST-TEST

1. List 4 methods for administering oxygen therapy.

   (1) _____

   (2) _____

   (3) _____

   (4) _____

2. List the 6 major organs of respiration.

   (a) _____ (b) _____ (c) _____

   (d) _____ (e) _____ (f) _____

3. What is an inflammation of the larynx called? _____

4. What is an inflammation of the bronchi called? _____

5. What is the diaphragm? _____

6. What is the instrument used to measure air volume in the lung?

   _____

7. Where is the respiratory regulatory center located? _____

8. What is the gas compound that stimulates the respiratory center? _____

   _____

9. What is the normal respiratory rate for an infant? _____

   For an adult? _____

10. How is oxygen carried in the blood? _____

11. List 4 common signs or symptoms of patients with respiratory problems.

    (a) _____

    (b) _____

    (c) _____

    (d) _____

12. Why is a humidifier used when oxygen is administered by nasal catheter?

    _____

13. Name the piece of oxygen equipment which designates (or registers) the amount of oxygen given to the patient. _____

14. Name at least 4 safety precautions you must observe when a patient is receiving oxygen therapy.

    (a) _____

    (b) _____

    (c) _____

    (d) _____

UNIT
29

15. List at least 6 nursing measures you must observe when caring for a patient who is receiving oxygen therapy.

(a) _____

(b) _____

(c) _____

(d) _____

(e) _____

(f) _____

16. List at least three indications for giving IPPB treatments.

(a) _____

(b) _____

(c) _____

17. List at least 4 common problems which may arise when a patient receives IPPB.

(a) _____

(b) _____

(c) _____

(d) _____

18. Why are hyperbaric oxygen chambers used? _____

_____

_____

_____

POST-TEST ANNOTATED ANSWER SHEET

1. cannula

   nasal catheter

   oxygen mask

   oxygen tent

   IPPB

   hyperbaric oxygen chamber (p. 583)

2. a. nose

   b. pharynx

   c. larynx (p. 595)

   d. trachea

   e. bronchi

   f. lungs

3. laryngitis (p. 595)

4. bronchitis (p. 596)

5. Large, flat muscle separating the abdominal and thoracic cavities (pp. 581 and 596)

6. Spirometer (pp. 582 and 596)

7. medulla, pons and chemosensitive cells (p. 582)

8. carbon dioxide (pp. 582 and 596)

9. 30 RPM; 14 to 18 RPM (p. 596)

10. hemoglobin (p. 582)

11. a. complain of suffocation, can't breathe

    b. restless and irritable

    c. decreased muscle and mental coordination

    d. dyspneic (pp. 582 and 583)

    e. cyanotic

    f. increased rate and depth of respirations

    g. may have syncope or vertigo

12. to moisten the air (pp. 581 and 583)

13. flowmeter (p. 584)

UNIT
29

14. a.   no smoking

    b.   no wool blanket

    c.   do not use electrical equipment near oxygen

    d.   secure oxygen tank to bed with restraining strap to prevent falling (p. 594)

    e.   use no lighted candles in religious activity

    f.   take temperature rectally

    g.   keep patient in oxygen tent from chilling by wrapping a cotton towel around his shoulders

    h.   do not give an alcohol or oil backrub with oxygen going

15. a.   keep breathing passageways open

    b.   place unconscious patient in Sims' position to drain throat secretions and prevent tongue from falling back into throat (p. 594)

    c.   change position frequently to avoid decubitus

    d.   give oral hygiene frequently

    e.   replace defective equipment at once

    f.   be familiar with equipment to reassure patient

16. a.   treat or prevent atelectasis or pulmonary edema

    b.   treat patients who don't breathe deeply (p. 593)

    c.   promote clearing of bronchial secretions

    d.   decrease breathing effort for weak patient

17. a.   gastric dilatation

    b.   pneumothorax

    c.   leaks in system

    d.   increased internal chest pressure, compressing blood vessels, decreasing heart output (p. 593)

    e.   contamination of equipment

    f.   rapid changes in vital signs due to some medications

18. To provide high oxygen concentration in the treatment of certain patients with infections or disorders which do not carry enough oxygen to the tissues. (p. 592)

PERFORMANCE TEST

1. You will correctly regulate the oxygen flowmeter to give 4 liters of oxygen per minute, and 10 liters of oxygen per minute. Be sure to have your instructor check you at each point. Practice recording activity in the nurse's notes.

2. You will demonstrate equipment used and discuss the purpose of the four major methods of oxygen administration.

PERFORMANCE CHECKLIST

OXYGEN THERAPY

USE OF OXYGEN THERAPY EQUIPMENT

The student will demonstrate the correct use of oxygen therapy equipment.

1. Wash hands, identify patient, and explain procedure.

2. Assemble appropriate equipment and position bed to working height.

3. For catheter:

   A. Measure catheter length for insertion (nose to ear lobe).

   B. Lubricate tip with water soluble lubricant.

   C. Insert catheter and check length by looking in mouth.

   D. Secure catheter with tape.

4. For cannula and mask:

   A. Place equipment in or over nose.

   B. Adjust head strap for comfort.

5. For tent:

   A. Place tent along top side of bed with regulating dials away from patient.

   B. Extend canopy arm.

   C. Plug in electrical cord (no frayed cords or wet hands).

   D. Turn on motor and set dials.

   E. Set temperature at $70°$F.

   F. Connect O_2 to wall outlet or O_2 tank.

   G. Arrange canopy over tent, secure bottom edge in cuff of drawsheet.

   H. Close zippered openings.

6. Regulate O_2 flow per physician's order.

7. Leave patient comfortable and in good body alignment.

8. Offer water and tell patient time of return.

9. Raise siderails if indicated and put hand call bell within reach.

10. Record activity on chart.

UNIT 29

REGULATION OF FLOWMETER

The student will demonstrate the proper method of regulating a flowmeter.

1. Wash hands.

2. Approach and identify patient, and explain procedure.

3. Check flowmeter to be sure humidifier bottle is 2/3 filled with water. If not filled, turn off O_2, remove jar, fill to 2/3 level, and replace jar on flowmeter.

4. Adjust flow by opening flow valve until gauge reads 4 LPM (to be checked by instructor).

5. Continue adjusting flow valve until gauge reads 10 LPM.

6. Adjust flow to read 4 LPM.

7. Record activity on nurse's notes.

Unit 30

CARDIOPULMONARY RESUSCITATION

I. DIRECTIONS TO THE STUDENT

View the film "Breath of Life" or one available to your agency through the local chapter of the American Heart Association. Take notes so that you will be able to perform the procedure in the skill laboratory. Complete the post-test, both written and performance, when you have finished this program.

II. GENERAL PERFORMANCE OBJECTIVE

Following this lesson you will be able to recognize the symptoms of cardiac arrest and be able to start the emergency cardiopulmonary resuscitation technique.

III. SPECIFIC PERFORMANCE OBJECTIVE

When you have finished you will be able to:

1. Recognize and describe the signs and symptoms of cardiac standstill (cardiac arrest).

2. Provide a patent airway for the patient.

3. Initiate mouth-to-mouth resuscitation.

4. Initiate closed-chest massage.

(Steps 3 and 4 will be done only if your agency permits you to initiate these procedures. However, everyone should know how to do them in order to assist the nurse or doctor as needed throughout the procedure.)

IV. VOCABULARY

Some of the words used in this lesson may be new or unfamiliar to you. These have been listed below with their meanings. You should go over this list several times and when you see the word used in the lesson, refer to this section unless you are sure of its meaning.

cardiac board—flat board usually kept on cardiac arrest cart. It is placed under the patient's back, if he is in bed, to provide a firm surface for giving external heart massage.
CPR—abbreviation for cardiopulmonary resuscitation.
pupil—contractile opening in the center of the iris (the colored portion of the eye) which permits light transmission.
contracted pupils—pupils become smaller when exposed to light.
dilated pupils—pupils enlarge in darkness (both pupils should be equal in size).
resuscitation—act of bringing back to full consciousness (life).
sternum (breastbone)—flat, narrow bone in the midline of the thorax between the ribs.
trachea—windpipe.
xiphoid process—lowest portion of the sternum (breast bone).

V. INTRODUCTION

The sudden cessation (stopping) of heart action and respiratory action creates an "emergency situation" in which you might become involved whether you are at work, at school, at play, or at home. If you know the signs of cardiac standstill and respiratory collapse, you can give immediate attention. When you know the required procedures and have practiced them until you become skillful, you will be able to manage an emergency with calm, decisive action. Your skill will give confidence to others around you and ultimately you may save a life.

The procedure you are about to learn is one of the most rewarding activities you can experience. Learn well; the life you save may be a loved one.

Cardiac arrest, or cardiac standstill, results when the heart and lungs suddenly cease functioning. Unless you can reestablish breathing and heart action almost immediately, vital brain cells will die because of lack of oxygen, which, you remember, is essential for the cells to live. Brain tissue does not regenerate; if any of the cells die, that particular portion of the brain will cease to function. Of course, if only a few cells are destroyed, the damage will be minimal. If a large area is destroyed, however, the patient may be left with very limited capabilities. Thus the *speed* with which you act is vitally *important for* the *survival* of the patient in a productive life.

If the circulation of oxygenated blood is started within four minutes, there will be relatively little brain damage. A period of more than six minutes without oxygen flowing to the brain cells will cause irreversible destruction of the tissues.

Cardiopulmonary resuscitation is utilized to provide oxygen to the cells of the body. This is done by means of mouth-to-mouth resuscitation and external cardiac massage (compression).

In the event that you find a patient with no respirations, note the time (because time is of the essence), check to see if there is a pulse, and look for dilation of the pupils (pupils react to light if there is an adequate supply of oxygen to the brain). If you observe danger signals—no respiration, no pulse, and dilated pupils—then you must immediately initiate the cardiac arrest call. This information should be obtained when you first start to work in a new agency.

Now view the film; be alert for the signs of cardiac arrest and the action that must be taken to restore the patient to an active life.

ITEM 1. MOUTH TO MOUTH RESUSCITATION

Important Steps	Key Points
1. Note the time.	Search for signs of breathing. Feel for a pulse. Observe the pupils of the eye for dilation.
2. Remain with the patient.	Place him in the dorsal recumbent position; remove the pillow from the bed.
3. Summon help	Get help by pulling emergency call button in patient's room, calling nursing station through intercom system, shouting loudly, or using patient's telephone. Help will arrive soon with the emergency cart and supplies. Each agency has a special code for cardiac arrest which is used on the loudspeaker system: e.g., Dr. Heart wanted in Room 609.
4. Stand beside the patient's head and clear his airway.	Inspect his mouth for any obstruction. Remove foreign bodies with your index finger if they can be seen and easily dislodged. *Note:* If the patient is on the floor, you would kneel beside his head.

Important Steps	Key Points
5. Lift his head with your left hand.	When patient is relaxed, his tongue will fall back into the throat. Place your hand under his neck and lift upward.
6. Tilt patient's head backward to maximum extension with right hand. (Reverse hand positions in this and in steps 5 and 6 if you are left-handed.)	Place your left hand on his forehead and push downward. This will force the tongue forward from the throat and open the airway. This action alone may make the patient breathe. If he does not breathe spontaneously (on his own), you will have to give mouth-to-mouth resuscitation.
7. Pinch the patient's nose shut (with your right thumb and index finger).	This will prevent the escape of air through his nose when you breathe into his mouth.
8. Open your mouth wide.	
9. Take a deep breath.	
10. Place your mouth over patient's mouth. (Use Resuscitube, if available.)	*For an adult patient:* Make a good seal—fit your mouth tightly over his mouth. Your right cheek will rest tightly against his nose, giving a more secure nose seal.
	For an infant or small child: Place your mouth over his *nose and mouth.* Breathe in smaller amounts of air.
11. Blow your breath into his lungs through his mouth.	Blow enough air into his mouth to inflate his lungs about twice the size produced by the usual inspiration.
12. Remove your mouth and allow him to exhale.	This will give you some momentary rest.
13. Repeat breathing cycle at 12 times per minute for an adult. For a child, increase the rate to about 20 times per minute.	You can tell when the lungs are inflating because: a. You can *see* the chest rise and fall b. You can *feel* the lungs expand c. You can *hear* the air escaping during expiration (breathing out).

UNIT 30

If the patient does not start breathing after five lung inflations and if the pulse is absent and the pupils of the eye are dilated, then you must begin external cardiac compression or massage. You will be able to do this better if there is someone to assist you. Usually someone will have responded to your emergency call by this time.

ITEM 2. CARDIAC COMPRESSION

1. Maintain your breathing cycle with the patient; stand beside his head, facing toward his body.	The second worker will place a cardiac board under the patient to provide solid support during compression cycle. The cardiac board is usually carried on the cardiac arrest cart. Your agency may have some other provision for providing a firm surface for the patient when he is receiving the external cardiac massage. If a board is not available, place the patient in supine position on the floor.

Important Steps	Key Points
2. The second person positions himself at the patient's left side, chest level.	He will be standing beside worker number one, but will be out of his way.
3. Place heel of your right hand over the lower half of patient's sternum (breast bone).	Do not include the distal end of the sternum (xiphoid process). Proper positioning of hands will prevent internal injuries and/or broken ribs.
4. Place your left hand on top of your right hand. (Reverse hand positions if you are left-handed.)	Keep your *elbows straight.*
5. Exert a sharp downward force on the patient's chest.	The application of this force creates pressure which "pumps" blood into the arterial system. Since you are using the whole upper portion of your body, you will be able to exert 60 to 100 pounds of pressure on the patient's sternum, and the weight should depress the sternum 1½ to 2 inches. This action will gently massage the heart muscle which is located under the sternum and slightly to the left. (Permit the chest to rebound.)
6. Repeat the compression action (pressing down on the sternum) with an alternating relaxing stroke.	Maintain a steady rate at about 60 times per minute (almost the normal adult heart rate). You will compress the chest five times between each lung inflation. If one person is doing both procedures, the ratio is 2 ventilations to 15 compressions.
7. Continue procedure until patient revives or the physician pronounces the patient dead (or follow your agency practice).	This procedure is very tiring. Someone else may take over the compression by placing his hand over yours (in the same position); he gets into the cycle of depressing the chest; you can then withdraw your hand carefully while he continues the compression.
8. Record on patient's chart.	Note the time at which the procedure was initiated, how long it was carried out, and the end result. Chart example:

3:10 P.M. Patient found not breathing. No pulse, pupils dilated. Cardiac arrest procedure initiated.   J. Jones, SN

3:12 P.M. Dr. White and the Inhalation Therapy personnel responded. Cardiopulmonary resuscitation continued.

3:20 P.M. Began breathing on his own; pulse 60, pupils reacting to light, color pinking up.   J. Jones, SN

Note: Both procedures can be done by one person, although it is difficult and *very tiring.*

VI. ADDITIONAL INFORMATION

The American Heart Association has published a prepared statement which makes the procedure easy to remember:

Five Rules of Five

1. Start immediately—always in less than 5 minutes. The brain can survive without damage 4 to 6 minutes after breathing stops, only 2 to 4 minutes after circulation stops.

2. Open airway and inflate the lungs every 5 seconds.

3. After 5 good breaths if breathing does not resume, pulse is absent, and pupils dilated, begin external cardiac compression.

4. For effective Heart-Lung Resuscitation, inflate the lungs between each 5 compressions.

5. *Never* interrupt Heart-Lung Resuscitation for more than 5 seconds at any time.

If you wish further information on the subject, your instructor will provide additional reading materials. The American Heart Association has published pamphlets which may be of interest. Your instructor probably will have samples available for you.

U
N
I
T
30

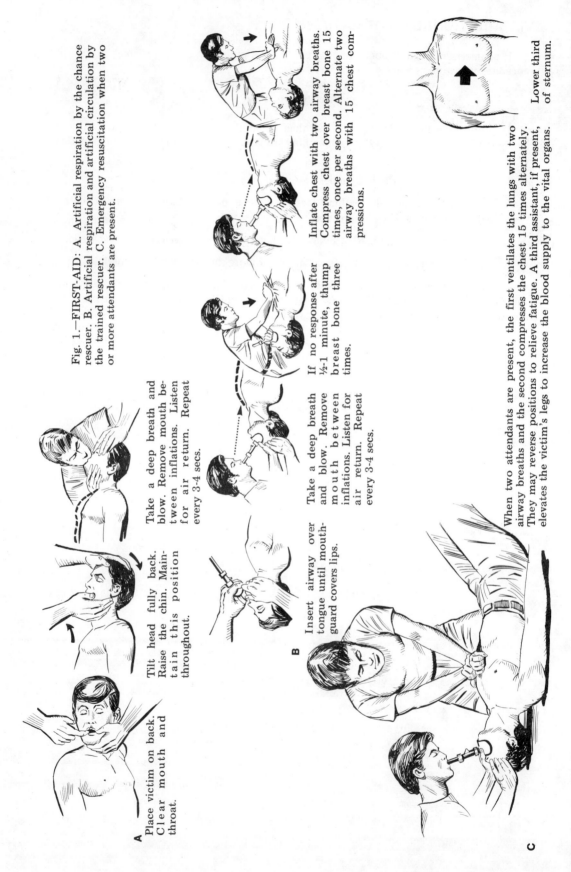

Fig. 1.—FIRST-AID: A. Artificial respiration by the chance rescuer. B. Artificial respiration and artificial circulation by the trained rescuer. C. Emergency resuscitation when two or more attendants are present.

A

Place victim on back. Clear mouth and throat.

Tilt head fully back. Raise the chin. Maintain this position throughout.

Take a deep breath and blow. Remove mouth between inflations. Listen for air return. Repeat every 3-4 secs.

B

Insert airway over tongue until mouthguard covers lips.

Take a deep breath and blow. Remove mouth between inflations. Listen for air return. Repeat every 3-4 secs.

If no response after ½-1 minute, thump breast bone three times.

Inflate chest with two airway breaths. Compress chest over breast bone 15 times, once per second. Alternate two airway breaths with 15 chest compressions.

Lower third of sternum.

C

When two attendants are present, the first ventilates the lungs with two airway breaths and the second compresses the chest 15 times alternately. They may reverse positions to relieve fatigue. A third assistant, if present, elevates the victim's legs to increase the blood supply to the vital organs.

POST-TEST

To be completed before a demonstration for your instructor.

1. List the 3 steps to determine if life is threatened or "sudden death" is imminent:

    (a) _____

    (b) _____

    (c) _____

Multiple Choice: Circle the letter of the correct answer.

2. How long a period of time can pass without oxygen before irreversible changes occur at the cellular levels of the human brain or brain damage occurs?

    (a) One to two minutes

    (b) Four to six minutes

    (c) Fifteen to twenty minutes

3. Lack of circulation causes the pupils of the eye to:

    (a) dilate

    (b) constrict

4. The first step in the management of any unconscious victim is to:

    (a) stop the hemorrhaging

    (b) provide warmth

    (c) establish an open airway

    (d) compress the chest for heart massage

5. To initiate artificial ventilation, the patient is placed in which of the following positions?

    (a) flat and prone

    (b) supine with chin on chest

    (c) supine with chin straight up and head lifted back

    (d) Sims position with head tilted back

6. In artificial resuscitation, an adult patient should receive how many breaths per minute?

    (a) 26 per minute

    (b) 12 per minute

    (c) 8 per minute

7. Artificial ventilation is continued until:

    (a) spontaneous breathing occurs

    (b) a pulse is present

    (c) pupils constrict

8. External cardiac massage refers to:

    (a) circular motions over the heart

    (b) squeezing the heart between the lower end of sternum and spine

    (c) squeezing the heart between the upper end of sternum and spine

9. Pressure is applied by

   (a) the heel of one hand

   (b) the fingers of both hands

   (c) the heels of both hands overlapping

10. For cardiac massage the patient should be:

    (a) in prone position on solid surface

    (b) in supine position on soft surface

    (c) in supine position on solid surface

11. Enough pressure should be applied to push the sternum down:

    (a) 6 inches

    (b) 1/2 inch

    (c) 1½ to 2 inches

12. The minumum number of compressions per minute for adults is:

    (a) 120 per minute

    (b) 60 per minute

    (c) 30 per minute

13. One person providing artificial ventilation and circulation should establish the following pattern:

    (a) 15 compressions, then 2 ventilations

    (b) 60 compressions, then 1 ventilation

    (c) 15 ventilations, then 2 compressions

14. When two persons provide CPR, the ventilator should interpose ventilation between:

    (a) every 3rd to 4th heart compression

    (b) every 10th to 11th heart compression

    (c) every 5th to 6th heart compression

POST-TEST ANNOTATED ANSWER SHEET

1. Respirations stop; no heartbeat; pupils dilated. (p. 604)

2. b   (p. 604)

3. a   (p. 604)

4. c   (p. 604)

5. c   (p. 604)

6. b   (p. 605)

7. a   (p. 605)

8. b   (p. 606)

9. c   (p. 606)

10. c   (p. 605)

11. c   (p. 606)

12. b   (p. 606)

13. a   (p. 606)

14. c   (p. 608)

U
N
I
T
30

PERFORMANCE TEST

In the practice lab, you will correctly perform either mouth-to-mouth resuscitation, or closed chest massage on the mannequin, Resusci-Annie. This will take you some time to practice so that you will obtain the correct results. When you have practiced sufficiently so that you can carry out the procedure quickly and correctly, ask your instructor to check your performance.

PERFORMANCE CHECKLIST

CARDIOPULMONARY RESUSCITATION

PERFORMANCE OF MOUTH-TO-MOUTH RESUSCITATION

The student will demonstrate the procedure to follow in performing mouth-to-mouth resuscitation.

1. Note the time.

2. Observe patient for signs of pulse and respiration.

3. Observe pupils of eyes for dilation.

4. Summon help (perform simultaneously with the above steps).

5. Position patient for resuscitation (place in dorsal recumbent position).

6. Remove obstructions from patient's airway, i.e., chewing gum, false teeth, or other materials which may be obstructing airway.

7. Hyperextend patient's neck (attempt to form a straight passageway).

8. Seal patient's nose with thumb and index finger.

9. Take a deep breath.

10. Place own mouth over patient's mouth.

11. Exhale into patient's mouth.

    A. Observe patient's chest (inflate the lungs about twice the usual inspiration).

    B. Observe abdomen for distention (raise abdomen, place free hand on top of the bubble and press down firmly, forcing air into lungs).

12. Remove mouth from patient's mouth, allowing patient to exhale.

13. Repeat cycle approximately 12 to 15 times per minute for an adult, and approximately 20 times per minute for a child.

14. *Note:* When applying procedure to an infant, the following adaptations should be made:

    A. Place mouth over the mouth and nose of patient.

    B. Exhale smaller amounts of air (puffs of air).

EXTERNAL CARDIAC MASSAGE

Demonstrate the proper procedure for cardiac massage.

1. Assume that artificial respiration procedures have been initiated.

2. Maintain patient's respiration.

3. If required, place patient on cardiac board or a non-compressible surface such as the floor.

4. Position self appropriately (patient's side, chest level).

5. Place heel of one hand over lower half of patient's sternum.

6. Place remaining hand on top of first hand.

   A. Make sure to keep elbows straight.

   B. Do not permit fingers to contact the chest wall.

7. Exert sharp downward force on patient's chest (depress sternum approximately 1½ to 2 inches).

8. Permit chest wall to "rebound" to a normal position.

9. Repeat process approximately 60 times per minute.

10. Continue procedure until patient is revived or physician terminates the activity.

11. Record the activity on patient's chart.

Verbal question

In the event that one individual must perform both artificial respiration and external cardiac massage, what is the rhythm of action?

Response

External cardiac massage 15 times, break to cycles of artificial respiration, followed by 15 chest compressions. This procedure is repeated as required.

UNIT
30

NOTES

Unit 31

ASSISTING WITH PROCEDURES

Assisting with hot and cold applications

I. DIRECTIONS TO THE STUDENT

You are to proceed through the lesson using this workbook as your guide. You will need to practice the tasks and procedures using the different types of equipment with the mannequin (Mrs. Chase) or student partners in the skill laboratory. After you have completed the lesson and practice of the procedures, arrange with your instructor to take the post-test.

For this lesson you will need the following items:

1. This workbook

2. A pen or pencil

3. Hot water bottle and cover

4. Ice cap and cover

5. Heat cradle

6. Mannequin (Mrs. Chase)

7. Electric heating pad

If at all possible, the following equipment should be available for demonstration and practice purposes:

1. Hypothermia machine

2. Aquathermia machine

3. Ultraviolet lamp*

4. Infrared lamp*

Please read the following paragraphs carefully. They will tell you what you will be expected to know and how you will be expected to assist in giving the appropriate heat or cold treatment which is ordered for the patient. If you feel that you have the necessary skills and would be wasting your time studying this material, discuss this with your instructor. You would then arrange to take the performance test. All students are expected to demonstrate accurately the skills required in the performance test and to take the written post-test.

II. GENERAL PERFORMANCE OBJECTIVE

Upon the completion of this lesson, you will be able to apply heat and cold as treatments for the patient's condition accurately, effectively, and safely.

---

*For demonstration purposes only

III. SPECIFIC PERFORMANCE OBJECTIVES

Upon the completion of this unit, you will be able to:

1. Apply heat locally to a portion of the patient's body using in a safe manner a hot water bottle, a heating pad, a heat cradle, or aquathermia pad.

2. Apply cold locally to a portion of the patient's body, efficiently and safely, using an ice cap, ice pack, or a hypothermia machine.

3. Assist in setting up and operating the hypothermia/hyperthermia machine for the general application of heat or cold to the patient's body correctly, efficiently, and safely.

IV. VOCABULARY

aquathermia—a small, electric, jarlike container that is used to hold an alcohol-distilled water solution. It has outlets to permit circulation of the fluid through tubes and a hollow vinyl pad (K-pad).

autonomic nervous system—peripheral (outer surface of a body) and visceral (internal organs) nervous system that regulates the internal conditions of the body as well as the sensations in the skin and muscles.

Central Service (CS)—a supply area in the hospital that provides sterile and unsterile equipment and supplies used in the care of patients.

cornea—glasslike coating of the eye that covers the iris and the pupil and permits light to enter the eye. In health, it is clear and transparent.

electrolyte—a solution that is a conductor of electricity. Electrolytes are essential for normal body functioning.

hypothermia—body temperature below the normal range (hypo- = less, below; -thermia = temperature).

hyperthermia—body temperature above the normal range (hyper- = more, above).

infrared lamp—a special device which has light rays beyond the red end of the visible light spectrum.

light spectrum—light is the sensation produced by electromagnetic radiation which strikes the retina of the eye, and spectrum refers to the length of the light ray.

metabolism—the entire process by which the body is nourished, maintained, and provided with energy (involves transforming a substance, such as a food, from the time it enters the body until the waste products are excreted).

suppuration—the formation of pus.

systemic—relating to the whole system; the whole body.

toxin—a poisonous or noxious substance.

ultraviolet lamp— a special lamp which emits light rays outside the visible spectrum at the violet end.

V. INTRODUCTION

The application of heat or cold to the skin surface is important in treating certain infections and traumatic conditions. Usually a physician's order is indicated before using any of these treatments because of the related and opposing effects produced elsewhere in the body.

In order to understand the use of heat and cold applications and their effect on the body, you need to know some of the principles involved. The following are some of the principles and procedures that are described in this unit.

1. Heat causes dilation of blood vessels and increases the supply of blood to the area.

2. Heat stimulates metabolism and the growth of new cells and tissues.

3. Cold causes contraction of blood vessels and decreases the supply of blood to the area.

4. Cold retards metabolism and decreases cell activity or growth.

5. Applications of heat and cold to portions of the body cause autonomic nervous system responses throughout the body.

6. Because the blood volume of the body is constant within a closed system, an increase in the blood supply to the skin causes a decrease of blood supply to other portions of the body; conversely, a decrease in the blood supply to the skin increases the blood supply elsewhere in the body.

7. As a conductor of heat and cold, water is more effective than air.

The dilation of blood vessels caused by heat application and the constriction of vessels from application of cold are shown in the figures below.

These principles help to explain the effects of heat and cold on the body. Let us consider heat first. Heat is applied to the skin surfaces to provide general comfort and to speed up the healing process. The elevated temperature or fever that so often accompanies an illness or infection is the body's way of combating the illness and promoting the healing process.

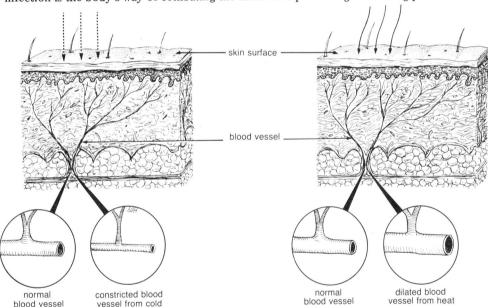

skin surface

blood vessel

| normal blood vessel | constricted blood vessel from cold | | normal blood vessel | dilated blood vessel from heat |

Effect of cold application.   Effect of heat application.

Heat dilates the blood vessels in the area of the heat application. This brings more blood to the area, which also means that more nutrients (food) and oxygen are made available to the tissues. The dilated blood vessels carry away toxins and excess tissue fluid. This helps to reduce swelling that causes pressure on nerve endings, and so pain is also reduced. The dilated blood vessels and the increased blood supply in the area of heat application cause the skin to appear pinkish or reddened, although this color would be hard to detect in dark-skinned or black patients. Heat is used to decrease inflammation and to promote the formation of pus (suppuration).

Cold applications are used to prevent or reduce swelling, to stop bleeding, and to decrease suppuration. When cold is applied to the skin surface, it contracts the muscles, which in turn squeeze the blood vessels to reduce the blood supply further. The blood vessels themselves contract, the diminished blood supply reduces the nutrients and oxygen to the cells, and cell activity is cut down. Since cold applications slow the metabolism of the body, the body can be cooled for prolonged surgery to decrease the stress of trauma and blood loss.

U
N
I
T
31

Prolonged cold reduces sensation and therefore lessens pain. However, if cold continues to interrupt the circulation, it can lead to necrosis (death of tissue), as seen in severe frostbite. When a cold application is removed from the skin, there occurs a secondary reaction as the circulation returns to normal. The blood vessels dilate and give the skin a warm, glowing pink color.

Heat and cold treatments can be either dry, as with hot water bottles, heating pads, and ice caps, or they can be moist, as with baths, soaks, and compresses. Moist applications have a more effective action, because water is better than air as a conductor of heat and cold. Dry heat is tolerated better than a moist heat application of the same temperature which may cause pain or burning.

Applications of heat and cold to the skin activate the autonomic nervous system. The nerve endings in the skin send a message to the control center in the brain, for example, that heat has been applied. In an effort to maintain the body temperature at an even level, the control center acts to dilate the blood vessels and increase the circulation to the area. Other blood vessels to the internal organs are constricted so that the temperature of those organs is maintained to prevent disturbance of other delicately balanced body functions. Although the procedure of applying heat or cold to the body is relatively simple, the effect on the body is much more complex.

Heat and cold can be applied to large or small body areas. A general application is one which is applied to the entire body; a local application is one which is used on a specific part of the body. The following figures show some examples of general and local applications.

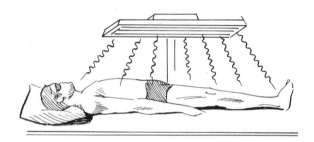

Example of general temperature application.

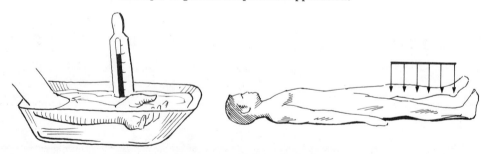

Examples of local temperature applications.

ITEM 1.   APPLICATION OF THE HOT WATER BOTTLE *

Important Steps	Key Points
1. Wash your hands; approach and identify the patient.	Explain the reason for using this treatment.
2. Obtain the hot water bottle from the supply area.	The location may vary from agency to agency; it could be Central Service, utility room, nurse-server, etc.

---

* Use of hot water bottles has been outlawed in some places for safety reasons. Follow applicable regulations.

Important Steps	Key Points
3. Obtain the protective cover from the supply closet.	If a cover is not available, use a pillow case. Some agencies use disposable protective covers (follow your agency procedure).
4. Take the hot water bottle to the sink and fill it 1/3 to 1/2 full with hot water (some agencies recommend filling 1/2 to 2/3).	Do not fill it so full that it is cumbersome and heavy. Lay the bottle on a flat surface and press on the outside to remove the excess air. In other words, expel excess air until the water comes to the mouth of the water bottle, and then put on the screw-top (or clamp shut with special closure tab). There will probably be water clinging to the outside of the bottle; use a paper towel to wipe it dry. Check the temperature of the bottle by placing it against the inner aspect of your forearm. If it feels comfortable to you, then it will be safe and comfortable for the patient. Now put the bottle in the flannel cover or the pillow case. Fold the pillow case around the bottle so that it appears as a neatly wrapped package. (This will give added thickness to the cover and avoid an accidental burn to the patient.)

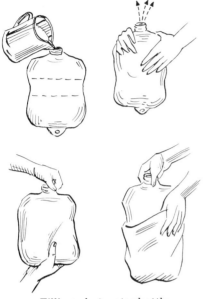

Filling a hot water bottle.

Important Steps	Key Points
5. Take the hot water bottle to the patient.	Tell him why he must use it in relation to his injury or infection and answer his questions. If you are unable to do so, ask your charge nurse to explain further to the patient.
6. Put the hot water bottle on the affected area.	If it has to be immobilized, wrap a piece of sheeting or towel around the area. Wrap firmly, securely, and with even pressure to make sure that the bottle will remain on the affected part.
7. Return to the patient at frequent intervals.	Check to see that the hot water bottle is effective. Observe the skin for an increase or decrease in redness, heat, swelling, pain, and blood circulation. As the water becomes cool, empty it. Refill it with hot water, if treatment is to be continued.
8. Remove the hot water bottle.	Do this when the treatment is completed or if the redness, swelling, or pain increases. Report immediately to your charge nurse. Put the cover in the laundry bag for dirty linen, or discard it in the wastebasket if it is disposable.
9. Return the hot water bottle to the central processing department for cleaning.	Most agencies no longer clean equipment on the unit. If this is done in your agency, follow the procedure for cleaning the hot water bottle with germicidal solution.
10. Return it to the proper storage place.	You may take it to Central Service or to the designated storage area on the unit.

Important Steps	Key Points
11. Leave the patient comfortable and safe.	Make sure that he is settled in good body alignment. Raise the siderails if indicated. Attach the call signal within his reach. Arrange the bedside table for his convenience.
12. Obtain the chart and record all pertinent information on the nurse's notes.	Charting example: 9:00 A.M. Hot water bottle applied to right knee.　　　　　　　　　　J. Jones, SN

ITEM 2.   ADMINISTRATION OF A DISPOSABLE HOT PACK

This new product eliminates the inconvenience of the reusable hot water bottle. An equally important advantage is that its one-time use decreases the probability of cross-infection; a further benefit is minimal danger of burning the patient because the temperature is scientifically controlled.

The disposable lightweight hot pack is a prefilled plastic package containing an exact amount of interreacting ingredients which, when combined by striking, squeezing or kneading, produce a sustained temperature. Most of the manufacturers color-code the hot packs by using a red package.

The packages come in a variety of sizes and shapes. The packages are made to conform to the body contour (shape) when applied. Sizes range from 4½ to 11½ inches for perineal applications, to 6¼ X 7½ inches and 7½ X 9½ inches for applications to reduce general swelling and pain. The temperature ranges from 101°F. to 114°F.; the action lasts from 20 to 60 minutes, depending on the size of the pack and the manufacturer's instructions. You must therefore check the specific directions on the product used by your agency.

Like the cold packs, most of these hot packs are applied directly to the skin surface. If the package is punctured and the contents leak onto the patient's skin, wash thoroughly and quickly with water to remove the chemical from the skin. Dispose of the punctured bag and obtain a new pack.

Important Steps	Key Points
1. Obtain a hot pack from the storage area.	Select the size according to the body area to be treated (small or large). The prepared packet is a single-use, self-contained unit containing a precise amount of chemical compound and solution which when combined in the package create a controlled heat.

DISPOSABLE HOT Pack
TO ACTIVATE
MIX CONTENTS
Patient_____ Rm _____

2. Wash your hands.	
3. Approach and identify the patient.	Check his identification band. This step is particularly important here since heat treatments may be contra-indicated for some conditions.
4. Explain the procedure.	Gain the cooperation of the patient.

Important Steps	Key Points

5. Mix the contents of the package.

This is done by a striking, squeezing or kneading motion. The action breaks the internal chambers to permit the contents to mix.

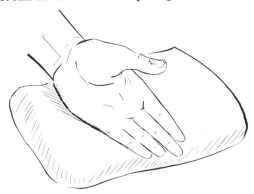

6. Continue to shake, squeeze, or knead the package vigorously.

This assures complete mixing of the chemical contents. The specific action taken in this step will depend on the product your agency uses.

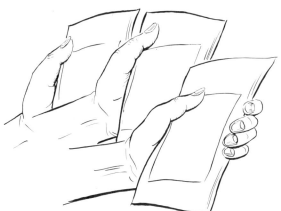

7. Apply the package to the designated area.

The pack can be applied directly to the area of treatment, e.g., over an abscess on the inner aspect of the right arm. You may need to immobilize the package on the area by wrapping a towel securely around the arm (covering the hot pack) and securing it with a safety pin or tape, according to agency procedure.

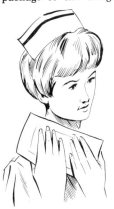

8. Return to the patient at frequent intervals.

See that the heat is working. Observe the patient's skin for an increase or decrease in redness, swelling, pain, and blood circulation. The same general principles and safety precautions for using heat applications apply for this disposable pack as those you learned in the introduction to this unit.

Important Steps	Key Points
9. Replace as needed.	The heat effect should be produced by the packet for *20 to 60 minutes.* Dispose of the packet when it becomes cold. Replace it with a new one PRN.

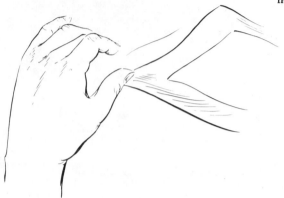

Important Steps	Key Points
10. Record the treatment on the patient's chart.	Charting example: 10:10 A.M. Disposable hot pack applied on the inner aspect of the right forearm. K. Dworsky, SN

ITEM 3. ICE BAG OR ICE COLLAR

Important Steps	Key Points
1. Wash your hands; identify the patient.	Explain what you are going to do.
2. Obtain the ice bag from storage area.	Some agencies have ice bags which are pneumatically sealed with a liquid solution inside. They are stored in the freezing unit of a special refrigerator. When the ice melts, the ice bag is returned to the refrigerator for refreezing. Be sure the outside of the bag is cleaned with a germicidal solution *before* returning it to the freezer.
3. Obtain a protective cover from the storage area.	If a cover is not available, use a pillow case (some agencies use disposable covers).
4. Take the ice bag to the utility working area.	Get a pan of ice cubes or crushed ice from the ice maker. Many hospitals have an ice machine either on the unit or in a centrally located area. If you use ice cubes, make sure the edges of the cubes are not sharp. If sharp-edged ice is used, it may puncture the ice bag. Fill the ice bag 3/4 full. Lay it on a flat surface and press on the outside to expel the air from it, so that the bag will be flexible and will fit the contour of the affected area without difficulty. Seal or close the bag. Water may cling to the outside of the bag; use paper towels to wipe it off. Check the bag for leakage. (If there is a leak, return ice bag to the supply room for repair, and obtain a

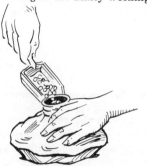

Filling ice bag.

Important Steps	Key Points

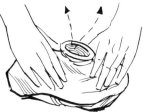

Expressing air from bag.

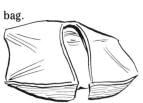

Ice bag with cover.

new bag.) Wrap the bag with the special cover. The bag is covered to protect the patient's skin. Remember, as the ice melts, droplets of water will appear on the outside of the ice bag and the cover may become wet. Therefore, it is suggested that a plastic cover or wrap be put around the bag before you wrap it in cloth.

5. Take the ice bag to the patient.

Explain why the ice bag is to be placed on the injured or infected area. Answer questions. If you cannot answer, refer to your charge nurse immediately. Put the bag on the affected area. If it must be immobilized, use a sheet or towel to apply the bag to the area. Wrap it firmly, securely, and with an even pressure.

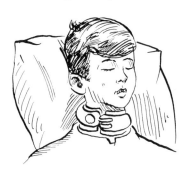

Ice collar.

6. Return to the patient at frequent intervals.

Check to see if the ice bag is effective. Observe the skin area for increased or decreased redness, swelling, pain, numbness, and blood circulation. Remove at once if these signs or symptoms occur. Report immediately to your charge nurse.

7. Remove the ice bag when the treatment is completed or if the skin becomes more red or painful.

Put the linen cover in the soiled laundry hamper (or down the linen chute). Discard the plastic and disposable covers in the wastebasket.

8. Wash, rinse, and dry, or return the ice bag to central processing room.

If you must clean the ice bag on your unit, follow your agency procedure for cleaning, disinfecting, drying, and then returning it to storage.

9. Leave the patient comfortable and safe.

Remember the safe, comfortable bed positions. Raise siderails if indicated. Attach call signal within patient's reach. Leave the bedside stand conveniently close.

10. Obtain the chart.

Record all pertinent information on the nurse's notes. Charting example:

11:00 A.M. Ice collar applied to throat.

J. Jones, SN

U
N
I
T
31

ITEM 4. ADMINISTRATION OF A DISPOSABLE COLD PACK

The disposable lightweight cold pack is a prefilled plastic package containing an exact amount of interreacting ingredients. When these ingredients are mixed by striking, squeezing, or kneading (depending on the manufacturer's instructions), they produce a sustained, controlled temperature. Most of the manufacturers color-code the cold packs by use of a blue package.

The packages are manufactured in many sizes and shapes and conform readily to the body contour (shape) when applied. Sizes range from 4½ × 11 inches for tonsillectomies or perineal packs to 6¼ × 7½ inches for small areas needed for emergency room treatment of burns, sprains, epistaxis, fractures, etc. The larger pack (7½ × 9 inches) can be used to reduce swelling in IV infiltrations, following dental extractions, and postoperatively to reduce swelling at a surgical site.

The temperature range is from 50°F. to 80°F. Because of the controlled temperature, the possibility of a freeze burn to the patient is almost nil. The action lasts from 30 minutes to 4 hours, depending on the size of the pack and the specific product used. Therefore, extreme caution must be taken to *read* the directions for the product used in your agency. There are variations in size, temperature control, length of action, and method used to initiate the reacting ingredients.

Some cold packs may be reused by placing them in a special refrigerator-freezer. However, disposable packs are generally designed for one-time use.

Most of the packs are intended to be applied directly to the skin surface. The outer covering of the pack is a special material which absorbs perspiration and prevents the cold, damp feel of plastic. Again, there may be a slight variation in this procedure, depending on the manufacturer (check your agency's supply).

Since the pack is usually meant for one-time use, it is an excellent preventive of cross-infection. If the pack is punctured and the contents leak out, thoroughly and quickly wash the patient's skin with water to remove any of the harmful chemical ingredients. Dispose of the punctured bag and replace it with a new pack.

Important Steps	Key Points
1. Obtain the cold pack from the storage area.	Select the size according to the patient's needs (i.e., the area to be treated, small or large).
	The prepared package is a single-use, self-contained unit which contains a combination of precise ingredients within an insulated wrap which delivers a controlled cold temperature after being altered by a special procedure.

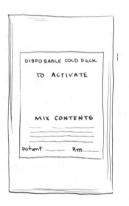

2. Wash your hands.

3. Approach and identify the patient.	Check his identification band to assure that you are treating the right patient. Cold applications may be contraindicated in some conditions.
4. Explain the procedure.	This is done to gain the patient's cooperation and to keep him from being apprehensive.

Important Steps	Key Points
5. Mix the contents of the package.	This is done by striking, squeezing, or kneading the package. (The method varies, depending on the specific manufacturer's product used in your agency.) The force will break the internal chambers and cause the chemicals to mix and create the cold temperature.

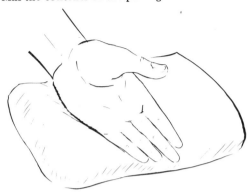

6. Continue to shake, squeeze or knead the package vigorously.	This will assure complete mixing of the contents for delivery of the precise cold temperature required.

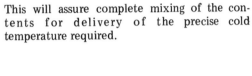

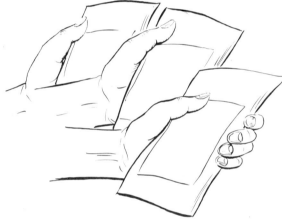

U
N
I
T
31

7. Apply the package directly to the designated area.	You may need to fasten the package to the area by means of a towel secured around the extremity or by wrapping an elastic bandage or towel around it (loosely) to hold it in place.

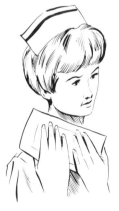

8. Return to the patient frequently.	Check to see that the cold pack is working properly. Observe the patient's skin for an increase or decrease in redness, swelling, pain, or blood circulation. The general principles for use and safety for cold applications should be followed for this disposable pack.

Important Steps	Key Points
9. Replace as needed.	The cold effect should remain for 30 minutes to 4 hours, depending on the size of the pack and its manufacturer. Dispose of the pack in a waste container when it becomes warm.

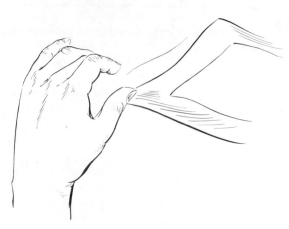

10. Record the treatment.	Charting example: 2:10 A.M. Cold pack applied to perineum. <div align="right">P. Shaw, SN</div>

ITEM 5.   ELECTRIC HEATING PAD

Important Steps	Key Points
1. Wash your hands; approach and identify the patient.	Explain what you will be doing.
2. Obtain the electric heating pad from the storage area.	The pad is usually made of rubber or plastic asbestos. *Note:* If the patient's own personal electric pad is used, it must be checked by your agency Maintenance Department to assure that it meets agency safety standards.
3. Obtain protective cover.	It should cover the entire pad.
4. Check the pad.	Put the plug into an electric outlet. Turn the regulating button to high so that the heating mechanism can be checked. The pad should become hot immediately. Caution: be aware that abusing electrical appliances can cause short-circuits which are very dangerous; they can electrocute you or the patient. Also, fires can be caused by short-circuiting equipment. *Do not use* heating pads if the cords are frayed, worn, or haphazardly repaired. *Do not use electric pad in or near water.*

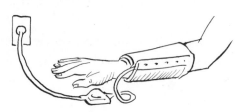

Heating pad.

5. Take the electric pad to the patient's bedside.	Give a detailed explanation to the patient, stressing all the safety measures to observe while the electric pad is being used, e.g., excess heat may lead to burns, protective coverings used to avoid blistering patient's skin.
6. Put the electric cord in an electric outlet as close to the patient as possible.	In this way you will avoid the danger of persons tripping over the cord and hurting themselves.

Important Steps	Key Points
7. Place the covered electric pad on the patient's injured area.	Turn the control button to *low. A low degree of heat should always be used when the electric pad is used for the patient.* Immobilize the pad if necessary by using sheeting wrapped around the pad and the injured area firmly, securely, and with an even pressure.
8. Return to the patient at frequent intervals.	Check to see that the appliance is effective. Observe the skin area for increased or decreased redness, pain or blood circulation. If the pain increases, remove the heating pad and report immediately to your charge nurse.
9. Remove the electric heating pad when the treatment is completed.	Place your hand on the *plug* and pull it from the electric outlet. Remove the protective cover from the heating pad and put it in the soiled laundry hamper or chute, or discard it in the wastebasket. *Do not yank or pull the cord from the outlet by holding on to the cord. You may flip the cord in the air and hurt yourself or the patient. Also, you may pull the plug and the cord apart. Do not handle electric equipment with wet hands.*
10. Leave the patient comfortable and safe.	Make sure the call light and bedside stand are nearby.
11. Obtain the chart.	Record all pertinent information on the nurse's notes. Charting example: 4:10 P.M. Electric heating pad applied at low temperature on anterior aspect of lower left leg. J. Jones, SN

U
N
I
T
31

ITEM 6. HEAT CRADLE

The heat cradle is made of metal bands, soldered and shaped in the form of a "half-moon," like the cradle used to keep the bedding off the patient's legs. An electric socket with a cord is attached to the center top band at the highest point. A 25-watt electric bulb is used. The heat from the bulb produces the warmth necessary for the treatment. When in use, the cradle is covered by a sheet or the top bedding so that the heat is kept within the area. The size of the cradle permits air to circulate and there is no weight directly on the patient's body to cause discomfort. This method of heat application is generally used on the lower trunk and extremities to promote healing of wounds and to increase the circulation.

Important Steps	Key Points
1. Obtain the heat cradle from Central Service.	
2. Wash your hands; approach and identify the patient.	Explain what you plan to do.
3. Take the cradle to the patient's bedside and place it on the bed over the area requiring the treatment.	Pull the curtains around the bed to provide for privacy while setting up the heat cradle. Fold back the top covers, but avoid undue exposure of the patient. For heat treatment of the lower extremities, place the cradle over the feet and legs. Plug the cord into an outlet near the bed.

Important Steps	Key Points

Important Steps

Key Points

(Make sure the cord does not droop or lie on the floor where someone may trip over it or pull on it so that the cradle is pulled off the bed.) Turn on the light and make sure the bulb is not more than 25 watts.

4. Prepare the patient for the treatment.

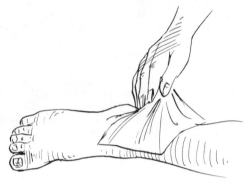

Check for dressing.

The heat cradle treatment may be ordered for a specified period of time or on a continuous basis. Check the physician's order for length of treatment. Also check the area for need of dressings. For dry heat and no dressings, the body part is exposed. If dry or moist dressings are required, these should be applied. You should wrap the affected area with plastic sheeting and cover with a towel if moist dressings are used.

Replace the top covers. *Make sure the sheets do not come near or in direct contact with the light bulb.* The heat from the bulb could burn a hole in the sheets and start a fire. Position the patient in good alignment, and adjust the position of the bed for his comfort.

5. Return to the patient at frequent intervals.

Observe the condition of the skin, noting decreased or increased circulation, swelling, temperature, or pain. Note the condition of the dressings. It may be necessary to add saline (a weak salt solution) or water to keep the dressing moist. (Usually this is done with a basin of water and an irrigating syringe.) Leave the heat cradle in place for the *ordered* length of time.

6. Remove the cradle.

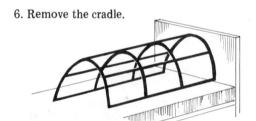

After treatment, place the cradle in a safe place in the patient's room if the treatment is to be repeated at intervals during the day. *Do not* set it on the floor; even though it looks clean, the floor has many organisms on it. When you return the heat cradle to the patient's bed, you could be bringing many new germs directly to the weakened patient, and a secondary infection could occur.

7. Leave the patient comfortable and safe.

Offer the bedpan/urinal. Adjust the bed and siderails. Attach call light within easy reach. Position patient in good body alignment.

8. Wash, rinse, and dry the cradle per agency procedure when the treatment is completed, return it to Central Service for cleaning and storage.

9. Obtain the chart.

Record all pertinent information in the nurse's notes, e.g., time, duration, type of treatment, and the results. Charting example:

7:00 P.M. Heat cradle applied to legs for 30 minutes.   J. Jones, SN

7:30 P.M. Heat cradle removed. Skin looks pink, swelling and pain have increased.

J. Jones, SN

ITEM 7. HYPOTHERMIA AND HYPERTHERMIA TREATMENT (FULL-BODY)

Hypothermia, or lowering of body temperature below the normal range, is a useful technique to decrease the rate of metabolic processes in the body. It is used to reduce high fevers, to control gastrointestinal hemorrhages, to prevent cerebral edema (swelling of the brain) in head injuries or surgeries, and for certain types of surgery. Usually the body temperature is reduced only a few degrees by cooling the body surface, but for surgical operations it may be reduced to 25°C. (77°F.) or even lower. Cooling may be achieved by cooling the body surface, or by cooling the blood directly.

Hyperthermia may be used to increase the body temperature after it has been lowered by hypothermia. It may also be used to increase the metabolic rate in the body.

The Aquamatic K Thermia Machine, a refrigerated unit with cooling blankets (or pads) attached to it, is used to raise or lower body temperature in a safe, simple, but precise manner. It controls body temperature in neurological (nervous system), cardiovascular (heart and circulatory), and thoracic (chest) surgical procedures. It is also used as a quick means to lower and regulate fevers or high temperatures due to infections and post-operative and traumatic conditions. It is both a labor-and time-saving device in caring for adult and child patients.

An electronically controlled freezing and heating unit, the machine contains a 20 per cent ethyl alcohol and distilled water solution. This solution circulates through the freezing or heating unit to produce the desired temperature, which is controlled by the automatic or manual control device on the machine. The solution also circulates through hollow cordlike vinyl Aquamatic K Pads which are placed in direct contact with the patient's skin. In this way the body temperature is controlled at an even and desired degree.

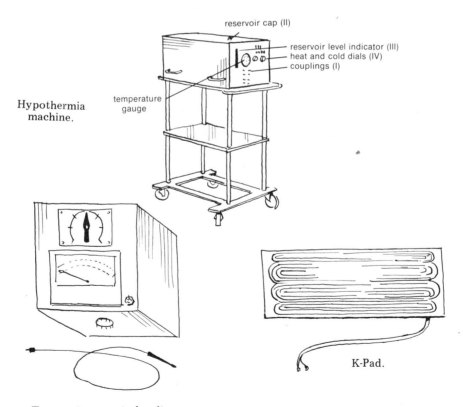

reservoir cap (II)

reservoir level indicator (III)
heat and cold dials (IV)
couplings (I)

Hypothermia
machine.

temperature
gauge

Temperature control unit
with thermistor probe.

K-Pad.

U
N
I
T
31

To Initiate Use of Hypothermia Machine

Important Steps	Key Points
1. Obtain the Aquamatic K Thermia Machine and take it to the patient's bedside.	Bring the machine from the supply area, including all its parts: the main refrigeration unit on a stand, temperature control box, thermistor probe, a gallon of 20 per cent ethyl alcohol and distilled water solution, vinyl body-sized or small-sized K-pads, and the manufacturer's complete instructional manual. (Size will depend on usage, size of patient, and area to be treated.)
2. Wash your hands; approach and identify the patient.	Explain the procedure to him.
3. Unit preparation.	
a. Plug electric cord into wall outlet.	All Roman numerals in the following instructions refer to the two sets of sketches appearing on the next two pages.
b. Select the number and size of K-pads to be used.	This will depend on the size of the patient and whether treatment is local or general.
c. Attach pads to unit (I).	There are 8 plugs for the pads clearly marked on the machine. Protective couplings remain on any plug not used. (Coupling caps dangle on a chain when not attached to outlets.)

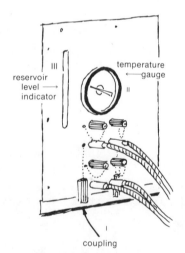

Couplings and plugs
of machine.

d. Fill reservoir (II) with distilled water to denatured alcohol. (Remove cap on top of machine before filling.)	See your equipment operating instructions; there are minor variations among manufacturers.
e. Observe reservoir level indicator (III) as a guide to how much fluid is needed and fill at least half full.	
f. Set cool and heat dials at 80°F. (IV).	
g. Turn on pump by pushing "HEAT" button (V).	This will pump fluid from the reservoir into the pads.
h. After a few minutes, check reservoir level indicator (III).	More fluid may be added because some was used in filling the pads.

Important Steps   Key Points

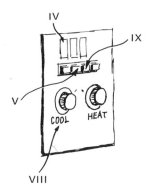   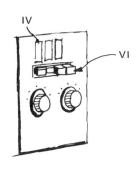

Regulating controls.

i. Turn off pump by pushing "OFF" button (VI) before adding fluid.

It may be necessary to turn the machine off and on several times until the pads are filled.

j. *Tighten* reservoir cap (II) when pump is turned *off*.

Loosen the reservoir cap (II) ¼ of a turn when pump is *running* to prevent a vacuum from developing.

k. To cool water, set "COOL" dial (VIII) to desired temperature and push "COOL" button (IX).

The *blanket* temperature will be adjusted from 40° to 50°F. initially, then adjusted to patient's temperature. Remember, this 40° to 50°F. is the temperature in the blanket, not the patient's temperature.

Note: The patient's body can be warmed and body temperature raised. Set the "HEAT" dial to the desired temperature and push the "HEAT" button.

4. Place pads on the patient (for full-body cooling).

a. Put one body-sized vinyl pad under the patient so that the pad comes in direct skin and body contact.

Some agencies may recommend placing a sheet between the pad and the patient's skin. Check your agency procedure.

b. As you remove the patient's gown, put the second body-sized vinyl pad on top of the patient.

Be sure to keep him covered with a blanket or top bedding to protect his modesty.

c. Do not expose the patient unnecessarily.

d. Put a sheet over the top of the patient and the pad.

This will prevent the cooled or heated air from escaping.

e. Optimum body temperature control is maintained by having as much of the body covered with the pads as possible.

Once the patient is on the cooling blankets, his temperature will begin to drop. It may take several hours to reduce the temperature as low as necessary; the doctor prescribes the temperature he wants and the length of time the temperature is to remain at that level. Check reservoir fluid level frequently. Refill PRN.

5. Attach the thermometer unit to the hypothermia unit at the marked connection.

The thermometer unit may be separate from the hypothermia unit. Check your agency equipment. Remove the thermistor probe from

U
N
I
T
31

Important Steps	Key Points

its plastic container. Insert the thermistor probe into the appropriate outlet in the control box shown below.

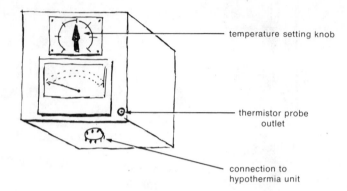

temperature setting knob

thermistor probe outlet

connection to hypothermia unit

Temperature control unit.

6. Place the thermistor probe into patient.

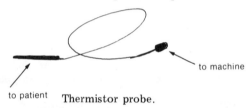

to machine

to patient   Thermistor probe.

Insert the free end of the thermistor probe into the patient's rectum. (It is most often used rectally, but check with the physician for proper place of insertion.) *Remember, the thermometer machine will not work if the probe is not in the patient.* (The continuous, automatic temperature of the patient is recorded on the patient temperature indicator scale shown above.)

7. Set dial (see foregoing sketch) for temperature limits between $40°$ and $100°$ F., at the desired temperature for the patient.

8. Set the automatic heat/cool button (IV in sketch on page 631).

Push the heat/cool button on the hypothermia unit. When the unit is working, the indicator light will go on. The electronic control device will automatically provide the heating and cooling control within the safety limits set on the temperature dial. The patient's temperature is indicated by the patient temperature indicator scale. Check the patient's skin condition at frequent intervals. Observe for circulation problems: increase or decrease in redness, numbness, swelling, or pain. If the patient's temperature must be reduced more rapidly than the machine alone can do it, place an alcohol-soaked sheet between the patient and the top vinyl pad, and the cooling process will speed up. Place the small K-pads in specific arterial areas of the body, e.g., groin, armpits, neck.

9. Safety factors.

    a. Keep the 20 per cent alcohol and distilled water mixture at minimal level.

Check the liquid level gauge at frequent intervals. (Refer to equipment manual for specifics.)

    b. Keep the unit on a stand in an open area so that air in and around the unit circulates freely.

Important Steps	Key Points

c. If oxygen is used, keep it at least 3 feet away from the unit.

d. Use heavy extension cords.

e. Remember that other electrical appliances may cause interference.

Refer to the manufacturer's instruction manual for other safety factors.

f. Prevent the patient from shivering during the cooling process.

Report any shivering to the team leader or nurse in charge. The shivering action increases the metabolic rate which produces heat. Shivering can be controlled by various medications. Charting example:

11:30 P.M. Hypothermia machine applied. Temperature set at 60°F.   J. Jones, SN

To Remove the Hypothermia/Hyperthermia Equipment

Important Steps	Key Points

1. Remove electric cord plug from room outlet.

2. Remove thermistor probe from the patient and wipe it clean with a tissue.

3. Disconnect thermistor probe plug from the unit.

Put it in a safe place, to be returned with the rest of the equipment to the storage area for cleaning. These probes are frequently lost in the linens. They are costly, so be careful.

4. Disconnect the vinyl pads from the coupling outlets in the unit.

• 5. Replace the caps to the coupling outlets in the unit.

6. Remove the pads from the patient.

7. Take the equipment to a sink or utility area and wash it with soap and water or a germicidal solution, or return it to central processing area for cleaning and storage.

8. Return it to the supply area.

Return *all* the equipment to the supply area or the proper storage place. Be sure that all parts of the hypothermia unit are returned. This is an expensive piece of equipment which will not operate effectively without all of its parts.

9. Leave the patient comfortable and safe.

Place the bedside stand, fresh water (if permitted), and the call signal so the patient can reach them without strain or discomfort. Adjust the bed to the low position and raise the siderails. Remember to utilize proper body alignment and movement for yourself and the patient. Provide for the general comfort of the patient. Take and record his vital signs frequently. If the patient has an indwelling catheter, be sure an accurate I and O is taken

Important Steps	Key Points
	and recorded. Reassure your patient, if he is conscious, by your quiet presence and quiet conversation.
10. Obtain the patient's chart.	Record all pertinent information concerning this task in the nurse's notes; include time treatment ended, vital signs, and patient's general condition.
	Note: Always use manufacturer's instruction manual when necessary.
	Charting example:
	11:30 P.M. Hypothermia unit removed. Patient comfortable and quiet. Temperature 97°F.
	J. Jones, SN

ITEM 8. AQUATHERMIA PAD (HYPOTHERMIA/HYPERTHERMIA LOCAL TREATMENT)

The Aquamatic K control unit is a small jarlike plastic unit operated by electricity. There is a temperature gauge on one side and two coupling outlets at the base. The top has a wide mouth with a lid on it so that distilled water can be poured into it. The vinyl Aquamatic K-pad (called K-pad for short) is attached to the coupling outlets at the base of the control unit. The water is heated and circulated through the unit and the pads in a manner similar to the hypothermia body unit. The pad is placed directly on the patient's injured area for a continuous heat treatment.

Important Steps	Key Points
1. Obtain the Aquamatic K-pad and control unit, and take it to the patient's bedside.	Bring it from the supply area (it will include the jarlike container, control unit, vinyl K-pad, and a bottle of distilled water), and place these articles on the patient's bedside stand.
2. Wash your hands; approach and identify the patient.	Explain what you will be doing.
3. Unscrew the reservoir cap on the top of the control unit.	All parts are easily visible. Review the equipment operations manual before proceeding. This unit works like the hypothermia machine except that the temperature equipment is applied to a local area for treatment.
4. Fill the unit 2/3 full with distilled water.	
5. Tilt the control unit slowly from the side to let air bubbles escape.	
6. Plug unit into the electrical outlet.	
7. Fill the K-pad with water by sliding the switch on the right to the "on" position.	Allow it to run at least 2 minutes.
8. Switch the unit off and tilt the control unit again to let air bubbles escape.	
9. Refill the reservoir to the cap level.	
10. Replace the cap, but loosen it 1/4 turn.	

Important Steps	Key Points
11. Set the desired temperature by inserting a special key into the center of dial.	Turn the dial until the indicator points to the desired temperature on the dial. Keep the key attached to the machine for PRN changes in temperature.
12. Check the operation of the unit; set the temperature at 105°F.	The pad should feel warm within 1 to 2 minutes. This is a delicate instrument; be sure it is not dropped or bumped.
13. Explain the task to the patient.	When you think he understands, proceed with the task.
14. Place the pad on the patient's injured area.	Secure the pad with sheeting or a bathtowel if necessary. Wrap it around the outside of the pad and the injured extremity firmly, evenly, and securely. Secure it with a safety pin or tape. Be sure not to puncture the K-pad with a pin because the fluid will leak out. Be very careful when you use this pad for diabetics, infants, and patients who have circulatory problems. The temperature should never be set in the red area (105° to 115°F.) If oxygen is used at the same time, keep it at least 3 feet from the unit to prevent possible fire or explosion from a spark generated by the electric motor.
15. Check the injured area at frequent intervals.	Note increased or decreased swelling, redness, circulation, pain, and numbness. Record on patient's chart as necessary.
16. Remove the equipment.	Remove the electric plug from the electric outlet in the room. *Do not yank or pull the cord; put your hand on the plug and pull the plug.* Unwrap and remove the sheeting and the K-pad.
17. Take the equipment to a sink or utility area and wash it with soap and water or a disinfectant solution.	*Do not immerse electric jarlike unit in water. Do not autoclave.*
18. Return the equipment to the supply area.	Return all the equipment to the supply area or to the proper storage place.
19. Leave the patient comfortable and safe.	Place the bedside stand, fresh water, and the call signal so the patient can reach them. Adjust the bed to the low position and raise the siderails.
20. Record all pertinent information concerning this task in the nurse's notes, e.g., time started, location of pad, time finished, general condition of the patient.	

UNIT 31

ITEM 9. IMPORTANT CONSIDERATIONS

1. Physician's orders

When electric or non-electric appliances are used for heat or cold in patient care, it is imperative to remember that an order must be written by the physician on the patient's chart before any appliance can be used. The order must state the kind of appliance, how often, and how long it is to be applied for the designated treatment.

2. Safety to the Patient

When electric or non-electric appliances are used for heat or cold in patient care, the patient's safety is of utmost importance. Do not use electric appliances close to open oxygen unless they are well-insulated and the electric outlets and plugs are far enough away so that it is impossible for electric sparks to ignite the oxygen and cause a fire. Do not permit the patient to put the plug in the electric outlet. Do not permit the patient to handle the temperature control. Do not permit the heat or cold pad to be used without a cloth cover. When heat or cold is applied to the *unconscious* patient, remember to be doubly aware of inadvertently burning or causing numbness to the patient. He *cannot* tell you whether the pad is too hot or if he is in pain or discomfort.

3. Safety to the Worker

When the electric appliance is used, be aware that it is dangerous to put the plug in the electric outlet in a dark room. Use a light to find the outlet; do not try to locate the outlet using your hand as a guide. Do not handle the plug or put it in the electric outlet when you have wet hands. Do not remove the plug from the outlet by pulling at the cord. Be aware of the cord; it may be stretched across a walking area on the floor. Do *not* trip over it and hurt yourself.

4. Cost to the Patient

All appliances obtained from Central Service are rented for the patient in most agencies. Some agencies have a daily treatment rate which includes the cost of all treatments and equipment needed to provide them. A requisition slip is usually sent to Central Service requesting the item; it is dated and stamped with the patient's name and hospital number. When the appliance is no longer needed, the requisition slip may be returned with it to Central Service. (Check your agency for specific procedure.) When the patient's needs have been met, the appliance must be returned to Central Service so that it can be reprocessed for the next patient. Do not keep it longer than necessary; the patient may be charged for something that he is not using.

5. Care of the Equipment

Initial care of the equipment is usually accomplished by the health workers in Central Service. When it is being used by the patient, it is maintained by the health worker who is responsible for the patient's care. It must be kept clean and in good working order. When necessary, report needed repairs to the proper person, and replace it immediately (send to Central Service). If equipment is faulty, do not express your concern or annoyance verbally in the presence of the patient or his family. This will only cause unnecessary apprehension or fear.

CONCLUSION OF THE UNIT

You have now concluded the lesson on Assisting with Hot and Cold Applications. When you have practiced the procedures so that you know them, arrange with your instructor to take the post-tests. You will be expected to demonstrate your skills in carrying out the required tasks as well as knowledge of the effects of heat and cold on the body.

VI. ADDITIONAL INFORMATION FOR ENRICHMENT

Other types of heat appliances which may be used are the ultraviolet and infrared lamps. Usually these treatments are given by the physical therapy staff, but you should know about them. The ultraviolet lamp projects heat rays and produces some chemical reactions which inhibit the growth of bacteria; it is also used for the heat it produces. The ultraviolet light seems to be effective in stopping rickets (a vitamin D deficiency disease).

The infrared lamp projects invisible heat rays beyond the red end of the light spectrum. The wavelength is below 477 billion vibrations per second, or longer than those at the other end of the spectrum. These rays are readily absorbed by the tissues. Infrared lamps are used for the relief of pain caused by arthritis and rheumatic conditions. Other heat sources are the sun, the electric arc, and the incandescent lamp.

Use of these two types of lamps is usually reserved for the professional health workers in the Physical Therapy Department. Great caution must be observed when these lamps are used and the patient must be under constant supervision to avoid severe burns. The heat rays from the lamps are like the rays of the sun, but the heating method is subtle (quietly active) because the light rays change to heat in the tissue.

Like sun rays, the lamps act on the skin and tissue. If you have experienced a sunburn, you can understand the possible dangers from these lamps. When the ultraviolet lamp is used, specially fitted dark glasses or protective eye coverings are worn by the patient to protect his eyes, particularly the cornea. When the light rays turn to heat rays, the corneal tissue could be destroyed. (The eye tissue would be coagulated, like the white of an egg when it is cooked.)

The lamps can be and are used for superficial and deep heat therapy, under the supervision of the physical therapist. If the patient is over-exposed to the lamp rays, tissue damage can be extreme—a third-degree burn will result. The skin area first becomes red, blistered, swollen, and burned so that the tissue eventually sloughs off. When this happens, there is danger of a systemic (general, throughout body) infection and an electrolyte imbalance due to the loss of fluid through the open wound. Symptoms to be noted accompanying the burn are nausea, headache, vomiting, and possible kidney malfunctions (anuria). For these reasons, the lamps are used only in the Physical Therapy Department or by specially trained personnel.

Several precautions must be taken when giving these treatments:

1. Apply to the local area only.

2. Observe the time elements very rigidly. The time of the treatment may be as limited as 1 to 2 minutes.

3. Know the heat method you are using, its expected results, and the complications which could arise from improper use.

4. Follow directions explicitly for applying the procedure, e.g., time, location, distance from light to skin surface.

5. Stay with the patient and observe his reactions closely.

U
N
I
T
31

POST-TEST

Multiple Choice. Select the best answer for each of the questions and place an X before your choice.

1. A local application of heat to the upper back would cause:

_____ A. a numbness or loss of sensation.

_____ B. a bluish, mottled color of the skin.

_____ C. dilation of blood vessels elsewhere in the body.

___✗___ D. increased circulation of blood in the area.

2. Metabolism and growth of new cells are stimulated by:

_____ A. oxygen

_____ B. cold

___✗___ C. heat

_____ D. light

3. A hot water bottle is filled only 1/3 to 1/2 in order to:

___✗___ A. make the bottle lighter and less cumbersome to use.

_____ B. keep it from getting too hot and burning the patient.

_____ C. assure that it is refilled frequently as it cools.

_____ D. make it easier to expel the air from the bottle.

4. Heat makes the blood vessels:

___✗___ A. dilate.

_____ B. contract.

_____ C. increase.

_____ D. decrease.

5. Hypothermia can be defined as:

_____ A. decreased blood supply to a part of the body.

___✗___ B. a decrease in the temperature of the blood.

_____ C. an increase in the temperature of the body.

_____ D. freezing of a part or all of the body.

6. Infrared and ultraviolet lamps are used under the supervision of the physical therapist because:

___✗___ A. heat from the light rays produced can cause serious burns.

_____ B. someone must observe the patient frequently.

_____ C. the rays can coagulate albumin, or the white of an egg.

_____ D. the lamps must be a certain distance from the patient's skin.

7. A patient can tolerate the dry cold of an ice bag for a longer period of time than a local bath of ice-cold water because:

_____ A. the nerve endings are numbed by the ice bag.

_____ B. the intensity of dry cold is greater than wet cold.

_____ C. dry cold reduces the contraction of muscles.

_____ D. water is a better conductor of cold than air.

8. The temperature indicated by the COOL dial or button on the hypothermia machine is used to regulate the temperature of:

_____ A. the fluid in the reservoir.

_____ B. the patient's body.

_____ C. the fluid in the K-pads.

_____ D. the air in the room.

9. When you are working with electrical equipment, such as the electric heating pad or the hypothermia machines, you should always avoid:

_____ A. using the equipment when oxygen is being used in the same room.

_____ B. touching the controls without an order from the doctor.

_____ C. using a cover between the electrical pad or machine and the patient's skin.

_____ D. plugging the cord into an outlet with wet hands.

10. A cold application causes which of the following effects:

_____ A. an increase in the metabolic rate of the body.

_____ B. a decrease in the blood supply to the area.

_____ C. a reduction in excess tissue fluid, or swelling.

_____ D. more rapid removal of toxins and waste products.

Completion. The following statements describe a condition or a situation in which heat or cold may be used. For each statement, you are to indicate which of the following would be used, based on your understanding of the principles involved, and then write the word in the space provided. Please indicate whether

Heat
Cold
Either

would be the best answer.

either 1. to reduce pain in the knee.

cold 2. to reduce swelling of the brain following an injury.

heat 3. to increase the relaxation of muscles.

cold 4. to control a nose bleed and reduce blood loss.

heat 5. to reduce stiffness in the joints of the fingers.

heat 6. to promote healing of an ulcer of the foot.

cold 7. to reduce pain and swelling after a tooth is pulled.

heat 8. to help bring a boil to a head, to increase suppuration.

cold 9. to reduce swelling from a bump on the forehead.

cold 10. to prevent the rupture of an infected or suppurating appendix.

POST-TEST ANNOTATED ANSWER SHEET

MULTIPLE CHOICE

1. D   Page 616, 617

2. C   Page 616, 617

3. A   Page 619

4. A   Page 616

5. B   Page 616, 629

6. A   Page 637

7. D   Page 618

8. C   Page 630

9. D   Page 635, 636

10. B   Page 617

COMPLETION

1. either   Page 617

2. cold   Page 617

3. heat   Page 617

4. cold   Page 617

5. heat   Page 617

6. heat   Page 617

7. cold   Page 617

8. heat   Page 617

9. cold   Page 617

10. cold   Page 617

PERFORMANCE TEST

In the classroom, or your skill laboratory, your instructor will ask you to perform the following activities without reference to any source material. You will need the mannequin or another student to take the part of the patient.

1. Given a patient who has a swollen, stiff, and painful right shoulder, you are to apply a hot water bottle (or disposable hot pack) to the part without danger of burning the patient even if the bottle should leak or break.

2. Given a patient with a circulatory disease of both legs, you are to apply a heat cradle that will be used indefinitely in a manner that will provide for the patient's comfort and safety.

3. Given a patient who has just had his tonsils removed, you are to apply an ice collar (or disposable cold pack) to his throat in a manner that will provide for the patient's comfort and safety.

4. Given a patient who is suspected to have cerebral edema (swelling of the brain), you are to set up the hypothermia machine to control the body temperature at $95°$F.

   If the machine is not available in your agency, describe the steps of the procedure that you would use.

PERFORMANCE CHECKLIST

ASSISTING WITH HOT AND COLD APPLICATIONS

APPLICATION OF A HOT WATER BOTTLE TO THE RIGHT SHOULDER

U
N
I
T
31

1. Wash hands.

2. Approach and identify patient.

3. Obtain hot water bottle and cover from storage.

4. Fill hot water bottle 1/3 to 1/2 full with hot water.

5. Expel excess air from bottle before securing top.

6. Test temperature of bottle against inner aspect of arm.

7. Put cover on bottle.

8. Take hot water bottle to patient and explain why it is being used.

9. Place bottle snugly against patient's right shoulder.

10. Make sure patient is comfortable.

11. Record pertinent information on patient's chair.

USE OF A HEAT CRADLE OVER THE EXTREMITIES

1. Wash hands.

2. Approach and identify patient.

3. Obtain heat cradle and bring it to bedside.

4. Provide for patient's privacy by pulling curtain.

5. Fold back top covers without undue exposure of patient.

6. Place heat cradle over patient's legs.

7. Plug in cord and turn on light.

8. Check wattage of light, and length and position of cord.

9. Inspect legs for need of dressings.

10. Replace top covers over heat cradle but away from light itself.

11. Position patient in good alignment.

12. Adjust bed for patient's comfort.

13. Tell patient that he or she will be checked at frequent intervals.

14. Record pertinent information on patient's chart.

APPLICATION OF ICE COLLAR TO THE THROAT

1. Wash hands.

2. Approach and identify patient.

3. Obtain ice collar and cover from storage.

4. If freeze pack is available, put cover on it, or

5. Fill ice pack about 3/4 full with ice.

6. Expel air from pack and wipe outside dry, after closing top.

7. Wrap ice collar in cover or towel.

8. Apply ice collar securely to patient's throat.

9. Inform patient that it will be checked frequently.

10. Make sure patient is comfortable.

11. Record pertinent information on patient's chart.

SET UP HYPOTHERMIA MACHINE AND CONTROL TEMPERATURE OF 95° F.

1. Wash hands.

2. Approach and identify patient, and explain procedure.

3. Obtain hypothermia machine with all its parts and take it to bedside.

4. Prepare hypothermia unit:

    A. Plug in cord.

    B. Select two large K-pads and attach them to unit.

    C. Fill reservoir with fluid.

    D. Turn cool and heat dials to 80°, then turn machine on by pushing HEAT button.

    E. Turn machine off before adding more fluids.

    F. Tighten cap on reservoir.

G. Set COOL dial between 40° and 50° for blanket temperature, and push COOL button.

5. Prepare patient:

   A. Place one large K-pad under patient.

   B. Place second large K-pad over patient, and remove his gown.

   C. Place sheet over upper pad on patient.

6. Attach thermometer unit to hypothermia unit.

7. Insert thermistor probe into patient's rectum.

8. Set desired temperature of 95° F. on thermometer unit.

9. Set automatic heat/cool button.

10. Provide for patient's comfort and report any shivering.

11. Inform patient that his temperature and adjustment of blanket temperature will be checked frequently.

12. Record pertinent information on patient's chart.

NOTES

Operation of patient turning frames

I. DIRECTIONS TO THE STUDENT

You are to proceed through this unit using the workbook as your guide. You will need to practice setting up and operating various patient turning frames in the classroom or the skill laboratory using the mannequin (Mrs. Chase) or a student partner in the role of the patient. After you have completed the lesson and your practice of the procedures, arrange with your instructor to take the performance test.

For this unit you will need the following items.

1. This workbook

2. A Foster or Stryker turning frame and accessory parts

3. A Circ-O-lectric bed and accessory parts

4. Sheets, bath blanket, and safety pins

Please read the following paragraphs carefully. They will tell you what you will be expected to know and how you will be expected to set up and operate the turning frames in order to care for the patient. If you feel that you have the necessary skills and would be wasting your time studying this material, discuss this with your instructor, and arrange to take the performance test. All students are expected to demonstrate their skill in setting up and operating the turning frames safely and efficiently.

U
N
I
T
31

II. GENERAL PERFORMANCE OBJECTIVE

Upon completion of this unit, you will be able to set and operate the Circ-o-lectric bed and the Foster or Stryker turning frame correctly, efficiently, and safely.

III. SPECIFIC PERFORMANCE OBJECTIVES

When you have finished this lesson, you will be able to:

1. Set up a Stryker (or Foster) frame and assist in transferring the patient onto the frame in an accurate, efficient, and safe manner which does not cause additional apprehension or injury to the patient.

2. Turn the patient on a Stryker (or Foster) frame from the supine to the prone position with the use of the anterior frame so that the patient is held securely and safely during the movement.

3. Set up and operate the Circ-o-lectric bed and assist in transferring the patient onto the bed in an accurate, efficient, and safe manner which does not cause additional apprehension or injury to the patient.

4. Operate the Circ-o-lectric bed accurately and rotate the patient from a supine to a vertical standing position and then to a prone position, using the anterior frame so that the patient is held securely and safely during the movement.

IV. VOCABULARY

gatch—the mechanism which allows a portion of a bed to be raised and held in a sitting position.
immobilize—to make or fix a part of the body so that it cannot move.
orthopedics—the prevention or correction of deformities and the treatment of diseases of bones and joints.
paraplegia—paralysis of the lower portion of the body and both legs.
perineal—refers to the perineum, located between the vulva and the anus of the female, and between the scrotum and the anus of the male.
pubis—the lower anterior part of the innominate bone in the pelvis.
quadriplegia—paralysis of all four extremities (arms and legs).
vertigo—dizziness.

Review. You should also review the following words to make sure you know their meanings.

abduction—moves away from the midline.
adduction—moves toward the midline.
anterior—the front side.
buttocks—the seat, rump, or gluteal prominence.
flexion—to bend or to fold; to decrease the angle of a joint.
posterior—the dorsal or back side.
prone—lying on stomach, or with face downward.
supine—lying on the back with face upward.

INTRODUCTION TO SPECIAL TURNING FRAMES

In the hospital, certain patients with orthopedic conditions (disease, surgery, or fracture of bones or joints) must be kept immobilized in order that healing may occur. Other patients may be immobilized or unable to move because of their disease or physical condition. As an example, the patient with a fracture or injury to his spinal column may need to be immobilized so that his spine can heal. At the same time, the patient needs to change position at frequent intervals to relieve pressure, to promote circulation, and for his own comfort. As you know, any position that is maintained for a long time becomes unbearable. In order to maintain the immobilization of part of the patient's body and yet provide for turning, various types of turning frames or beds may be used. The more common types that you may see or use are the Stryker frame, the Foster frame, or the Circ-o-lectric bed.

Patients who may need to use these special turning frames include those who have paraplegia, quadriplegia, spinal fusion, multiple fractures of the spine or long bones, acute arthritis, severe dermatitis, genito-urinary disorders, and other diseases which cause immobility or paralysis.

In this unit, you will become familiar with the various types of turning frames, how to set them up, and how to operate them in order to provide care for the patient.

ITEM 1.   THE PSYCHOLOGICAL NEEDS OF THE IMMOBILIZED PATIENT

How would you feel if you were unable to turn yourself and had to be confined to a narrow bed for days, weeks, or even longer? How do you think you might express your feelings and with what emotions? What fears do you think you might have? The immobilized patient has many apprehensions as well as his great need for physical care. His behavior and his willingness to cooperate in the treatment are related to the manner in which his psychological needs are met, as well as to the physical care that he receives. Let's consider some of these psychological needs.

He has a need to express his feelings. The immobilized patient should be encouraged to discuss his immobilization and how it affects him. He needs someone to listen to him. His emotional response can be varied—ranging from fear, anger, and hostility to depression or withdrawal. When the patient expresses his emotions, you should accept his right to do so and yet not take it personally, even when it seems to be directed toward you.

The patient has a need to know. He should be told the reason for the use of the equipment. It is no longer adequate to say that it has been ordered by the doctor or some other authority figure; people want to know "why" as well. Just because we know that a treatment is beneficial or good for a patient does not mean that he knows it or is willing to accept our word for it. The patient needs to know why a turning frame must be used for him. Some of these reasons might be as follows:

1. To change his position at frequent intervals with minimum pain or discomfort.

2. To relieve pressure on parts of the body.

3. To increase circulation.

4. To maintain the immobility of the affected part so that healing can occur.

5. To increase his comfort, well-being, and activities.

He must be considered as a whole person. Even though he may be greatly restricted in his physical activities and dependent on others for his care, his mind is usually not impaired. He should be encouraged to use his intellectual abilities. He is not just a body lying on a turning frame, but a person who belongs to a family, to a community, and who has a purpose in life.

He also needs safety and protection. The immobilized patient must be sure that those who care for him know how to use the equipment correctly and safely. His apprehension and fear for his own safety are greatly increased by the fumbling and gropings of workers who do not know how to operate the turning frames.

And finally, the patient has a need to make decisions, to determine what is to happen to him. He even has the right to refuse to be put on the turning frame. Whenever possible, the patient should be involved in planning for his care and allowed to make decisions about many things, such as the time of his bath, the foods he wants to eat, his bedtime, and other various activities within allowable and recognized boundaries.

The psychological needs of the immobilized patient, or the patient who may need to use a turning frame, are very important. Usually this patient has a serious injury or illness which might leave him greatly impaired and which requires a longer period of hospitalization than for most other patients. So, in addition to knowing how to set up and operate the equipment, you should know how the patient might respond to these activities.

ITEM 2. THE STRYKER FRAME AND THE FOSTER FRAME

The Stryker frame consists of a canvas-covered frame on which the patient lies. It is attached to a metal frame on wheels. The canvas-covered frame is connected at a pivot joint, so that the entire frame turns when the patient is turned from his back to his abdomen and vice versa. When turning the patient, a second canvas covered frame is placed on top of the patient and the two frames are secured with the patient between them like a sandwich. Safety belts are used to hold them together.

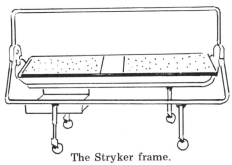

The Stryker frame.

The posterior frame on which the patient lies when he is in a supine position is prepared by covering it with canvas sections: one from the top of the frame to the pubis; a small middle section that can be removed for the use of the bedpan, and one that extends from mid-thigh to the foot end of the frame. The canvas sections are covered with folded bath-towels and drawsheets which are pinned on the underside.

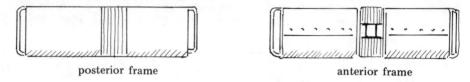

posterior frame   anterior frame

Preparation of the turning frame.

The anterior frame is usually prepared in a similar manner, except that one section extends from the shoulders to the pubis in order to allow space for the head. A narrow section is used to support the forehead. The lower section extends only to the ankles so that the feet can be properly aligned when the patient is lying on his abdomen.

With the patient strapped securely between the anterior and posterior frames, one nurse can safely turn the patient in the Stryker frame by loosening a spring lock at either end of the frame. The frame will automatically trip the lock when it is turned, and again be locked in place. After the patient has been turned, the upper frame is removed. Armrests can be attached to the sides of the frame when the patient is in a prone position. The sketch below shows how the patient is turned to a prone position and shows the patient in a prone position.

When the bedpan is needed, the small canvas section across the middle of the frame is detached and the bedpan is placed as shown in the bottom illustration.

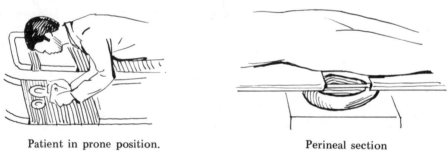

Patient in prone position.   Perineal section
                                              detached for bedpan use.

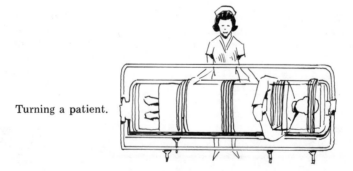

Turning a patient.

The Foster frame is similar to the Stryker frame except that it is bigger, more stable, and more expensive. It is used for the same purposes and the procedure of setting it up and operating it is almost the same as for the Stryker frame.

ITEM 3. PROCEDURE FOR SETTING UP AND USING THE STRYKER FRAME

Important Steps	Key Points
1. Obtain the frame.	The frame is usually kept in a supply area, and personnel from that area are usually responsible for assembling the equipment and bringing it to the patient's room.
2. Check to see that you have all the parts.	You should have the following parts: basic frame anterior and posterior frames four long stem pins canvas sections: 2 long, 2 short, and 2 narrow sponge pads: 2 long, 2 short, 2 narrow, 2 shoulder pads, and 1 abdominal pad footboard and 2 armrests tray table bedpan support 2 safety straps (webbed) with airplane buckles forehead strap or face mask cover for forehead strap or face mask spring clamps covers for sponge pads, or linen and safety pins to secure it
3. Prepare the posterior frame.	
a. Attach the canvas sections across the posterior frame and secure them with spring clamps.	Measure the canvas sections to fit the patient and fold the unneeded portion underneath. *Top section*—from top of patient's head to the pubis. *Middle section*—(perineal section) from the pubis to the upper third of thigh. *Lower section*—from upper third of thigh to bottom of frame.
b. Place sponge pads on canvas sections and cover them with bath blankets or sheets.	Make sure that all ends of the linen coverings are secured (pinned) so they won't catch or interfere when the frame is turned.
c. Place the posterior frame on the basic frame.	Tightly latch or screw the nuts in place at the pivoting joint.
d. Attach the footboard in the slat at the bottom of the posterior frame.	
4. Take the Stryker frame and its parts to the patient's room.	
5. Wash your hands.	
6. Approach and identify the patient, explain what is to be done, and enlist his cooperation.	Be sure to explain to the patient and his family the reasons why the turning frame is used and how it will benefit the patient.
7. Transfer the patient to the frame.	*A physician may be required to be present* when a patient is transferred to the frame.
a. Lock the wheels of the frame so that it will not move.	Leave folded bath blanket or sheet covering the patient to avoid exposing him.

UNIT 31

Important Steps	Key Points
b. Move all furniture and equipment away to provide a clear path from the patient's bed to the frame.	Reassure the patient during the transfer.
c. Secure additional help.	At least 3 or 4 people will be needed. Use at least a 3-man carry, and another to support the head if needed. Use good body alignment and smooth, coordinated movements. Lift and move the patient on signal.
8. Position the patient in correct body alignment on the frame.	
a. Head and neck are straight in line with the rest of the spine.	Usually no pillow is used, or a small one may be allowed. Avoid flexion of the neck.
b. The shoulders should be relaxed and flat against the frame.	
c. The back should be straight and flat against the frame.	A small pillow or pad may be used to support the small of the back, if it is needed.
d. The buttocks are supported by the perineal section except when the bedpan is used.	
e. The arms should be alongside the body, or supported on the armrests attached to the sides of the frame.	
f. The knees should be slightly flexed.	A small pillow or pad can be used under the knees unless contraindicated by the patient's condition.
g. The feet should be in good alignment, placed against the footboard, and supported laterally.	
9. Place the top covers over the patient.	These covers may have to be folded so that they do not drag on the floor. Make sure that they cause no pressure on the toes or feet.
10. Provide for the patient's comfort and care.	Leave the call light within his reach. The immobilized patient on the Stryker frame needs highly skilled and attentive nursing care. Unless acutely ill, he also needs diversional activities to help pass the time, such as reading or TV.
11. Move the regular hospital bed and tidy the room.	The regular bed may be moved out of the way in the room, or it may be taken out of the room by the housekeeping department in order to provide more space for the Stryker equipment. (Follow your agency procedure.)
12. Record the pertinent information on the patient's chart.	Charting example: 10:15 A.M. Transferred onto the Stryker frame under the direction of Dr. Jones. Color good. Cardinal signs stable. No complaints. M. Doe, RN

ITEM 4. TURNING THE PATIENT ON THE STRYKER FRAME

Important Steps	Key Points
1. Wash your hands; approach and identify the patient.	Read his name from his identification band so that he can confirm it.
2. Explain that you are going to turn him to the prone position.	The patient should be involved in planning a schedule in which he is turned every 1 to 3 hours.
3. Provide for privacy.	Pull the curtain around the Stryker frame or close the door of the room.
4. Check or prepare the anterior frame for use.	The anterior frame should have its three canvas sections padded and covered. There should be space at the top for the head and the forehead support, and space at the bottom for the feet.
5. Remove the top covers from the patient.	Pull the patient's gown down over his body to avoid undue exposure.
6. Attach the anterior frame in place over the patient.	Explain to the patient what you are doing as you go along.
a. Latch or screw the ends of the frame to the basic frame.	
b. Remove the armrests and place his arms along his sides.	
c. Adjust the forehead support or face mask to proper position.	
d. Wrap the safety belts around both frames and the patient; one around the chest and the other around the thighs.	
7. Turn the patient to a prone position.	As an additional safety measure, you should have an assistant to help you turn the patient.
a. One worker stands at the head and the other at the foot of the frame.	
b. Each worker will unlock the safety locks at each end of the frame with one hand, and with the other hand will hold the same side of the frame.	Explain to the patient and your assistant that you will be turning the frame to the right on the count of three.
c. On a signal, such as "1, 2, 3, turn," quickly and smoothly turn the frame clockwise until it locks in position.	The patient will now be facing the floor, or be in the prone position. Wait a few moments for him to become oriented. Stay close beside him, talking, comforting, and reassuring him.
8. Remove the posterior frame.	Place the frame so that it will be out of the way, and will not tip over or interfere with work in the area.
9. Adjust the patient's body alignment.	Check for alignment as in Step 8 of Item 3. Also check for pressure, particularly around the ankles, when in the prone position.
10. Provide for the patient's comfort and welfare.	Put the top covers over the patient again. Leave the call signal within his reach. Provide other assistance and diversional activities as may be needed.

Important Steps	Key Points
11. Report and record on the patient's chart.	In some hospitals or agencies, turning the patient on a schedule is recorded as a treatment, e.g.:

"Turn q 2 h.

10 MD 12 BN 2 MD 4, 6, etc."

(The hours are marked through and initialed by the worker turning the patient.)

Note: To turn the patient from the prone to the supine position, the same procedure would be used as above, except that the posterior frame would be placed over the patient, and the turn would be made in the counterclockwise direction (left).

ITEM 5.   PLACING THE PATIENT ON THE BEDPAN

Important Steps	Key Points
1. Wash your hands, approach and identify the patient, and explain what you will do.	Usually the patient will request the bedpan when he needs it.
2. Place the patient in a supine position.	Both male and female patients may be able to urinate while in the prone position, but need to be in the supine position for a bowel movement. (Some women patients find it difficult to urinate while in a prone position.)
3. Put the bedpan support on the proper inserts of the basic frame, and place the bedpan on the support.	
4. Detach the perineal (middle canvas section) support and put it out of the way to prevent soiling.	
5. Clean and dry the patient's perineum after use of the bedpan.	The immobilized patient is unable to do this for himself. You will therefore wipe him with tissue and use soap, water, washcloth and towel if the patient is soiled. Leave the patient clean and dry. Return supplies to storage.
6. Empty and clean the bedpan, then store it for later use.	
7. Reattach the perineal section to the frame.	Bedpan support may be left in place for future use, but should be clean.
8. Provide for the patient's comfort and welfare.	

ITEM 6.   THE CIRC-O-LECTRIC BED

The Circ-o-lectric bed is an electrically operated circular frame used to turn and position a patient with restricted or limited body movement. The turning movement is in a vertical direction rather than from side to side as in the Stryker frame. It is used for patients who have any of the following: severe circulatory conditions, orthopedic problems, or other conditions requiring specific treatment.

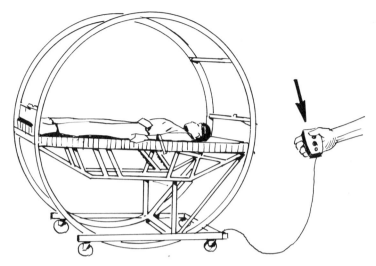

The Circ-o-lectric bed.

The bed is operated by an electric motor, which has hand controls that can be used by the patient when he is well enough. The worker can operate the bed by using a pushbutton on the control switch. The patient lies on a posterior frame which roughly forms the diameter of the circular frame. Before the patient is turned from his back (supine position), the anterior frame is placed over the patient's body and attached in place. The bed is then rotated forward to the "face" position until the patient is in a prone position. The posterior frame can then be raised in the frame so that it is not resting on the patient, as shown in the sketch below.

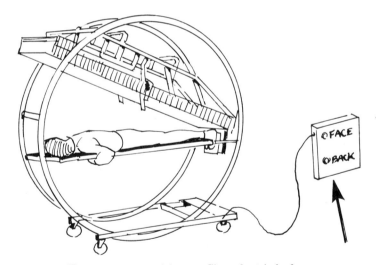

Face or prone position on Circ-o-lectric bed.

U
N
I
T
31

ITEM 7. PROCEDURE FOR SETTING UP AND OPERATING THE CIRC-O-LECTRIC BED

Important Steps	Key Points
1. Order the Circ-o-lectric bed.	The bed is generally obtained from the storage area and delivered by the Housekeeping Department. Usually the bed is set up before the patient is admitted to the room in order to

Important Steps	Key Points
	lessen the number of times the patient is moved. The regular bed can be stored until it is needed.
2. Check the parts and accessories for the bed.	Follow the manufacturer's instructional manual. The parts of the Circ-o-lectric bed that should be checked are: the basic frame, anterior frame, foam mattress, special sheet, safety or restraining straps, footboard attached to the frame, adjustable siderails, forehead and chin straps, and the accessory parts such as traction bars, suspension, and exercise apparatus.
3. Prepare the bed.	Place the plastic cover over the posterior frame and use spring clamps to hold it in place. Place the foam mattress on the frame. (Note that the mattress has a circular section that can be removed when the bedpan is in place.) Use the special sheet that fastens to the mattress with elastic bands. Lock the wheels to stabilize the bed during the transfer. *Note:* The nursing team may require practice in manipulating the bed, since it may have been some time since it was used for a patient.
4. Wash your hands.	
5. Approach and identify the patient.	The patient may be one who is to be transferred from a regular bed, or one who is admitted from Emergency, Surgery, or a special care unit. Read the patient's name aloud and have him or a co-worker verify it.
6. Explain the task to the patient and his family.	If at all possible, demonstrating the use of the bed before the patient is placed in it is helpful.
7. Transfer the patient to the Circ-o-lectric bed.	You will need additional help. *The presence of a doctor may be required.* You will need at least 3 or 4 people.
a. Clear all furniture and equipment away to provide a clear path to move the patient onto the frame of the bed.	
b. Transfer the patient using at least a 3-man carry.	Use good body alignment and smooth, coordinated movements. Lift and move the patient on signal.
8. Position the patient in correct body alignment on the frame.	Follow Steps 8 through 12 in Item 3, the Stryker frame procedure.

ITEM 8.   TURNING THE PATIENT TO A PRONE POSITION IN A CIRC-O-LECTRIC BED

Important Steps	Key Points
Follow Steps 1 through 6 in Item 4, Turning the Patient on the Stryker Frame.	
7. Turn the patient to the prone position.	Set or press the "face" position button on the control and put the bed in motion. Turn the patient gradually and slowly to prevent vertigo and loss of consciousness.

Important Steps	Key Points

8. Remove the posterior frame.

   a. Release the locks on the posterior frame and push the frame upward at the head end, until it locks in position over the patient (see sketch on page 648).

   b. Place the safety or restraining belts over the patient and hook them into the underside of the frame.   These are used to prevent a possible fall because the siderails cannot be used in the prone position.

Follow Steps 9 through 11 of Item 4.

Note: To turn the patient from the prone to the supine position, the same procedure is used, except that the posterior frame is placed over the patient, secured in place, and the "back" button is pressed on the control.

ITEM 9. USE OF THE BEDPAN IN THE CIRC-O-LECTRIC BED

Follow the same procedure as described in Item 5 for use of the bedpan on the Stryker frame, except:

   a. Remove the circular metal plate and the circular mattress section under the perineal area.

   b. Place the bedpan on the Evertaut fasteners so that it is held in place under the patient's buttocks.

   c. The bed may be tilted slightly or the head gatch elevated, if the patient's condition permits.

   d. The circular sections are replaced after the bedpan has been used.

U
N
I
T
31

ITEM 10. ADJUSTING THE POSITIONS OF THE CIRC-O-LECTRIC BED

When the patient is permitted unrestricted movements, the bed can be put in a sitting position. His hips should be centered over the point where the bed "breaks" for best body alignment when sitting.

Manual Gatching. The posterior frame has a lever on each side within easy reach of the patient. When one or both levers are pulled, the head and foot sections adjust in relation to the amount of effort exerted to sit up when the levers are depressed. This action is similar to that of adjusting seats in a bus or an airplane. Releasing the pressure on the lever locks the posterior section to the desired degree of gatch.

Electrical Tilting. After the bed is gatched, other positions can be obtained by tilting the bed forward or backward on the basic circular frame. When the bed is moving in the head-down position, automatic stops prevent it from going too far. The forward or "face" adjustments must be controlled by the patient or an attendant.

CONCLUSION OF THE UNIT

You have now completed the lesson on the operation of patient turning frames. After you have had sufficient practice with the equipment to become familiar with it and have some skills in performing the procedures, you should arrange with your instructor to take the performance test.

PERFORMANCE TEST

In your classroom or the skill laboratory, your instructor will ask you to perform the following skills accurately without any use of reference or source materials. You may need the assistance of other students in the procedures, and you may use the mannequin (Mrs. Chase) or another student to play the part of the patient.

1. Given a patient who is quadriplegic and paralyzed from the neck down, you are to set up a Stryker frame and assist in transferring him onto the frame as he arrives on the unit from Emergency so that the transfer is achieved safely and without injury to the patient or the workers.

2. Given a patient who has had surgery on his spine and who is lying in a supine position on a Stryker frame, you are to turn him to a prone position safely and without increasing his apprehension.

3. Given a patient in a Circ-o-lectric bed, you are to turn the patient from a supine (back position) to a prone position accurately and safely and align his body properly. (If a Circ-o-lectric bed is not available for your use, describe the steps of the procedure to your instructor.)

PERFORMANCE CHECKLIST

OPERATION OF PATIENT TURNING FRAMES

SET UP AND TRANSFER A PATIENT TO A STRYKER FRAME

  1. Obtain Stryker frame.

  2. Check to see if all the parts are present.

  3. Prepare posterior frame.

    A. Measure and attach upper, middle, and lower canvas sections to frame.

    B. Place the sponge pads on the sections and cover with linen so that all ends are secure.

    C. Place posterior frame on basic frame.

  4. Attach footboard.

  5. Take frame to patient's unit.

  6. Wash hands.

  7. Approach and identify patient.

  8. Explain to patient reasons for using Stryker frame.

  9. Obtain assistance to help transfer patient.

 10. Lock wheels of frame so it will not move.

 11. Clear furniture and equipment away between bed and frame.

 12. Place bath blanket or sheet over patient during transfer.

 13. Use at least a 3-man carry, lift on signal, and move patient to frame.

 14. Position patient correctly in good alignment on frame.

    A. Head and neck straight.

B. Shoulders flat.

C. Spine (or back) straight.

D. Arms supported.

E. Knees slightly flexed.

F. Feet against footboard and supported laterally.

15. Replace top covers on patient.

16. Provide for patient's comfort by giving signal cord, etc.

17. Tidy room.

18. Record information on patient's chart.

TURNING A PATIENT TO PRONE POSITION ON STRYKER FRAME

1. Approach and identify patient.

2. Explain what is going to be done.

3. Provide for patient's privacy by pulling curtains.

4. Check or prepare the anterior frame for use.

A. Provide space for patient's face.

B. Provide support for patient's forehead.

C. Provide space for bottom of frame and patient's feet.

5. Remove top covers, and smooth down patient's gown.

6. Place anterior frame correctly over patient's body.

7. Secure ends of frame to basic frame.

8. Remove arm support if these have been used.

9. Apply at least 2 safety belts, one around chest, another around thighs, and secure them snugly.

10. Have an assistant help to turn patient.

A. One at head and one at foot.

B. Unlock safety locks with one hand, hold frame with other.

C. Both turn in clockwise direction smoothly until locked in place.

11. Remove posterior frame.

12. Adjust alignment of patient's body.

A. Head and neck straight.

B. Shoulders flat.

C. Spine straight.

D. Arms supported.

E. Knees slightly flexed.

F. Feet against footboard, and anterior of foot protected from pressure.

UNIT 31

13. Provide for patient's comfort, leave call signal within reach, etc.

14. Report or record turning procedure.

TURNING PATIENT IN CIRC-O-LECTRIC BED TO PRONE POSITION AND ALIGN

1. Approach and identify patient.

2. Explain what is going to be done.

3. Provide for patient's privacy by pulling curtain, closing door.

4. Check or prepare anterior frame for use.

   A. Provide space for patient's face.

   B. Provide support for patient's forehead.

   C. Provide space for bottom of frame and patient's feet.

5. Remove top covers, and smooth down patient's gown.

6. Place anterior frame correctly over patient's body.

7. Secure ends of frame to basic circular frame.

8. Apply safety belts and secure them snugly around patient and both frames.

9. Turn patient slowly by pressing "face" button on control.

10. Remove posterior frame by pushing head end up until it is locked in place on frame.

11. Adjust alignment of patient's body.

   A. Head and neck straight.

   B. Shoulders flat.

   C. Spine straight.

   D. Arms supported.

   E. Knees slightly flexed.

   F. Feet against footboard, and anterior of foot protected from pressure.

12. Provide for patient's comfort, leave call signal in reach, etc.

13. Report or record turning procedure.

Application of restraints

I. DIRECTIONS TO THE STUDENT

Please read the following paragraphs carefully. They will tell you what you will be expected to know and how you will be expected to use restraints when caring for patients in your agency. You are to proceed through the lesson using this workbook as your guide. You will need to practice the procedures in the skill laboratory, using the mannequin (Mrs. Chase) or another student as the patient.

For this lesson, you will need the following items:

1. This workbook

2. A cloth limb-holder or wrist restraint

3. A restraint belt, or safety belt with buckle, 5 or 6 feet long

4. A body or jacket restraint

5. Roller gauze

6. ABD pads or wash cloth

After you have completed the lesson and your practice of the procedures, arrange with your instructor to take the post-test. If you feel that you have the necessary skills and would be wasting your time studying this unit, talk with your instructor. You would then arrange to take the post-test, in which all students are expected to demonstrate accurately the required skills.

U
N
I
T
31

II. GENERAL PERFORMANCE OBJECTIVE

Upon completing this lesson, you will be able to apply various types of restraints that will help to immobilize or support a part of the body.

III. SPECIFIC PERFORMANCE OBJECTIVES

When you have finished this unit, you will be able to:

1. Apply a wrist restraint or limb-holder to partially immobilize a patient's arm or leg in a way that does not interfere with his circulation or cause him injury.

2. Apply a body or jacket restraint to partially immobilize a patient who is in bed, or to support a patient in a chair or wheelchair, in a manner that provides for his safety and comfort.

3. Apply an elbow restraint safely and effectively on an infant or young child to prevent flexion of the elbow.

4. Apply a belt restraint or safety belt around a patient's waist in such a way as to give him a feeling of safety and security.

IV. VOCABULARY

discipline—training that corrects, molds, or perfects the mental facilities or moral character; to correct or train.

limb-holder—a cloth tie or restraint that keeps a limb (arm or leg) in a certain position or limits its full range of motion (sometimes called a soft restraint).

Posey belt—a commercially made restraint belt or strap.

punishment—act of subjecting to penalty, pain, loss, or other affliction for some offense or transgression.

restrain—to hold back from action, to check or keep under control, to repress, to deprive of liberty.

V. INTRODUCTION

In the field of health, restraints are used only as a safety measure. The most common safety needs of the patient are those to immobilize a part of his body wholly or partially, to assist in the support of part of his body, or to prevent possible harm to himself or to others. There are legal restrictions concerning the use of restraints that forcibly interfere with the patient's right to liberty, and these must be observed. Restraining a person (or patient) in a locked room, for instance, is subject to certain legal requirements.

Restraints may be indicated in the care of patients based on the patient's need for safety, or on the doctor's judgment of a need to limit the patient's movements for medical reasons. You need to know the principles involved in the use of restraints and the correct method of applying them. In this unit, you will learn procedures for using restraints on an extremity or on the body.

ITEM 1. PRINCIPLES RELATED TO THE USE OF RESTRAINTS

There are certain principles involved in the use of restraints for patient care in any health facility. These principles and the attitudes about restraints as described in this unit may differ from those taught or practiced by other workers in nursing. The emphasis here is on the patient and his needs, and how the use of the restraint will benefit him.

Principle 1. *The use of restraints must meet some need or help the patient.* The patient must have some safety need involving total or partial immobilization of a part of his body, support of part of his body, or prevention of harm to himself or others. If he is unable to handle these safety needs himself because of his mental or physical condition, and if other methods have been tried without effect, then the use of restraints may be indicated.

As an example: A patient may be receiving an IV in his left arm which is supported on a board. After he has had a medication for pain that dulls his awareness, he tries to pull out the IV with his other hand. As a safety measure, a loose wrist restraint might be applied to the right wrist which would allow some movement, yet not enough to reach the IV.

Another example: The ill patient who has periods of mental confusion (often seen in the elderly) may need a body jacket or safety belt when in bed or sitting in a wheel chair. Without the reminder of the jacket or belt, he might try to get up without assistance and suffer further injury.

Principle 2. *All restraints that limit movement or immobilize must be ordered by a physician.* Most agencies have specific policies and regulations about the use of restraints. You should check these. In every state, there are legal requirements and regulations about providing for the safety of patients, and limiting the patient's liberty or movements by forcible means. When the patient's movements must be limited for medical reasons, there must be an order for the restraint, either a specific written order, or an agency policy statement, which stipulates when and what kind of restraints may be used.

Principle 3. *Restraints must not be used as a means of punishing or disciplining the patient for his behavior.* The use of restraints or the threat of tying the patient down as a method of coercing, threatening, punishing, or disciplining, should not be tolerated in any health agency. When a bossy, dictatorial, "Do as I say, or else" approach is taken with the patient, it often leads to anger on both the part of the patient and the worker, and the probable use of force and restraints. The "caring for" and "caring about" approach to the patient would be more effective in understanding his need for our help.

Perhaps it would be better if health workers referred to restraints as "safety belts." The very word "restraint" conveys a sense of punishment or discipline.

Principle 4. *Restraints are applied snugly to a body part, but not tight enough to interfere with blood circulation.* Care must be taken when applying safety belts or restraints so that the patient's restless movement or tugging does not close off the circulation. Impaired circulation to the part will cause the following symptoms: coolness of the skin, a pallor or bluish color, numbness, and loss of sensation or movement. The restraint must be loosened or removed immediately and the part gently massaged to restore the circulation.

Principle 5. *The patient's position should be changed every 2 to 3 hours when restrained and active or passive exercise given; the restrained part is released unless contraindicated.* The change of position for the patient is necessary to relieve pressure, to increase circulation, to improve body functioning, and to make him more comfortable. Positioning, changing, and exercising the restrained part help to reassure the patient that the restraint is truly a safety measure and not a punishment.

ITEM 2.   TYPES OF RESTRAINTS AND SAFETY BELTS

Restraints come in many sizes and shapes. Increasingly, hospitals and health facilities are using commercially made restraints, of a strong cloth or canvas; the belts are usually webbing or tightly woven strong twill. Some agencies use folded sheets, bathrobe belts, woven strips of material or webbing, or gauze as a means of immobilizing a part of the body. A few examples of the commercial type of safety belt or restraint are described below.

Safety belt or restraint—made of webbing or twill with a buckle on one end. It is available in a variety of lengths, but is often 5 or 6 feet in length. Longer lengths are used to secure the patient on stretchers, when turning a patient on a Stryker frame, or on a Circ-o-lectric bed, and for other purposes. It is often used for patients in wheelchairs to provide safety. See the sketch below for the safety belt.

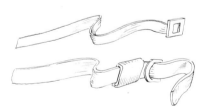

Safety belts.

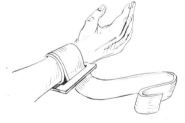

Limb-holder or
wrist restraint.

Limb-holder or wrist-type restraint (also called a soft restraint)—made of strong cloth about 3 inches wide with an 8 to 10 inch soft flannel padded end that is wrapped around the wrist or ankle. The padded end has a slit in it so the longer belt part can be drawn through it to encircle the wrist or leg. Some people may refer to it as a "Posey," which is the name of one of the leading manufacturers of restraints.

Body restraint—made of canvas or strong material; it has a short belt that buckles around the patient's body and is attached to the middle of a much longer belt which can be tied to the bed or around a wheelchair. (See the following sketch.)

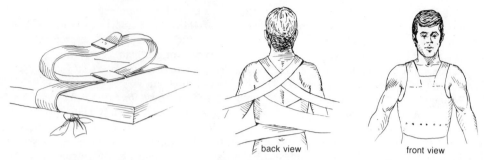

Body restraint.   Jacket restraint.

Jacket restraint—made of canvas or strong material; it has a portion that fits over the patient's chest with straps or belts that go over the shoulders and others that go around the waist. The straps or belts may be crossed or tied behind the patient's back. Generally used as a safety measure and to support the patient's trunk in an upright position while he is in a wheelchair. (See the sketch above.)

Elbow restraint—made of cotton or flannel; it is about 12 inches long, with slots in it where tongue blades can be inserted (or it has ribs that prevent bending) and has ties along one edge. This is used to restrain infants and small children from flexing their elbows to reach their face in cases of severe skin rashes or surgery of the face, such as the repair of a harelip. (An example of an elbow restraint is shown below.)

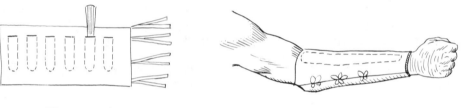

Elbow restraint.   Restraint on arm.

Leather restraint—made of leather with a buckle that has a locking device. A key must be used to unlock the buckle to remove the restraint. This is used only as a last resort when a patient is so disoriented that he becomes dangerous to himself, to other patients, or to the health workers. This type is being used less and less today, and always requires a doctor's written order when it is employed.

ITEM 3. PRECAUTIONS TO BE USED IN APPLYING RESTRAINTS

You should avoid tying unnecessary knots in restraints. In case of danger to the patient (such as a fire) or when emergency treatment is needed, restraints may have to be removed in a hurry. In such cases, you may have to cut the restraint if there are numerous knots, or if the knots are tied so tightly that it is difficult and time-consuming to untie them. A word or two about knots is therefore important.

Clove hitch—may be used to apply a wrist-type restraint to an extremity. The advantage of this knot is that it permits the patient some mobility while it will not cut off the circulation to the extremity. The clove hitch is made as shown at the top of page 663. Your observational skills are needed when you have any patient in restraints to assure that circulation in the extremity is maintained.

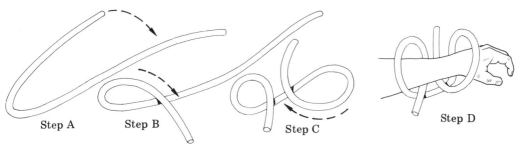

Step A   Step B   Step C   Step D

Square knot—may be used to secure the restraint to an extremity, or to secure the ends to the bed frame or the wheelchair. The advantage of the square knot is that it does not slip and will not tighten if pulled on. It also will not loosen when the stress or pull on the ties is released. The square knot is made as follows and as shown below. Take the left tie, pass it over, under, and across the right tie. It is now on the right side. Take the original right tie, pass it under, over and across the other tie. Place the first crossover where you want the knot to be located, and tighten the second crossover to form the square knot. (*Note:* the two crossovers form a partial loop at each end, and the ties on each side of the loop are in the same position; see step C.)

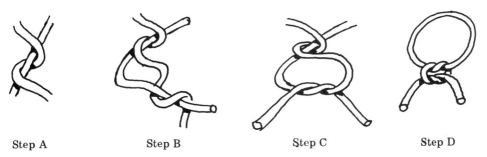

Step A   Step B   Step C   Step D

Half-bow knot—used to secure the restraint to the bed frame or the wheelchair. It is much easier to untie than the square knot, because you merely pull the loose tie end to remove the bow portion, and then loosen the crossover tie. It also will not slip even when stress or pull is exerted on the secured portion of the tie. You already know how to make the half-bow knot because you use it when tying your shoelaces, except that for a restraint you make only one loop in the bow.

These types of knots are likely to be the ones you will use to apply and secure restraints.

One final precaution should be noted before you begin practicing the procedures. When a restraint is secured to the bed frame, you should avoid tying it to the movable siderails or to the immovable portion of the bed. If the siderails are lowered, it may pull the restraint too tightly or cause strain on the patient's body where it is being immobilized. Raising or lowering the head of the bed may produce the same effects if the restraint is tied to the immovable portion of the bed frame.

UNIT 31

ITEM 4. APPLYING A LIMB-HOLDER OR WRIST-TYPE RESTRAINT

Important Steps	Key Points
1. Check for doctor's order or agency policy before restraints are applied.	This is a legal requirement when a patient's movement is to be restricted.
2. Wash your hands.	
3. Obtain the cloth restraint that is to be used, a limb-holder or Posey wrist restraint.	A charge may be made for the use of a restraint, depending on the policies of your agency.

Important Steps	Key Points
4. Approach and identify the patient.	Read the patient's name aloud so he can confirm it.
5. Explain to the patient what you plan to do and why.	The manner in which you approach the patient and explain the procedure may determine whether the patient will accept it or resist all efforts to apply it. Stress that the limb-holder or tie is used for his safety and as a reminder not to move his arms (or legs).
6. Apply the limb-holder to the wrist (or leg). Take the padded end and wrap it around the wrist. Pull the tie through the slit in the wrist portion. Attach the loose end to the spring frame of the bed, using a half-bow or a square knot.	If a commercially made limb-holder is not available, you can improvise: Use roller gauze, preferably 2 or 3 inches wide and at least 3 to 4 feet long. Use a wash cloth or ABD pad to wrap around the wrist. Tie the gauze around the wrist using a square knot, or fold the gauze in half and make a slipknot. Secure the loose ends to the spring frame of the bed.
7. Check the extremity distal to the restraint for adequate circulation.	Good circulation in hands and feet is indicated by warmth, normal color, and capability of movement.
8. Provide for the patient's comfort and welfare.	Place the signal cord where he can reach it even with his restrained hand. *Do not leave your patient unable to signal for you.* Adjust the position of the bed as allowed or desired. Make sure he is in good body alignment.
9. Assure the patient that you will return soon to check on the restraint and to change his position.	The patient needs assurance that you will not avoid him or neglect him. *Note:* If the patient were receiving an IV, you would be checking on him every 15 to 30 minutes to make sure that the IV has not infiltrated.
10. Provide care for the patient who has one or more extremity in restraint: Remove one restraint at a time; give active or passive exercise to the joints, and then replace the restraint. Change the patient's position every 2 hours. He can be placed on his side and the restraint attached to the other side of the bed, or the tie can be lengthened so that good alignment of shoulders and arms (or hip and leg) is maintained.	If his behavior is unpredictable because of confusion, mental illness, or disease of the brain, you should have an assistant to help you care for the patient when you release the restraint.
11. Remove the restraints when the time specified by the doctor has elapsed, or the need to immobilize has passed.	
12. Record the pertinent information on the patient's chart, including the time the restraint was applied, the type, the reason, and the time removed.	Charting example: 9:30 A.M. Soft wrist restraint applied to right wrist per doctor's order while IV running in other arm. M. Doe, NA 2:45 P.M. Wrist restraint on right wrist removed. M. Doe, NA

ITEM 5. APPLYING A JACKET RESTRAINT

The following procedure is used to apply a jacket restraint to a patient who is in a wheelchair. It could also be used for the patient who is in bed, although he would have to be turned from side to side, and wrinkles smoothed out.

Important Steps	Key Points

Follow steps 1 through 5 in Item 4.

6. Apply the jacket support or restraint to patient in a wheelchair:
   Place the front portion of the jacket over the patient's chest with the shoulder straps and side straps in place. Have the patient lean forward slightly while you stand behind the chair. You may need an assistant to help hold the patient so he won't fall if the jacket is being used to support his trunk in an upright position in the wheelchair.
   Reach for the lower side ties, cross them behind his back (smooth out wrinkles in his clothing) and tie them in a half-bow knot or square knot at the back of the wheelchair. Reach for the upper ties, cross them behind his shoulders (avoid wrinkles) and tie them in a half-bow or square knot behind the wheelchair.

Be sure that the wheelchair brakes are locked.

Follow Steps 8 through 12 in Item 4.

Charting example:

10:00 A.M. Up in wheelchair. Jacket restraint applied for safety.   M. Doe, NA

ITEM 6. APPLYING AN ELBOW RESTRAINT ON AN INFANT

Important Steps	Key Points

Follow Steps 1 through 4 in Item 4.

5. If necessary, prepare the elbow restraint.

You may have to slip a tongue blade into each of the insert pockets, unless the restraint has built-in rigid supports.

6. Apply the elbow restraint, one on each of the infant's arms.
   Wrap the restraint snugly around the arm with the ties on the outer edge. Tie the ties around the arm, using a half-bow knot. Pin an upper portion of the restraint to the baby's shirt.

This will prevent the restraint from working off the infant's arm. Be careful to keep your fingers between the area being pinned and the baby's skin to avoid sticking him with the pin.

Follow Steps 7 through 12 of Item 4.

Even though the baby will not know enough to expect you, you must return frequently to turn him, exercise his elbows, and provide care. Charting example:

1:00 P.M. Elbow restraints applied to both arms. Incision on upper lip dry and clean.
    M. Doe, NA

ITEM 7. APPLY A SAFETY BELT OR RESTRAINT STRAP

Important Steps	Key Points

Follow Steps 1 through 5 in Item 4.

6. Apply the safety belt or restraint strap around the patient's waist.

This can be done for the patient who is lying in bed, sitting in a wheelchair, or lying on a stretcher. It is not commonly used however for the bed patient because siderails are generally adequate to protect the patient from falling out of bed.

With the patient sitting in a chair, place the strap around his waist, bringing both ends behind the chair and tying them in a half-bow or square knot, or fasten the buckle, if there is one.

Or

Place the strap or belt completely around the patient's waist, cross the ends in the back, then bring both ends behind the chair and tie them in a half-bow or square knot, (or fasten the buckle).

Or

Place the strap around the patient's waist, tie it at one side in a square knot, bring the ties to the back of the chair and fasten them with a half-bow or square knot.

There are several ways to apply the safety belt or strap. You may find that one method works well for one patient and another method is better for a different patient.

Follow Steps 8 through 12, Item 4.

Even though the patient is sitting up, his position must be changed or his weight shifted frequently to relieve pressure. Charting example:

10:15 A.M. Up in wheelchair. Safety belt applied around waist.   M. Doe, NA

ITEM 8. CONCLUSION OF UNIT

You have now completed the lesson on Application of Restraints. After you have practiced the procedures to become familiar with them and gain some skills, arrange with your instructor to take the performance post-test. You will be expected to demonstrate accurately the procedures involved in providing for the patient's safety in a reassuring manner.

PERFORMANCE TEST

In the classroom, or your skill laboratory, your instructor will ask you to perform the following activities to demonstrate your skill without referring to any source material. You may use Mrs. Chase (the mannequin) or another student in the role of the patient.

1. Given a patient receiving an IV in the left arm who tries to remove the needle from the vein, you are to apply a limb-holder, or similar soft restraint, to the right wrist. You are to tie the restraint at the wrist with a knot so that patient's tugging on it will not cut off circulation to the hand.

2. Given a patient with a muscular disease involving the muscles of the trunk, you are to apply a jacket restraint to support his body while he is sitting in a wheelchair, using the method that provides the most safety for the patient.

3. Given a four month-old child who has a severe rash on his face and neck, you are to apply elbow restraints to both arms and describe the care you would give the child during the time the restraints are used. The care referred to would be in addition to bathing, diapering, feeding, or holding the child.

4. Given an elderly, slightly confused patient in a wheelchair who is not to bear any weight on the left leg, you are to place a safety belt or restraint strap around his waist and fasten the ends of it behind the wheelchair, using the method and knots of your choice from those described in the procedure.

PERFORMANCE CHECKLIST

APPLICATION OF RESTRAINTS

APPLYING LIMB-HOLDER TO RIGHT WRIST

U
N
I
T
31

1. Check for doctor's order.

2. Wash hands.

3. Obtain limb-holder or similar soft cloth restraint.

4. Approach and identify patient.

5. Explain what you are going to do and why.

6. Apply limb-holder or wrist restraint to right wrist correctly.

   A. Place padded end around wrist, or pad it.

   B. Pull tie through slit, or make slip or square knot in gauze or other cloth strap.

   C. Tie loose end to spring portion of bed.

   D. Make slip, square, or half-bow knots correctly.

7. Check wrist and hand to see if circulation is good.

8. Provide for patient's comfort and welfare.

   A. Adjust bed to allowed position.

   B. Leave signal cord within reach.

   C. Make sure patient is in good body alignment.

9. Explain to patient that he will be checked in two hours or sooner.

10. Record pertinent information on patient's chart.

APPLYING A JACKET RESTRAINT FOR SUPPORT OF PATIENT IN WHEELCHAIR

1. Check for doctor's order. (Some agencies may not require an order for support, but it would be better to have one.)

2. Wash hands.

3. Obtain jacket support or restraint.

4. Approach and identify patient.

5. Explain what is to be done and why.

6. Apply the jacket restraint to patient in wheelchair.

   A. Lock wheels of wheelchair.

   B. Have an assistant support the patient while jacket is being applied.

   C. Place large portion of jacket correctly over patient's chest with shoulder straps at top.

   D. Stand behind chair while assistant supports patient, cross lower side ties behind patient, and tie them behind wheelchair.

   E. Take shoulder straps, cross them behind patient's shoulders, and tie them behind wheelchair.

   F. Make square or half-bow knots correctly.

7. Provide for patient's comfort and welfare.

8. State that patient will be checked at specified time.

9. Record pertinent information on patient's chart.

APPLYING ELBOW RESTRAINTS TO A CHILD AND GIVING CARE WHILE RESTRAINED

1. Check for doctor's order.

2. Wash hands.

3. Obtain elbow restraints, and tongue blades, if needed.

4. Approach and identify patient.

5. Prepare elbow restraints by inserting tongue blades.

6. Apply elbow restraints, one on each arm.

   A. Wrap around arm leaving tie edge outermost.

   B. Wrap ties around arm and tie in half-bow knots.

   C. Pin restraint to baby's shirt without sticking baby.

7. Check circulation in hand.

8. Provide for child's comfort.

   A. Adjust bed, if necessary

   B. Check for good alignment of body.

9. State that child will be checked in two hours or less to do the following:

   A. Remove one restraint at a time and provide flexion exercise of elbow, then re-apply restraint.

   B. Change baby's position.

   C. Provide other care as needed.

10. Record pertinent information on patient's chart.

APPLYING A SAFETY BELT OR RESTRAINT STRAP AROUND WAIST

1. Check for doctor's order.

2. Wash hands.

3. Obtain safety belt or restraint strap.

4. Approach and identify patient.

5. Explain what you are going to do and why.

6. Apply safety belt or restraint strap around patient's waist while he is sitting in a chair.

   A. Place strap around patient's waist and back of chair, then tie or buckle it, *or*

   B. Place strap around waist, cross straps behind patient, and tie ends behind chair, or buckle, *or*

   C. Encircle strap about waist, tie it to one side in square knot, and then tie it behind chair.

   D. Make square or half-bow knots correctly.

7. Provide for patient's comfort and welfare.

8. State that patient will be checked in two hours or sooner.

9. Record pertinent information on patient's chart.

U
N
I
T
31

NOTES

Unit 32

APPLICATION OF BANDAGES AND BINDERS

I. DIRECTIONS TO THE STUDENT

Proceed through this lesson. After you have finished take the post-test, and practice in the skill laboratory. You will then demonstrate the application of common bandages and binders for your instructor.

II. GENERAL PERFORMANCE OBJECTIVE

Following this lesson, you will be able to apply clean bandages and binders.

III. SPECIFIC PERFORMANCE OBJECTIVES

When you are through with this lesson, you will be able correctly to:

1. Apply circular, figure 8, spiral, spiral reverse, and recurrent bandages.

2. Apply scultetus, straight abdominal, T-binder, double-T-binder, breast binders, and an Ace bandage.

3. Discuss with the instructor the reasons for which bandages and binders are applied.

4. Check for impaired circulation in an area which is wrapped with a binder or a bandage and take correct steps to remove the impairment as soon as discovered.

IV. VOCABULARY

A. Bandages

bandage — piece of soft material, like gauze, used to wrap, bind, support, provide warmth, protect, or immobilize a part, e.g., a leg bandage.

circular bandage — applied around and around a part. Each turn covers the preceding turn and holds it securely in place. It is fastened with tape, a special holding clip, or a safety pin.

elastic bandage — stretchable; when pulled tightly causes compression. Impaired circulation is a frequent problem with this type of bandage. (A commonly used elastic bandage is called the Ace bandage.)

figure 8 bandage — the turns cross each other like a figure 8; generally used over joints to retain dressings or to exert pressure in the case of sprains or hemorrhage.

recurrent bandage — used over the end of a stump, e.g., of an amputated (cut off) leg or finger.

reverse spiral bandage — special technique used in which a part of the bandage is folded back on itself to make it fit more uniformly (evenly). The reverse, or folding back, technique may be used as a part of each complete spiral or circular turn to make the bandage fit neatly over a difficult area, e.g., wrist, fingers or ankles.

roller bandage — continuous strip of soft material (commonly gauze or elastic material) used to bind up injured parts. It comes in widths of ½ inch to 6 inches, and lengths of 2 to 6 yards. The length and width you will use depend on the area to be bandaged.

spiral bandage — consists of a series of circular turns ascending (going up) a part, e.g., from the fingers to the wrist. Each turn is higher than the preceding one and overlaps the previous turn about half the width of the bandage.

triangular bandage — 3 cornered; it holds dressings in place. It is called a *sling* when used as a swinging bandage to support the forearm or elbow; it is most often used this way.

B. Binders

binder — bandage generally used to provide encircling support of the chest or abdomen; however, it can be used in other situations.

abdominal binder — a single width of soft material (18 to 24 inches and 3 to 5 feet long) used to provide strong abdominal support.

breast binder — usually a sleeveless, jacket-type, soft muslin binder used to hold breast dressings in place, support the breasts, or compress the breast as in the case of a new mother who is trying to dry up the milk in her breasts.

scultetus binder (many-tailed) — a succession of interlocking, overlapping bands used to enclose a part with rigid support, e.g., an abdominal girdle-like support following an abdominal operation.

T-binder (sanitary belt) — shaped like a letter "T," it is used to hold in place perineal pads (peri-pads) as well as rectal or perineal dressings.

T-binder, double — shaped like a letter T except that it has two tails TT; commonly used for male patients who have had rectal or perineal surgery, to hold the dressings in place.

General rules for determining length and width of roller bandages:

Type	Length	Width
head bandaging	6 yards	2 inch
body bandaging	10 yards	3 to 6 inch
leg bandaging	9 yards	2 to 4 inch
foot bandaging	4 yards	1½ to 3 inch
arm bandaging	7 to 9 yards	2 to 2½ inch
hand bandaging	3 yards	1 to 2 inch
finger bandaging	1 to 3 yards	½ to 1 inch

V. INTRODUCTION

Bandages and binders are used for the following purposes:

1. To apply pressure (compression) to stop bleeding or swelling, and to assist in absorption of tissue fluids.

2. To provide for immobilization of an injured part, e.g., a fractured (broken) arm.

3. To hold dressings in place.

4. To protect open wounds from contaminants.

5. To apply warmth to a joint, e.g., for persons suffering from painful joints due to arthritis.

6. To provide support and to aid in venous (return blood flow) circulation, e.g., bandaging leg of patient suffering from varicose veins or limited circulation in the extremities (arms or legs).

Bandages and binders are made from many kinds of soft materials such as muslin, gauze, flannel, rubber, and elastic fabric. There are a number of commonly used bandages and binders; you should be familiar with their names and know how to apply them correctly. These bandages, and combinations of them as described in this unit represent the most generally applied types. The specific method used will not only depend on the part to be bandaged, but on the purpose of the bandage, e.g., support, immobilization.

Bandages and binders should be applied so that they provide even pressure to the area. If a joint is involved in bandaging, it should be supported in its normal position with a slight flexion of the joint. Both the bandage and binder should be attached securely to avoid friction or rubbing of the underlying tissue which could cause severe irritation. However, great care must be taken not to make it too tight so that circulation is cut off. It must be tight enough to stay in place, but *not so tight as to cut off circulation!* Do you remember the signs and symptoms of impaired circulation from the unit "Special Skin care"?

At least 4 signs of impaired circulation are: _____ , _____ , _____ , and _____ . It is helpful if you can leave the tips of the fingers and toes visible on a bandaged extremity so that you can watch for a darkening color of the nailbeds to determine if the circulation is impaired.

A bandage or binder should be applied over a clean, dry area. Remember that microorganisms grow in warm, damp areas. Be sure that skin surfaces are not bandaged directly together — they will sweat and provide a moist environment in which microorganisms can grow. Always put some kind of padding (4 X 4 or ABD Bandage) between adjoining skin surfaces before bandaging or binding. It is also wise to pad over a bony prominence before bandaging to avoid friction which could lead to excoriation of the skin. If left unattended for several days, such an irritation could become a decubitus ulcer.

If a bandage or binder is applied to the dressing of a draining wound, it must be changed frequently to keep it as clean and dry as possible. This reduces the chance of pathogenic organisms getting into the wound and setting up an infection. Discard the soiled dressing, return the binders to the laundry for washing and reprocessing, or discard if your agency uses disposable items.

You will be expected to apply the following bandages and binders safely and correctly. With your partner in the skill laboratory you will practice the following procedures.

ITEM 1: THE APPLICATION OF A CIRCULAR BANDAGE

Apply a clean dressing to an abscessed area on the posterior aspect of the right middle arm.

Important Steps	Key Points
1. Obtain your supplies.	Get the type and amount of bandage needed to complete the procedure. Wash your hands.
2. Approach the patient and explain what you are going to do.	Check his identification band. Gain his cooperation by explaining that you will be applying, or changing, his bandage. Tell him why it is being done, e.g., support, immobilization, to hold a dressing in place. You can get this information from your team leader.
3. Wash area to be wrapped, if area is soiled.	Remember that microorganisms grow in dark, moist, dirty places. You may use soap and water or an antiseptic cleansing solution (check your agency rules).
4. Elevate area to be wrapped.	If it is an arm or leg, raise it so that it is at the same level as the heart. It should be elevated in this manner at least *15 minutes before* applying the bandage. This will restore equal circulation in the limb. If you should wrap a leg that has

Important Steps	Key Points
	been hanging over the side of the bed (called a dependent position), the limb may swell and become edematous (filled with tissue fluid). This condition is caused by restricting the circulation in a limb which had excessive circulation because of the dependent state. To prevent this from happening, place the limb comfortably in a horizontal position for at least 15 minutes. *Note:* To bandage a leg, have patient in supine position.
5. Place the patient in a comfortable position.	The position should also be convenient for you when you work with him. The patient may be sitting or lying prone, depending on where the bandaging is required. Adjust the patient to your comfortable working height (remember your body alignment).
6. Stand directly in front of the patient.	This will make it easier for you to see what you are doing.
7. Begin applying bandage over wound on inner aspect of mid right arm.	Stand close to the working edge of the bed, with the patient lying close to the right side of the bed. Ask him to raise his right arm slightly (about 6 to 12 inches) from the bed, palm upward, so you can wrap the arm. If the patient is unable to lift his arm, you may need some assistance. Be sure the area of application is dry and clean.
8. Hold the roll of bandage in your right hand so that it unwinds from the top (reverse hand positions if you are left handed).	Make two initial circular turns around wound area to secure in place. Secure the proximal (free) end to the arm directly over the site. Hold bandage in place with your left thumb on top of the bandage and the anterior surface of the arm, and your left index finger on the posterior side of the arm. For the patient's comfort, the beginning (initial) and terminal ends of the bandage are *Not* to be placed directly over the wound, a bony prominence, or inner aspect of a limb, or over a part the patient will lie on.
9. Unroll the bandage.	Unwind it toward the right, around the patient's arm. Hold bandage with moderate tension. If you hold the bandage too loosely while wrapping, it will come off easily. If the bandage is wrapped too tightly, it will cut off the patient's circulation. You will have to practice wrapping until you can judge the proper tension to use.

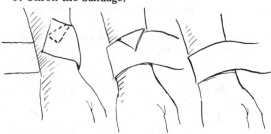

Anchoring a bandage.

| 10. Each circular turn goes directly over the preceding turn. | Each successive turn anchors (holds in place) the underlying layer of bandage. Continue unrolling bandage from right to left around the arm. (Reverse hand positions if you are left-handed.) Use only as many circular turns as needed to hold the dressing in place or to |

Important Steps	Key Points
	immobilize the part. You may need to cut off a portion of the bandage with your scissors. (Remaining portion may be used for later changes.)
11. Secure terminal end of bandage.	You can use tape, special metal clips, or a safety pin. Usually the circular bandage is used to keep a dressing in place. Place patient's arm in comfortable position.
12. Tidy the work area.	Return unused supplies to storage area. Dispose of soiled bandages in waste container. Place call light, bed controls, and bedside stand conveniently for the patient (check every 30 minutes for 3 times after application; if circulation is impaired, remove bandage immediately and rewrap).
13. Record on patient's chart.	Chart the time, type and location of bandage applied. Charting example:
	10:10 A.M. Dressing changed on right arm. Large amount of purulent, foul-smelling discharge. J. Jones, RN

To remove a roller bandage from a patient's arm or leg, cut the bandage off with your scissors. Be careful not to injure the tissue under the dressing with the tip of the scissors; to prevent this from happening, insert your left index finger under the bandage and elevate it slightly. With the scissors in your right hand, cut the bandage free slightly to the side of your left finger.

Cutting the bandages off will usually save time and avoid fatigue for the patient. However, you may want to save the bandage for re-use if it is not soiled. If so, carefully unwind the bandage from left to right. Roll it as you unwind; this will prevent it from becoming soiled and tangled as it is removed.

ITEM 2: THE APPLICATION OF A FIGURE 8 BANDAGE

This type is applied at the elbow and knee joints, ankles and wrist. It is used to retain a dressing, apply pressure or support, and to immobilize a joint.

Important Steps	Key Points
Follow Steps 1 through 9 of the spiral reverse procedure. Use successive spiral turns until you reach the elbow. Then proceed in the following manner.	
10. Make an initial circular turn directly over the elbow.	
11. With the next turn, wrap in a spiral upward motion just above the elbow, above the first circular turn.	Flex joint and wind from right to left, coming across the back of the arm in a downward fashion. Cover the preceding layers about half the width of the bandage.
12. Wrap the next spiral turn in a downward motion just below the first circular turn.	Cover each preceding layer, overlapping by a half. Be sure no skin shows between successive layers.

U
N
I
T
32

Important Steps	Key Points
13. Continue alternating the upward and downward spiral turns above and below the elbow, i.e., crossing the elbow alternately above and below.	These turns are called oblique (slanting or diagonal) turns. Continue in this manner until there is 4 to 6 inches of bandage above and below the elbow or until you believe the bandage is secure.
Now follow Steps 11 through 14 of the spiral bandaging procedure.	Charting example:
	3:15 P.M. Dressing changed on right hand. No discharge noted. Wound healing well.
	J. Jones, RN

ITEM 3: THE APPLICATION OF A SPIRAL BANDAGE

This procedure may be used to apply an Ace bandage to the leg (commonly used for the treatment of varicose veins).

Important Steps	Key Points
Follow Steps 1 through 6 for the circular bandage procedure.	
7. Begin applying the bandage on the patient's right arm. 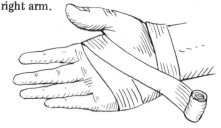	Start as you did for the circular bandage. Anchor at the wrist with two circular turns. Hold the roll in your right hand to unwind downward from right to left around the arm. Secure bandage on back of arm with your left index finger, and on the front of the arm with your left thumb. (Reverse hand positions if you are left-handed.) See figure in Step 10 if wrapping a leg.
8. With next turn, wrap in a downward spiral motion between thumb and index finger forward across palm of hand, and then bring bandage in upward motion posterior to anterior around wrist.	Wrap at least twice in this manner to hold bandage securely during hand and arm movement. *Note:* If applying a spiral bandage (i.e., Ace bandage) to a lower extremity, begin with the 2 circular turns just above the ankle. Then use the figure-8 bandage around the foot and ankle to provide security so that the bandage will not come loose during patient movement. Then proceed spiral bandaging up the leg. Always secure a spiral bandage with a figure-8 motion across the nearest joint, i.e., the thumb, ankle, knee, and elbow.
9. With each succeeding turn of the bandage, angle slightly upward around the arm.	The direction is upward and circular, like a spiral staircase, in the same direction as the blood which is returning to the heart. Each turn is parallel to the preceding turn and covers (overlaps) about 1/2 to 2/3 the width of the bandage. The spiral bandage is usually applied on the legs, arms, and fingers.
10. Wrap bandage evenly and smoothly.	Hold the appendage (limb) firmly and wrap it securely. Take care not to wrap it so tightly that you cut off the patient's return circulation. As you wrap, ask the patient how it feels. Loosen it immediately if he says it is too tight. Signs of impaired circulation are cyanosis or

Important Steps	Key Points
	pallor, cold, tingling sensation, and swelling. If you are applying the bandage over a wet dressing, you must wrap loosely to allow for shrinkage of the bandage as it dries.
11. Continue wrapping in the spiral fashion.	Wrap until the part is thoroughly covered. Do not use excessive bandage. Do not waste motions or material while wrapping.
12. Secure the terminal end of the bandage. 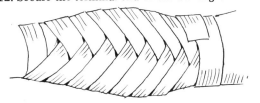	Use tape, clips, or safety pins. As before, do not start or finish the bandage over wounds, bony prominences, etc. (Review Step 10 in preceding item.)
13. Make the patient comfortable.	Check circulation flow by looking at the color of his fingers and fingernails, and feeling the temperature of the fingers. They should feel as warm as the fingers on the other hand. *Note:* Ace bandages are rewrapped at least every eight hours.
14. Tidy the work area.	Dispose of waste materials. Return unused supplies to storage area.
15. Record on patient's chart.	Chart time, type, and location of bandage. Charting example: 8:00 A.M. Right leg rewrapped with Ace bandage. Toes warm and pink. J. Jones, SN

Note: An elastic stocking may be ordered instead of the Ace bandage. Read directions on package before applying. Frequently observe circulation in toes after application.

ITEM 4: THE APPLICATION OF A SPIRAL REVERSE BANDAGE

This type is used to wrap an extremity that has varying thicknesses (such as the thin ankle portion which rises to a thick area like the calf of the leg). This method of bandaging provides a means to make a secure, smooth, even-fitting bandage on an extremity.

Important Steps	Key Points
Follow Steps 1 through 8 of the spiral bandage procedure as though you were wrapping the left leg. Always start a bandage with at least 2 circular rounds to fasten the initial end securely.	
9. Make a spiral reverse turn. 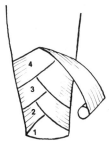	This is done at the place on the leg where the bandage no longer will lie smoothly as you continue around the leg. Place your left thumb on the upper edge of the anterior turn; hold the bandage firmly. Unwind the roll of bandage about 4 to 6 inches, turn your hand downward (pronated) so that the bandage is now folded over your thumb in a downward direction toward the lower edge of the previous layer. Continue unrolling the bandage to the right and then to the left on the underside of the leg, covering about 1/2 to 2/3 of the previous lap.

Important Steps	Key Points
10. Continue making spiral reverse turn.	Wind bandage in the same manner, and place like the previous layers until the bandage will once again lie smoothly as you unroll it in a spiral direction. Then follow Steps 11 through 14 of the previous procedure. Charting example:

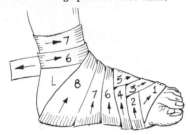

9:25 A.M. Spiral reverse bandage changed on right foot. Patient states the warmth of the dressings minimizes the pain in the ankle.

J. Jones, RN

ITEM 5: APPLICATION OF THE RECURRENT BANDAGE

This bandage is applied to hold pressure dressings in place over the tip end of a finger, toe, fist, or stump of an amputated extremity to prevent bleeding or edema.

Important Steps	Key Points
Follow Steps 1 through 10 of the circular bandage procedure.	
11. Turn bandage roll and bring forward over tip.	Hold the top layer of bandage securely on the anterior leg with your left thumb at the highest (proximal) edge of the circular bandage. Continue unrolling the bandage downward over the tip of the stump toward the back. Continue to the highest point of the circular bandage layer at the center of the posterior aspect of the leg. Hold the bandage firmly at this spot with the left index finger.
12. Bring the roller bandage downward over the tip of the stump and forward up to the same level as the previous layer.	Move each successive turn alternately to the left, then to the right of the first layer over the tip of the stump (in a somewhat spiral manner). Continue wrapping until the stump end is well covered, overlapping each layer about 1/2 to 2/3 the width of the previous layer. Continue to hold succeeding layers securely in place with your left thumb and index finger. (Reverse hand positions if you are left-handed.)
13. Secure ends with several circular turns. 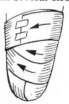	When the stump is smoothly, evenly, and totally covered, once more reverse the direction of the roller bandage and make at least two circular turns to cover the gathered ends which you have been holding securely between your left thumb and index finger. Secure final end with tape, a clip, or a safety pin.
Complete the procedure by following Steps 12 and 13 of the circular bandaging procedure.	Charting example:

11:00 A.M. Right AK stump bandage removed. Wound cleansed with antiseptic. Wound appears to be healing well. No drainage noted. Bandage replaced.   J. Jones, SN

Note: This is the type of bandage used on the stump of an *above-the knee (AK) amputation (below the knee amputation is identified as BK amputation).*

ITEM 6: THE APPLICATION OF A SCULTETUS (MANY-TAILED) BINDER

The scultetus binder is designed to provide abdominal support following an abdominal operation, post-delivery, or post-paracentesis. The binder is made by sewing heavy flannel strips 3 to 4 inches wide and 4 feet long in overlapping layers of 1/2 inch. The middle third section of the strips is sewed together, leaving about 20 inches free on each end.

Important Steps	Key Points
Follow Steps 1 through 3 in the circular bandage procedure.	
4. Move patient to distal side of bed.	This makes it easier for you to work. To avoid straining your back muscles, you must stand close to the bed facing the patient at his hip level. The height of the bed should be comfortable for your work. Fold back the top bedding, exposing only the portion of the body you are working on. Remember the patient's modesty and his need for privacy. (Siderails should be in place if you have to roll the patient.)
5. Ask patient to raise his hips.	Quickly slip the scultetus binder under the hips, the top edge at waist level. The solid portion of the binder should be centered under the patient's body; the many-tailed ends lying flat on the bed extending straight out from the patient. If the patient is unable to raise his hips, have him roll to his side away from you. Place solid portion of binder on bed, centered on area which his hips will rest. Return him to the supine position.
6. Begin application by bringing the *bottom tail* across the abdomen. 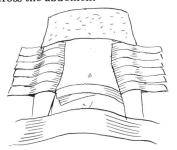	You will begin in the direction the tail is going, to provide for smooth, successive spiral-type layers with a 1/2 inch overlap of each layer. Pull tightly. If the end is too long, you may need to fold the free end back on itself, just far enough so it fits smoothly. *Note:* Incorrect placement of the overlaps causes pressure and discomfort for the patient.
7. Proceed toward the waist, slanting each succeeding tail slightly upward.	Alternate strips (tails) first from one side of the abdomen, then the other side.
8. Secure final tail with safety pin. 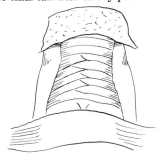	This type of abdominal bandage provides good support for the patient. If you have pulled it securely enough as you criss-cross each strip and then firmly pinned it, the patient will be able to move freely about (even walk) without having the bandage come undone.

UNIT 32

Important Steps	Key Points
Follow Steps 12 and 13 in the circular bandaging procedure to complete the action.	Charting example: 8:00 A.M. Scultetus binder reapplied after bath. The additional support is comforting to the patient. J. Jones, SN

ITEM 7: THE APPLICATION OF A STRAIGHT ABDOMINAL OR CHEST BINDER

The exact type of binder (scultetus or straight) will depend on what is available, the purpose for which it is intended, and possibly the size and shape of the abdomen or chest.

Important Steps	Key Points
Follow Steps 1 through 4 in the scultetus binder procedure. Pull back the top bedding to expose only the area with which you are working. Remember the patient's modesty.	
5. Ask patient to raise his hips or chest. 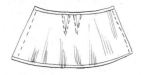	Quickly slip the binder under the hips or chest if applying a breast binder. Center it under the patient's body. The lower edge of the abdominal binder should come well below the curve of the buttocks (rump). (If it is a breast binder, the lower edge comes to the waistline.) For the breast — fold the binder so that it laps well over the largest part of the breast.
6. Fasten lower edge first with safety pin.	Pull binder very tightly. Keep your hand between the patient's skin and binder to prevent sticking the patient with the pin (much as you do when diapering a baby).
7. Continue straight up the midline.	Pull edges tightly with about a 3-inch overlap. Secure every 3 to 4 inches with a safety pin.
8. Make darts in the binder. 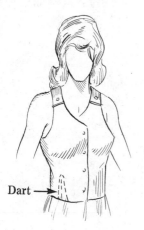 Dart ➝	Because of the contour (shape) of the chest or abdomen, it is often difficult to make the binder lie flat without puckering; therefore, a few darts at the waistline will help to make the binder fit more snugly. With safety pins, take up the slack in the material and secure the tuck with a safety pin. Pin perpendicularly. Make a "V" dart, starting with a large tuck at the midline, and decreasing the size a few inches inward to make the binder fit neatly. You may need a tuck on each side of the midline. The darts in these binders serve the same purpose as darts when you are sewing a blouse. If the breasts are very large, be sure to pad under the breasts before applying the chest binder. This will prevent perspiration resulting from the two skin surfaces being held tightly together. Some physicians may specify that the abdominal binder be applied in the female by securing it downward from the waistline so that the abdominal organs are pushed against the uterus (womb) to control uterine bleeding. Check with your agency. *Note:* Breast binders may not be used in your agency. Check your agency procedure.

Important Steps	Key Points
Follow Steps 12 and 13 in the circular bandaging process to complete this procedure.	Charting example: 4:40 P.M. Breast binder changed. No drainage noted. No complaints of pain or discomfort. <div align="right">J. Jones, SN</div>

ITEM 8: APPLICATION OF A T-BINDER OR A DOUBLE T-BINDER

These binders are primarily used to keep peri-pads or rectal and perineal dressings in place. (The double T-binder is used for the male patient.)

Important Steps	Key Points
1. Obtain supplies.	Select binder, peri-pad and dressings. Wash your hands.
2. Approach the patient and explain what you are going to do. 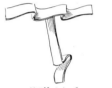 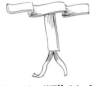 "T" binder Double "T" binder	Identify the patient by the identification band. Note that the male patient may be somewhat embarrassed and may wish to apply the binder himself. If the patient is able, permit him to do so. Stand by to give assistance if needed, however. Explain why you are using this type of binder. Fold back top bedding to expose the area you are working with. Avoid undue exposure or chilling the patient.
3. Ask patient to raise hips.	Quickly center the binder under the patient's back at waist level. Be sure the tail (or tails) lie smoothly under the patient toward the bottom of the bed. Secure band around waist firmly with a safety pin.
4. Apply peri-pad or dressing to rectal or perineal area.	Avoid touching the side of the pad or dressing that will come in contact with the patient's skin.
5. Secure the pad in place.	Fasten by bringing the free end of the T forward between the legs and secure it snugly at the waist with a safety pin. *Note:* The double-tailed binder is usually used for the male patient. Bring each tail or strip forward between the legs. Extend the right tail to the right of the external male organs and secure snugly to the waist band just to the right of the midline with a safety pin. Bring the left tail forward up between the legs, to the left of the external male organs and attach snugly to the waist band slightly to the left of the midline with a safety pin.
6. Leave patient comfortable.	Adjust the top linen neatly over the patient. Leave him in a comfortable, well-aligned position. Place call light, bed controls and bedside stand conveniently within reach of the patient. Tidy the room. Dispose of waste materials. Return unused supplies to storage area. Wash your hands.

UNIT
32

Important Steps	Key Points
7. Record on patient's chart.	Chart the time, type and location of dressing; describe drainage if any was present (sanguinous — bloody, or serous — thin, watery). Charting example: 9:45 A.M. Peri-pad changed. Large amount of foul-smelling sanguinous drainage present. J. Jones, SN

ITEM 9:   APPLICATION OF A SLING (TRIANGULAR) BANDAGE

This bandage is commonly used to support an injured arm. It can be made from a piece of cloth 30 to 40 inches square. Fold diagonally in half to make a double triangle. You can cut it across the center fold if you want a single thickness.

Important Steps	Key Points
1. Obtain the supplies from store room.	Wash your hands.
2. Approach the patient and explain what you are going to do to enlist his cooperation.	Identify the patient by checking his identification band. Quickly demonstrate how you will be applying the sling. Adjust his bed to working height. Have him sit on the edge of the bed facing you.
3. Put one end of the triangle over the shoulder on the uninjured side (1). 	For this lesson, we will say it is the right arm that is injured. Therefore, the end of the triangle will be placed over the patient's left shoulder.
4. Place the point (apex) (3) of the triangle toward the elbow.	Ask the patient to bend his injured arm horizontally across his body with his thumb up. Place the bandage under his arm flat against his chest.
5. Bring other end of the triangle (2) around his injured arm and up over his right shoulder (injured side). 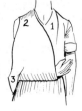	Have the patient keep his elbow bent at right angles across his lower chest.
6. Tie the two ends of the triangle together with a square knot.	Make the knot to one side of the neck so that it will not be uncomfortable if the patient lies down (or from the continuing pull on the back of the neck when the arm is in the sling). Tie the knot securely so it will not loosen from the weight of the arm in the sling.

Important Steps	Key Points
7. Fold the apex (or point) of the triangle neatly over the elbow toward the front.	Secure it with a safety pin. 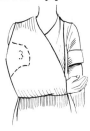
8. Adjust the height of the sling by adjusting the knot at the neck.	The hand should be slightly higher than the elbow (about 4 inches). This will prevent the fingers from swelling.
9. Check the circulation in the fingers frequently.	Observe the color of the fingernail beds; they should be pink. Feel the fingers; they should be the same temperature as the fingers on the good hand. If fingers are cold and pale, report immediately to the charge nurse.
10. Tidy the work area.	Dispose of waste materials in the wastebasket. Return unused supplies to storage area.
11. Record on patient's chart.	Chart the time and type of bandage. Comment about the appearance of the extremity. Charting example: 3:10 P.M. Sling applied to right arm. Fingers warm and nailbeds pink. No pain reported by patient. J. Jones, SN

U
N
I
T
32

POST-TEST

1. List 3 purposes for which bandages and binders are used.

   (1) _apply pressure_

   (2) _provides immobilization_

   (3) _holds dressings in place_

2. The skin should be _clean_ and _dry_ before applying bandages or binders. Why? _to prevent pathogenic organisms from getting into the wound & causing infection_

3. Circulation distal to the bandage or binder should be checked every _30_ minutes.

4. _fingers_ and _toes_ are good indicators of impaired circulation.

5. Describe a scultetus or many-tailed binder as to shape and where and why applied. _provides support by a succession of overlapping bands applied to abd area._

6. Describe usage of a triangular bandage. _used to hold dressing in place. Called a sling when used to support forearm_

7. Describe the use of the T-binder and double T-binder. _Binder - shaped like a T single or double T is used to hold rectal & perineal in place._

POST-TEST ANNOTATED ANSWER SHEET

1. To apply pressure, provide immobilization, hold dressings in place, protect open wounds from infection, apply warmth to a joint, provide support, and aid circulation. (p. 672)

2. Clean; dry; to prevent pathogenic organisms from getting into the wound and setting up an infection. (p. 673)

3. Every 30 minutes multiplied by 3. (p. 675)

4. Fingers; toes. (p. 673)

5. A many-tailed abdominal girdle-like support; provides support through a succession of overlapping bands. (pp. 672 and 679)

6. Triangular in shape and is used to hold dressings in place. It is called a sling when used as a support for the forearm. (pp. 672, 682 and 683)

7. Binder-shaped like a single or double T, and is used to hold rectal or perineal dressings in place. (pp. 672, 681, and 682)

PERFORMANCE TEST

In the skills laboratory, with a partner, you will correctly apply two of the following types of binders or bandages:

1. Scultetus binder.

2. Breast binder.

3. Triangular bandage.

4. Figure 8 bandage.

PERFORMANCE CHECKLIST

APPLICATION OF BANDAGES

1. Identify patient

2. Wash hands

3. Explain procedure to patient

4. Identify proper bandage for use

5. Obtain proper materials

6. Identify proper location

7. Anchor bandage properly

8. Follow specific sequential wrapping procedures

   A. Smoothness

   B. Overlap

   C. Tension

      1. Pain

      2. Decrease temperature

      3. Color change

      4. Insufficient tension; wrap falls off

9. Secure (anchor) tail of bandage

10. Chart appropriately

Unit 33

PRE-OPERATIVE
CARE OF A PATIENT

I. DIRECTIONS TO THE STUDENT

This lesson includes the psychological and physiological preparation of the patient for surgery. Proceed through all the steps. When you finish, practice both the psychological and physiological preparation with another student or an instructor. Prepare to complete the post-test when you are through.

II. GENERAL PERFORMANCE OBJECTIVE

Upon completion of this unit, you will be able to prepare a patient for a surgical operation.

III. SPECIFIC PERFORMANCE OBJECTIVES

When you have finished this unit, you will be able to:

1. Provide the patient with privacy and safety during the pre-operative preparations.

2. Procure a surgical consent from the patient, if agency policy permits.

3. Explain to the patient the reasons for pre-operative laboratory procedures.

4. Safeguard the patient from any food or fluids in the specified period prior to surgery.

5. Provide the necessary personal hygiene as required during the pre-operative preparation.

6. Eliminate safety hazards to the patient after he receives the pre-operative medications.

7. Instruct the patient and family regarding the recovery and waiting rooms.

8. Complete a pre-operative checklist accurately.

IV. VOCABULARY

anesthesia — partial or complete loss of sensation with or without loss of consciousness, as result of disease, injury, or administration of drug.
    general — one that is complete and affects the entire body, with loss of consciousness.
    local — one that affects a local or specific area only.
    spinal — one that causes loss of sensation from the hips down, induced by injecting a drug into the lower end of the spinal column.
asphyxia (asphyxiation) — cyanosis due to interference with oxygen content of the blood. May be general (whole body) or local (part of body).

aspirate — to breathe in; to get foreign material in the lungs.

barbiturates — a group of drugs used as sedatives or relaxers.

bladder sphincter — plain muscle around the opening of the bladder.

catheter — a tube for evacuating or injecting fluids through a natural passage, i.e., a urinary catheter.

complete blood count (CBC) — measurement of the *numbers* and *kinds* of white blood cells (WBC) and red blood cells (RBC). (There may be certain agency differences — some may include a Hct (hematocrit) and/or a Hgb (hemoglobin).

cyanosis — slightly bluish-gray or purple discoloration of the skin due to a deficiency of oxygen and an excess of carbon dioxide in the blood. (Oxygen in the blood makes it look red and gives the skin a pink tone.)

hematocrit (Hct) — This test measures the volume percentage of erythrocytes in whole blood.

hemoglobin (Hgb) — the essential oxygen carrier of the blood. It is found within the red blood cells and is responsible for the red color of blood.

hemorrhage — abnormal discharge of blood, either external or internal.

laparotomy — the surgical opening of the abdomen; an abdominal incision.

mastectomy — excision or removal of a breast.

narcotics — group of drugs producing stupor, sleep, or complete unconsciousness; used to allay pain. (Regulated by federal laws.)

nasogastric tube — small tube that is passed through the nose (naso) down to the stomach (gastric) for the purpose of taking materials out of or putting materials into the stomach.

perineum (perineal) — in the female the area between the vagina and the anus.

prosthesis — artificial organ or part, e.g., artificial limbs, eyeglasses, dentures.

thoracotomy — surgical incision of the chest wall.

white blood count (WBC) — the laboratory count of the numbers of white cells in the blood; also called leucocytes, they fight infections. There are several types of leucocytes: lymphocytes, monocytes, granulocytes, eosinophils, basophils.

Prefixes and Suffixes for Surgery

cardio-: heart (as cardiac).

cephal-: relating to the head (as cephalic).

cyst-: bladder (as cystoscopy).

dent-: relating to teeth (as dental)

derma-: skin (as dermatitis)

gastro-: stomach (as gastrotomy).

glosso-: tongue (as glossopharyngeal).

hemato, hem-: relating to the blood (as hemoglobin).

hepa, hepar, hepato-: liver (as hepatitis).

nephro-: kidney (nephrosis).

oculo-: eye (as oculist)

oophoro-: ovary (as oophorectomy).

os-: mouth (as cervical os).

pulmo-: lung (as pulmonary).

vaso-: vessel, vein (as vasoconstrictor)

-cele: tumor, cyst; hernia (as appendectomy).

-ectomy: cutting out, cutting off (as appendectomy).

-oma: tumor (as hematoma)

-ostomosis, ostomy: to furnish with a mouth or an outlet (as colostomy).

-otomy: cutting into (as thoracotomy).

V. INTRODUCTION

Preparation for surgery usually starts the afternoon before the patient is to have his operation, although it can be done at any time, such as in an emergency.

Patients differ in their emotional reactions to surgery. We expect children to express their emotions directly by crying and trembling, but we expect adults to behave with dignity and restraint even in situations of stress.

What fears may the surgical patient have? _diagnosis._
thought of being unconscious and not knowing

Fear of the diagnosis is probably the greatest concern. Other fears include mutilation (e.g., the removal of a breast or the amputation of a leg); the thought of being unconscious and unable to know or control what is happening; fear of pain or death, fear related to separation from family, home and employment.

The surgeon usually speaks to the patient before surgery. It is very important for those giving the patient care to know what the physician has told the patient. With this knowledge, the nurse will be in a better position to help the patient to understand any points that are not clear, or to refer him to the doctor for further explanation, if she is unable to clarify for him.

Religious faith is a source of strength and courage for many patients. Opportunities for contact with a clergyman of the patient's faith and for the sacraments of his church are especially important during a crisis like an impending surgery.

When the patient is to have surgery, the physician will write orders for the immediate pre-operative preparation. In many hospitals, the writing of these orders cancels all previous orders. Be sure to check these orders carefully with the registered nurse.

After the physician tells the patient and his family that the operation is scheduled and gives them any other information that they may wish to have, the nurse may begin preparing the patient.

Consents

The patient is asked to sign a statement showing that he consents to have the surgery performed. If the patient is a minor or is confused or comatose, the next of kin with legal responsibility will be asked to sign the consent for the patient. This consent implies understanding of the nature of the surgery to be undertaken. If the patient has more than one operation or procedure during his hospital stay, he should sign permission for each of them separately. The patient is protected from having surgery for which he has not consented, and the hospital and the doctor are protected against claims that unauthorized surgery has been performed. The consent should be signed while the patient is alert. *Do not* wait until the patient has had his pre-operative medication. The procedure for witnessing of consents is established by each hospital. Be sure to review the policy of the institution before securing a consent. (Review the unit entitled Consents, Releases and Incidents, if required.)

Vital Signs

The patient's temperature, blood pressure, pulse, and respirations should be taken the day before surgery as well as the morning of surgery. They are taken the day before to see if any abnormalities exist which may be reason for delaying surgery. Review the lesson on Cardinal Signs, if necessary, before going on with this procedure.

Laboratory Procedures

Generally a patient will have blood drawn the day before surgery to determine his complete blood count (CBC), hemoglobin (Hgb), and hematocrit (Hct). The results of these studies help to determine if any infection may be present, as indicated by increased white blood count (WBC), and if the patient will be able to tolerate a minimal blood loss (hemoglobin and hematocrit). For major surgery, the physician often orders a blood typing and cross-match for a specific number of pints of blood he may give the patient in case of excessive blood loss during the operation. Blood is kept in a designated refrigerated place available if needed during the surgery or immediately after.

A *clean specimen* of urine will be obtained the day before surgery. Please review the lesson on collection of specimens for this process or procedure. Urinalysis will reveal the condition of the patient's kidneys.

U
N
I
T
33

X-Ray (Radiology) Procedures

A chest X-ray is also ordered pre-operatively to determine the condition of the patient's lungs. The result may influence the type of anesthesia used during surgery, as well as the type of pre-operative medication the physician will order.

Foods and Fluids

Unless the patient is on a special diet, or NPO, he may have a regular meal the evening before the operation. If the operation is scheduled for afternoon of the next day or if it is going to be done under local or spinal anesthesia, the physician may allow the patient to have a light breakfast and fluids until about six hours before surgery. The physician will order the patient to be *NPO*, which is *non per os* (Latin for "nothing by mouth"), at a specific time, usually at midnight before surgery. This means the patient may not even have a sip of water after that time. The accidental feeding of patients who are fasting (without food or water) before surgery is a serious error because it usually means that surgery must be delayed. Rescheduling the surgery is distressing to the patient, and prolongs his hospitalization and expense. *Always* report immediately to the team leader or RN if a patient who is NPO (which means ___nothing by mouth___) has accidentally taken any food or fluids. This is a safety precaution for the patient who may vomit during surgery and aspirate the vomitus (get it into his lungs). *This may be fatal to him.* In other words, the patient may vomit any food or liquid which is in the stomach at the time of surgery. Careful instructions given to the patient and his family clarifying why he may *not* have food or water are the most effective measures to avoid this mistake. Do not assume that removing his water pitcher and glass is enough. Place the "NPO for Surgery" sign on or over the patient's bed so that all persons caring for him are aware of it.

Elimination

It is most important that the patient empty his bladder just before surgery. Offer him a urinal (bedpan), or have him go to the bathroom if he has not had any pre-operative medication. Do not try to hurry the patient, because often the anxiety about surgery makes the bladder sphincter contract and requires more time than usual.

Turn on the bathroom cold water tap (hot water may cause the bathroom to steam and become too warm for the patient); the sound of the water (suggestion) may effect some relaxation of the bladder sphincter.

If the patient has an indwelling catheter, empty the catheter drainage bag immediately before he goes to surgery. If necessary, review the lesson on elimination of urine and catheters. Record the amount of urine removed on the proper record (i.e., nurse's notes, intake and output record).

Enemas are ordered usually for the evening (and in some cases the morning) before surgery. They are ordered so that the patient will be spared the strain and exertion of moving his bowels during the immediate post-operative period, which could cause hemorrhage in the operative area. Also, general anesthesia produces muscular relaxation and possibility of involuntary bowel movement during or immediately after the operation if the intestinal tract is not clear of feces. Review the lesson on Bowel Elimination to assist you with completion of this procedure.

Skin Preparation of the Operative Site

The purpose of skin preparation (commonly called a prep) is to make the skin as free of microorganisms as possible, thus decreasing the possibility during surgery of bacteria entering the wound from the skin surface. Skin preparation is usually performed the afternoon or evening prior to surgery. A wide area of the skin is prepared because this precaution further reduces the possibility of infection. Cleanliness of the skin and the removal of hair from its surface (without injury to or irritation of the skin in the process) are fundamental. Hair is shaved because microorganisms cling to it and may be a source of infection to the operative site.

Plain soap and warm water are often used for cleansing the skin. Antiseptic solutions are sometimes preferred because they are particularly effective in decreasing the number of microorganisms on the skin and thereby decrease the possibility of infection in the operative site. Each agency establishes its own "prep" procedure.

Personal Hygiene

Shampoo. Most patients will shampoo their hair prior to admission for surgery. If the patient has been hospitalized for some time pre-operatively, he may (if he is able and the doctor gives permission) have a shampoo at the hospital. Review the lesson on Care of the Hair for this procedure.

Bath. The patient should bathe thoroughly the evening before or the morning of surgery. If surgery is scheduled for very early in the morning, it is best to have the patient bathe the evening before. Review the lesson on Baths if necessary.

Nails and Hair. Details of personal grooming such as trimming the nails and shaving should be completed before surgery. All metal objects such as bobby pins should be removed from the hair; during surgery they may be lost or could injure the patient's scalp. Long hair may be braided to keep it neat and out of the way. Most hospitals provide turbans or some similar head covering for patients to wear to the operating room. These serve the double purpose of preventing the straying of loose hair in the operating room and keeping the patient's hair clean and in place during the operation and the recovery from anesthesia.

Attire. The patient is given a clean hospital gown. Review the lesson on Assisting the Patient to Dress and Undress, if necessary. If a female patient asks permission to wear her own gown or pajamas, explain that sometimes patients perspire a good deal and need to have their gowns changed while still in the recovery room. Also, her gown may be soiled or lost in the hospital laundry. Neither the operating room nor the recovery room has facilities to take care of a patient's clothing if it has to be changed while in one of these units. For added warmth, some hospitals provide patients with long, white cotton stockings or boots to wear to the operating room.

Prostheses. In most hospitals, the patient is asked to remove dentures so that they will not become broken or dislodged and cause respiratory obstruction during the administration of anesthesia. This includes all bridges, partial plates, and full dentures. Other prostheses such as glasses, contact lenses, or limbs must be removed before surgery. Be sure the small items are placed in a labeled container with the patient's name and room number. Dentures should be kept moist with water or a denture cleansing solution. All prostheses are costly and easily broken or lost; *take extra care to keep them safe.* You may find yourself paying for the patient's broken or lost dentures or glasses.

Mouth Care. All patients should have thorough mouth care before surgery; a clean mouth makes them more comfortable and prevents the aspiration of particles of food that may be left in the mouth. Chewing gum is not permitted since it too may be aspirated.

Makeup and Jewelry. Because the color of the face, lips, and nailbeds is watched carefully for cyanosis during surgery by the anesthesiologist, patients are asked to remove their makeup and nail polish. Cyanosis is a Greek word for the bluish-gray or purple color of the skin caused by a deficiency of oxygen and excess of carbon dioxide in the blood. Cyanosis may be caused by certain gases, drugs, asphyxiation or any condition interfering with the entrance of air into the respiratory tract or lungs.

Jewelry should be removed for safekeeping; a valuable ring might slip off the finger of an unconscious patient and be lost, or stones may be loose and fall out. If the patient prefers to leave his wedding band on, it may be taped to the finger, or a piece of gauze may be threaded under it and tied to the wrist (be careful not to tie it too tightly so as to impair circulation). Although taping the ring is the most common safeguard used, some patients are allergic to tape of any kind, and gauze would then be preferred.

The aforementioned policies for pre-operative preparation are designed for the safety of the patient and his property. Try not to lose sight of this reason, or to enforce meaningless rules as an assertion of authority or discipline. Sometimes exceptions can be made by the physician, if in doing so the patient will be spared acute embarrassment.

UNIT 33

Pre-operative Medication

Usually medications are given to help the patient relax before surgery. Barbiturates are often given the evening before surgery to help the patient to sleep. About an hour before surgery a narcotic, such as morphine or Demerol, is usually administered to relieve apprehension. Although he may awaken or be awake when he is taken to the operating room, the medication dulls the patient's awareness of the experience and makes it easier for him to relax and take the anesthetic.

Atropine may be administered with the narcotic to dry up (lessen) respiratory secretions, if a general anesthetic is to be given. This decreases the likelihood of respiratory complications resulting from aspiration of secretion. Atropine will make the patient's mouth feel very dry, and this should be explained to him.

Post-Operative Instructions for the Patient and Family

Instruct both the patient and his family that the patient will go to the recovery room following surgery. He will be in the recovery room until he is awake and responding. In the recovery room, the nurses will be checking his dressings and taking his blood pressure frequently.

The family should be directed to the area designated for those awaiting a patient in surgery. This ensures that the surgeon will see them as soon as he is able after surgery. If the surgical waiting room has no facilities, you may show the family where the cafeteria and restrooms are located.

Checklist for Pre-operative Care

Some hospitals place a checklist or reminder sheet on the front of the chart of each pre-operative patient. In some hospitals, you are required to initial and note the date and time of the activities you are responsible for performing in the pre-operative period.

Some of the items in this checklist may include:

1. Operative consent signed and on chart.

2. Blood report on chart.

3. Urine report on chart.

4. X-ray report on chart.

5. Identification wristband on patient.

6. Operating area prepared.

7. Enema(s) given.

8. Douche given.

9. NPO at ____ .

10. Tube inserted: Nasogastric _____ Catheter _____ Other _____

11. Jewelry: Removed _____

12. Prosthesis: What removed _____
        What remained on _____

13. Hair prepared or covered _____

14. Bathed and gowned for surgery _____

15. Voided or catheterized.

16. Morning T, P, R, B/P charted.

17. Pre-operative medication given.

18. Bed lowered and siderails up.

19. To surgery: Time _____ Date _____

Wristband checked by _____
(O. R. Personnel)

_____
(Floor Personnel)

The Day Before Surgery

You will explain to the patient what the pre-operative routine is. Wash your hands and identify the patient.

Important Steps	Key Points
1. Take and record vital signs.	See lesson on Cardinal Signs.
2. Collect urine specimen. 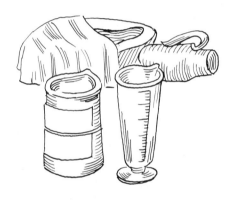	Inform the patient that a test of his urine is needed before surgery and that this is routine for all patients. Ask him, if he can, to void directly in specimen bottle. If not, provide him with bedpan or urinal. After he voids, transfer the urine to a specimen bottle. Label bottle with patient's name, room number, hospital number, name of doctor, age, sex, and date. If an addressograph stamp is available, stamp the label. Do not label the bottle prior to obtaining the specimen. Voiding directly into bottle or transferring urine may spill it and ruin the label. Make sure that your label matches the patient's identification band and that it is his urine. Incorrectly identified urine specimens *are* common. See that you do not make an error. Wash your hands.
3. Explain laboratory and X-ray procedures.	Explain to patient that a lab technician will be taking some of his blood for tests. These tests are done to ensure that his condition is safe for surgery. At this time, tell him that he will be going for a chest X-ray (a film of his lungs) and that it is routine. (Do not give specific times for these procedures because a change may produce more anxiety for him.) *Note:* In some agencies, the pre-op laboratory and X-ray work is done at the time of admission to the hospital *before* the patient is sent to his room. In this case, step 3 would be omitted.
4. Prepare a consent form (usually done by RN or ward clerk).	Consent forms are generally kept at the nursing station. In the area designated (usually upper left- or right-hand corner of the form), write or stamp patient's name, age, sex, room number, hospital number, doctor's name, and date. Ask RN to check for accuracy when you are completing the surgeon's name and kind of surgery.
5. Obtain patient's signature on consent form. (Usually, consents are witnessed by RN or designated person. Check your hospital's policy before securing the signature for consent.)	Take the consent form, pen, and a clipboard or some stable backing, for the consent form to the patient's bedside. (It is easier for him to sign if the consent is placed on a stable surface.) Ask him to read the consent carefully. Do not

UNIT 33

Important Steps	Key Points

try to answer questions you are unsure of; refer these to the RN who will notify the doctor if necessary. Ask the patient to sign his full name. You may sign as witness with your full name, *if agency policy permits.*

6. Explain food and fluid restriction.

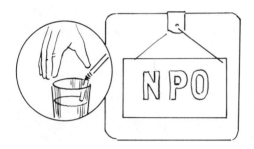

If patient is on a regular diet, he will receive a regular dinner the evening before surgery. If not, he will receive his "special diet" the evening before surgery. Explain that after midnight, his water pitcher will be removed and he may not have anything to eat or drink, not even a sip of water. This is to ensure an empty stomach at the time of surgery. If surgery is scheduled late or if a local anesthesia is to be administered *and* the doctor *ordered* it, explain that he may have a light breakfast or liquids until a specific time, and then will be NPO.

7. Give an enema, if ordered.

Review lesson on enemas (Bowel Elimination). Explain that an enema is given to remove contents of lower bowel for the purpose of: (a) preventing incontinence during surgery and (b) straining during post-operative period.

8. Explain skin preparation.

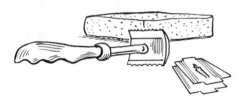

Tell the patient that some time during the evening before surgery, an OR technician or other designated person will come in to clean and shave the area surrounding the site of the incision. The purpose of this is to remove as many bacteria as possible in order to prevent infection of the operative site. Remember from your unit on Hair Care that bacteria cling to the shafts of hair.

9. Provide personal hygiene.

If the patient wishes a shampoo, and an order is obtained, give the shampoo, utilizing the lesson on Care of the Hair. Remove nail polish if worn. Use acetone or nail polish remover; explain that the anesthesiologist checks the color of the nails as an indication of the amount of oxygen the patient is getting. If surgery is scheduled for very early in the morning, the patient may wish to take a bath the night before; see that this is made possible.

The Day of Surgery

Important Steps	Key Points

1. Wash your hands, approach the patient, identify him and explain what you are going to do.

2. Take patient's vital signs and record them.

Take his temperature, pulse, blood pressure, and respirations according to the lesson on Cardinal Signs, and record them on the nurses' notes on the patient's chart.

Important Steps	Key Points
3. Give A.M. care.	Assist the patient to wash his face, hands, and to clean his teeth. If dentures are worn, ask him to remove and place them in a labeled denture cup. (Use the same procedure for partial plate or bridges.) Make sure that the denture cup is clearly labeled, with the patient's name and room number on it.

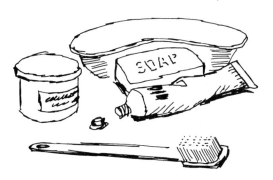

4. Give hair care.	Brush the patient's hair neatly. If it is long, you may braid it for neatness. If the hospital requires a turban or head covering, place it around the hairline. Secure headpiece by taping it.
5. Dress the patient in a hospital gown.	Assist him to remove his own pajamas and put on a hospital gown. Review the lesson on Assisting the Patient to Dress and Undress, if necessary. Explain that the hospital gown is used in case it is soiled by perspiration or drainage, and also to ensure that the patient's belongings will not be lost.
6. Remove the patient's makeup and jewelry.	Tell her not to use makeup because it becomes smeared by perspiring during surgery. Also, the anesthesiologist is better able to check the skin color if it is not covered with makeup. Ask patient to remove her jewelry so that it is not lost during surgery. Put the jewelry in the place provided for safekeeping. If patient wants to keep a wedding band on, either tape it to the finger or thread a gauze strip under the ring and tie the gauze around the wrist securely, but not so tight as to stop circulation.
7. Encourage voiding (just prior to pre-operative medication).	If the patient is able, assist him to the bathroom or assist him with bedpan or urinal immediately before pre-operative medication. A full bladder in surgery can easily be cut; thus it is extremely important that *the bladder be empty*. Explain that the medication will make him sleepy and he will not be allowed out of bed after his injection because he may fall and hurt himself.
8. Apply safety measures after pre-operative medication.	Following pre-operative medication, place the bed in low position with siderails up. Remove all smoking articles to ensure safety.

UNIT 33

Important Steps	Key Points
9. Give recovery room information. 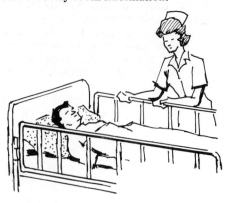	The patient and his family should be told that he will be in the recovery room until he is awake. *Do not* give any definite period of time because if the time is extended, it will increase everyone's anxiety. Explain that in the recovery room the patient's dressings, blood pressure, and general condition will be checked frequently.
10. Direct family to waiting room facilities.	Show the family where the waiting area for surgery and the restrooms are located. Also, tell them where coffee, tea, or food may be purchased.
11. Complete checklist.	Check each item for which you are responsible; write your initials and the time. Notify RN when completed. Record in the appropriate place on the nurses' notes or the surgical checklist.
12. Assist with transfer of patient to the OR cart. 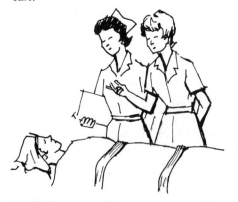	When OR orderly comes to take the patient to surgery, check the name of the person he is to pick up; check the chart for the correct person, and then check the patient's wristband. *All of these must match.* Assist in moving the patient from bed to cart, using proper body alignment, balance, and movement. When he is on the cart, secure the straps for safety. Sign off the chart in nurses' notes "Patient to surgery," time, date, your first initial and last name, and category. *Both* you and OR personnel must sign the checklist at the bottom, indicating that both of you have identified the patient's wristband. You may go with the orderly to the OR area with a female patient if this is the agency policy. (Females must be accompanied by another female while being transported within the hospital.)

V. ADDITIONAL INFORMATION FOR ENRICHMENT

Pre-operative care is very essential to the patient. It can be used as an opportunity for teaching good health practices which he should observe after surgery. It also provides an opportunity to answer some of his questions and lessen his fears.

You may wish to know more about pre-operative care for a specific patient. Your instructor will give you additional reading assignments. In some agencies you may observe surgery when it is performed on your patient. This, of course, requires permission from your instructor, charge nurse, and operating room supervisor. (Check your agency regulations on this matter.)

POST-TEST

1. Define the following:

   a. aspirate _to breathe in_

   b. cyanosis: _bluish color to skin due to lack oxygen_

   c. general anesthesia: _complete & effects the whole body_

   d. spinal anesthesia: _numbness from waist down_

   e. bladder sphincter: _plain muscle around the opening of bladder_

   f. CBC: _complete blood count_

   g. prosthesis: _any false limbs, organs, dentures etc._

2. List three kinds of fear or concern a person may have about surgery.

   (a) _pain_

   (b) _death_

   (c) _fear of diagnosis_

3. Complete the following:

   a. Skin preparation is usually carried out the _evening_ before surgery.

   b. Hair is shaved because _microorganism_ readily cling to it.

   c. Enemas are ordered pre-operatively to _prevent strain on bowels_ immediately after surgery and _during accident_ during surgery and in the recovery room. _involuntary B.M._

   d. Patients are ordered NPO usually from 6 to 10 hours before surgery to prevent _vomiting_ and _aspirating_ during surgery.

   e. The anesthesiologist checks the color of the _nailbeds_ and _face, lips_ for cyanosis during surgery.

   f. Pre-operative policies are designed for the safety of the _patient_ and his _belongings_

   g. Consents should be signed by the patient _before_ receiving the pre-operative medication.

4. List three safety precautions that must be carried out after the patient has had his pre-operative medication.

   a. _siderails up_

   b. _bed in low position_

   c. _remove smoking articles_

POST-TEST ANNOTATED ANSWER SHEET

1. a.   aspirate: to breathe in, to get foreign materials in the lungs (p. 688)

   b.   cyanosis: a lightly bluish-gray or purple discoloration of the skin due to a deficiency of oxygen and an excess of carbon dioxide in the blood. (p. 688)

   c.   general anesthesia: One that is complete and affecting the entire body with loss of consciousness. (p. 687)

   d.   spinal anesthesia: one that causes loss of sensation from the hips down, induced by injecting a drug into the lower end of the spinal column. (p. 687)

   e.   bladder sphincter: plain muscle around the opening of the bladder. (p. 688)

   f.   CBC: complete blood count; includes RBC, WBC, possibly Hgb and Hct. (p. 688)

   g.   prosthesis: artificial organ or part, i.e., artificial limbs, eyeglasses, dentures, etc. (p. 688)

2. Fear of diagnosis, mutilation, pain, death, of being unconscious and unable to control self. (p. 689)

3. a.   Afternoon or evening prior to surgery, although it may be done at any time (as in emergency). (p. 690)

   b.   microorganisms (p. 690)

   c.   prevent patient from strain and exertion of moving his bowels following surgery; and decrease possibility of involuntary bowel movement during the operation because of relaxed muscles. (p. 690)

   d.   vomiting, aspirating (p. 690)

   e.   nailbeds, face, lips (p. 691)

   f.   patient and his belongings (p. 691)

   g.   before (p. 689)

4. a.   raise siderails (p. 693)

   b.   lower bed to low position

   c.   remove smoking articles

PERFORMANCE TEST

1.   Complete nurses' notes and pre-operative checklist from the following situation. Read through the case and record the appropriate information on the nurses' notes and on the pre-operative checklist.

A young woman, 26 years of age, was admitted by stretcher to room 223 at 0745 A.M. She was complaining of severe pain over the entire abdomen. The intern ordered an ice bag to be applied to the abdomen. The TPR were: (rectal) 101.4° F. — 92 — 22. At the time of admission, the patient was unable to void; however, two hours later she voided 400 cc. A urine specimen was sent to the laboratory. The lab technician drew blood for a CBC. When Dr. Smith called at 0930, the patient was still complaining of pain and was extremely nauseated although she had not vomited. Dr. Smith visited shortly thereafter to examine the patient and to write the history and physical reports. He then scheduled the patient for an appendectomy for 6:30 that evening. The consent for surgery was signed by the patient.

The OR technician performed the surgical skin prep and a cleansing enema was given by the nurse's aide. Since her pre-op medication was ordered to be given by the RN at 5:00 P.M., the patient was prepared for surgery at 4:30 P.M. The TPR remained the same as it was on admission with a B/P of 124/72. The patient voided at this time. She had no dentures but she did remove her contact lenses, hair pins, and nail polish. A solid gold watch and $20.00 in four bills were placed in a valuables envelope and locked in the nurse's station.

The pre-op medication was given at 5:00 P.M., and the bed was placed in low position with siderails up. The patient slept until 6:25 P.M., at which time she was taken to surgery via stretcher.

2.   With a partner in the skill laboratory, prepare the patient for a cholecystectomy, which is scheduled for tomorrow at 9:00 A.M. Follow the steps outlined in your procedure. Record your activities on practice nurses' notes.

PERFORMANCE CHECKLIST

PRE-OPERATIVE CARE OF A PATIENT

1. Complete pre-operative entry in nurses' notes, observing following rules:

   A. Legibility

   B. Print or write with blue ink; sign each entry with handwritten signature and title.

   C. Date and time of entry, effect; record results for each activity.

   D. Do not skip lines.

   E. Correct error with one line through error, with error notation written above.

   (1) If a whole page needs retyping, it is included as a permanent part of the chart.

   F. Describe clearly and concisely the appearance, behavior, character, and drainage of excreta, type, location, and duration of pain.

   G. Use standard abbreviations.

   H. Enter each pre-op activity with complete description, time, date, and signature.

   I. Sign specimens out to laboratory in stated manner (from unit on Elimination) and follow other laboratory and X-ray procedures.

   J. Chart prep, noting time, type, and by whom.

   K. Chart disposal of valuables.

2. Complete pre-operative checklist with required information on form (observing above rules).

PREPARATION OF PATIENT FOR A SURGICAL PROCEDURE

Day Prior to Surgery

1. Wash hands; identify patient, and explain procedure.

2. Take vital signs.

3. Collect urine specimen.

    A. Correctly label specimen and attach label to prepared requisition.

    B. Provide for transmittal of specimen to lab.

4. Explain laboratory and X-ray procedures which will occur.

5. Prepare surgical consent form and obtain patient's signature.

6. Explain food and fluid restrictions.

7. Give enema.

8. Explain "prep."

9. Provide for personal hygiene, e.g., shampoo, shower, oral hygiene, removal of nail polish.

10. Chart activities in patient's chart.

Day of Surgery

1. Wash hands, identify patient, and explain procedure.

2. Take vital signs.

3. Give A.M. care, care for hair, and dress patient in hospital gown.

4. Remove makeup and jewelry.

    A. Place valuables in secure place (with family; in agency's safe).

5. Have patient void (should be able to explain why this is necessary).

6. Apply safety measures (bedrails up, bed in low position, and smoking articles removed).

7. Explain Recovery Room Procedure to patient or family.

8. Direct family to waiting room.

9. Complete Pre-operative checklist

10. Assist in transfer of patient to OR stretcher.

Unit 34

PREPARATION OF CONSENTS, RELEASES AND INCIDENTS

I. DIRECTIONS TO THE STUDENT

Obtain sample packet of consent, release, and Incident Report forms from your instructor. Proceed through this lesson. When you are through, complete the post-test.

II. GENERAL PERFORMANCE OBJECTIVE

You will be able to obtain consents and releases and complete Incident Reports according to legal requirements.

III. SPECIFIC PERFORMANCE OBJECTIVES

Upon completion of the Unit, you will be able:

1. To recognize the circumstances and procedures which require consents or releases and to prepare appropriate reports.

2. To explain the purpose and meaning of consents and releases to patients and other persons and obtain a legally valid consent or release from a patient or guardian.

3. To recognize an incident, and to report and record incidents in the proper manner.

IV. VOCABULARY

biopsy — excision of a small piece of tissue for the purpose of examination and diagnosis.

bone marrow — soft tissue (spongy) in the hollow of long bones. The center bone marrow is yellow and is chiefly fat; the surrounding tissue is called the red bone marrow because it manufactures red blood cells.

lumbar puncture — the act of puncturing (with a needle) the subarachnoid space in the lumbar region (middle back) of the vertebral column, usually between the third and fourth lumbar vertebrae. The puncture is done for diagnostic or treatment purposes, e.g., injecting an anesthetic.

radiology — branch of medicine which deals with X-rays and other radiations for the purpose of diagnosis or treatment.

V. INTRODUCTION

What is the Purpose of Consents and Releases?

The purpose of releases and consents is the protection of the patient's rights. In treating a patient without a valid consent, the hospital (as a business organization), the physicians, and the hospital employees place themselves in a position of liability (responsibility by law). To reduce or eliminate the possibility of a patient bringing a legal suit against the hospital, physicians and employees, the patient or his *legal* designate (guardian) signs an agreement (consent, release) for treatment. This agreement also protects the patient from having any treatment for which he did not sign. For the above reasons, the relationship between hospital and patient is contractual. (A contract is a binding agreement between two or more parties.)

ITEM 1: COMMON TYPES OF CONSENTS

Usually the general admission procedure includes an *Admission Agreement*. This agreement provides for nursing care, medical treatment (other than surgery or surgical procedures), and release of information (to insurance companies, workmen's compensation insurance, etc.) It generally has paragraphs about the patient's valuables and his financial agreement with the agency. This agreement is usually executed with several copies, one of which is given to the patient and another placed in the patient's chart. In some agencies, there is a waiver clause in certain Admission Agreements giving the agency (and patient) the *right* to settle grievances out of court. This is done to speed up legal proceedings and to decrease court costs. This Admission Agreement form is filled out by the admitting office personnel.

Consent to Operation and Administration of Anesthetics (sometimes called a Surgical Consent): This form is used for every surgical procedure. The patient authorizes a particular physician(s) to perform a specific operation. It also allows for the administration of anesthesia and for the services of pathology and radiology.

Depending on agency policy, this form may also be used for procedures which may be carried out in the patient's room under local anesthesia and for the services of pathology and radiology.

These forms are usually initiated by the nurse in charge of the patient's pre-operative preparation (as specified in the agency procedure manual). The form is completed as a routine step in the pre-op preparation; however, many physicians write a specific order to obtain a signed consent. In the case of a surgical procedure, the surgeon states exactly what the procedure will be. This information is entered in the appropriate blank on the operation consent form.

In an *emergency situation* where the patient is unconscious, no family is present, and immediate surgery is indicated if the life is to be saved, the consent for operation can be signed by two physicians. In this case, however, the form would be initiated by the nurse.

The above two consent forms are the most commonly used. Others include:

1. *Consents for use of experimental drugs or treatments.* The agency form is always used. It may be initiated by the doctor or nurse. Usually there is an agency procedure to be followed when using experimental drugs or treatments.

2. *Refusal of drugs, treatments and other procedures.* The agency form is used and is usually initiated by the nurse.

3. *Consent for photograph.* The agency form is used and is usually initiated by the nurse or representative of the public relations department.

4. *Permit for using patient's own electrical appliances.* The agency form is used and is initiated by the nurse.

5. *Release of body to the mortuary.* Agency form is initiated by the nurse.

6. *Autopsy permit.* Agency form is initiated by the nurse upon the order of a physician. Some agencies have the physician obtain the "Next-of-Kin" signature. Follow agency procedure.

7. *Authorization for consent to treatment of minor.* Agency form is initiated by nurse.

ITEM 2: COMMON TYPES OF RELEASES

Leaving Hospital Against Medical Advice form is used whenever a patient demands to be discharged from a hospital *against medical advice* (AMA). This form is generally made out in duplicate and must be offered to the patient, even if you believe he won't sign it. Encourage him to sign. If he does not, a notation must be made on the patient's chart to that effect. AMA discharges are reported at once to the attending physician, the nursing office, and administration. Every reasonable effort should be made to avoid this action by the patient.

Release from Use of Siderails form is used when a patient refuses to follow agency policy regarding the use of siderails; the patient must sign this release. If the patient refuses to have his siderails up as per policy, make every effort to remove safety hazards. Lower the bed, move objects that would be harmful, and check the patient frequently.

Record on the patient's chart that he has been instructed about siderail regulations but refuses to cooperate (release signed or not signed), and that the doctor, nursing office, and administration were informed (if indicated by your agency policy).

ITEM 3: WHO MAY SIGN CONSENTS OR RELEASES?

Generally, any *adult* may sign a consent or release if he is not under a guardianship (as in the case of incompetency). An adult is any person, male or female, who has reached the age of 21 years (many states now moving to 18 years), who has contracted a valid marriage, or, in some states has been designated as an emancipated minor.

Minors are persons who fail to meet the criteria of adulthood, as stated above. Minors may be treated when the authorization to treat the minor has been signed by his parent or *legal* guardian. An emergency situation, e.g., life or death, may be handled differently as prescribed by agency policy. Every parent of a minor child left in the care of baby sitters, in school, or on vacation should give written permission for treatment of the child in case of illness or injury at a time when the parent cannot be reached. This would avoid the many hours spent by treatment facilities trying to obtain a legal authorization to treat.

The patient should first read the consent or have it read to him, so that he knows what he is signing. Ask the patient to explain what he is signing, *not* "Do you understand?" Frequently patients say they understand when they do not because they wish to avoid embarrassment. If the patient still does not understand after explanation, postpone his signing of the consent until the doctor can explain. All dates, times, and signatures must be in ink, including witnesses' signatures. Follow your agency policy regarding the witnessing of consents. Usually there are specific regulations as to who may sign documents as a witness, e.g., RN only, admitting clerk, notary public.

Consents and Releases

Important Steps	Key Points
1. Obtain form and equipment: consent, pen, and surface (e.g., clip-board) to write on.	If you are responsible for securing consents, make sure that patient's name, age, sex, room number, physician, and type of surgery or procedure are correct before you take it to the patient. This preliminary information can be completed on the form before taking it to him for signature. Forms are usually stored in a designated place in the nurse's station.
2. Wash your hands, identify the patient, and explain the procedure.	Give the Consent form to the patient to read, or read it *fully* to him. Make sure he understands the form. Ask him to explain what he understands the form to say. Clarify if he does not understand.

UNIT 34

Important Steps	Key Points
3. Obtain his signature.	Ask the patient to sign his full name in ink in the appropriate space. You write the date and time in the space provided. If the patient refuses to sign the consent, refer to your charge nurse. She will notify the physician and await his order. The final determination about the consent is the responsibility of the physician.
	Note: If the patient cannot write his name but can make an "X", you will need two witnesses.
	If you obtained the patient's signature, you *must* witness his signature. Sign your full name and title with a pen. This form becomes a part of the patient's chart or record. See sample Surgical Consent at the end of this unit.
4. Place completed consent or release on patient's chart.	See sample forms in your packet.

ITEM 4.   INCIDENT REPORTS

Incident Reports are made out if there is an error in treatment or a patient accident occurs. They are not part of the patient's chart as are consents and releases but are intended for the hospital administration and attorneys. They alert the hospital administration to the possibility of litigation (law suits).

What Constitutes an "Incident"?

The following generally constitute incidents that are reportable:

1. Patient falls.

2. Patient is burned.

3. Articles are lost inside patient, e.g., following a surgical operation.

4. Personal articles are lost or damaged.

5. Medication errors.

6. Errors in patient identification, e.g., giving the treatment to the wrong patient.

7. Injection injuries, e.g., needle injury to a nerve during medication injection.

8. Treatment injuries.

9. Thermometers broken in patient's mouth, rectum, bed, etc.

Who Completes Incident Reports?

The nursing personnel most familiar with the incident, or who observed its happening, should complete the account of the incident according to the agency policy.

If an incident occurs, provide emergency and safety measures for the patient; call for help, either verbally or by patient call bell. Your team leader will notify a house physician or the patient's own physician.

After patient comfort and safety are provided, try to obtain the patient's account of the incident. You will need this to complete the report. Carry out doctor's order for care if incident necessitates follow-through, e.g., patient falls and breaks an arm — doctor orders an X-ray.

Incidents: Immediate Procedure

Important Steps	Key Points
1. Provide for patient's safety and comfort.	Call for help verbally or by signaling with the patient's call bell. Do not try to move patient by yourself because you may hurt the patient and yourself. Remove any safety hazards such as broken glass. Provide for his warmth.
2. Return patient to bed.	Do this as soon as possible. Get assistance as needed. Make patient comfortable. Follow doctor's orders if given, e.g., call for an X-ray or discontinue a blood transfusion.
3. Complete Incident form.	Ask team leader for assistance in completing your history of the incident and other patient information. Charting should be clear, concise, and accurate.
4. Secure patient's report of incident.	After patient is calmed or has been seen by a physician, you may ask him to relate what happened to cause the incident, if he is aware there was an incident. Write this information in the space provided in the report. It is desirable (when appropriate) to quote patient's own words. You will start the comment on the form: "The patient states that . . . . "
5. Place completed form on patient's chart.	Physician will sign in the appropriate place; one section is forwarded to the nursing office, one to the administration, and one remains on patient's chart.

VI. ADDITIONAL INFORMATION FOR ENRICHMENT

Consents, Releases and Incident Reports provide important safety aspects for the patient, you, and your agency. Adhere to the agency's established policies.

VII. APPENDIX

Sample Consents, Releases, Incident Reports.

UNIT
34

POST-TEST

Check all of the following statements that are *true*.

_____ 1. A new consent must be obtained before an operation can be performed by a physician other than the one originally named in the consent for the operation.

_____ 2. A consent usually is not required when a patient is admitted to a hospital only for observation.

_____ 3. A consent for treatment of a married woman who is under 21 years of age must be obtained from her husband.

_____ 4. A minor may legally consent to his own treatment if an emergency exists and his parent or guardian is not available.

_____ 5. A physician does not incur liability if he performs emergency surgery on an unconscious patient without a consent other than the general admission agreement.

_____ 6. A specific consent must be obtained for a blood transfusion.

_____ 7. A specific consent must be obtained for photographing a patient.

_____ 8. A patient must sign a release before he can leave a hospital against the advice of his physician.

_____ 9. When a patient signs a release from use of siderails, this relieves the nurse of responsibility for his safety in bed.

_____10. An occurrence is classed as an incident only if it involves actual or possible injury to a patient or other person.

_____11. When an incident involves a patient, a copy of the Incident Report must be entered in his records.

12. What is the purpose of a consent or release?
_____ *to protect patient & hospital's rights* _____

13. Suppose a patient fails to understand the form. You try to explain, but he says he still does not understand. What do you do?
_____ *Refer to the doctor & wait until* _____
_____ *he understands* _____

14. If the patient refuses to sign the form even though he understands, how far should you go in trying to persuade him? What do you do when his guardian or relative refuses to sign? *Do not try to persuade him.*
_____ *Refer to doctor.* _____

15. Name two common types of consents.
(1)__*Surgery*_____ (2)__*admission*_____

16. Name two common types of releases.
(1)_____*AMA*_____ (2)__*Body to mortuary*___

17. Define an adult (as it relates to signing consents and releases).
_____ *age 21 or marriage,* _____*mentally competent*_____
_____ *license* _____

18. List four instances which constitute an "incident."

(1) _patient is burned_

(2) _patient falls_

(3) _Medication errors_

(4) _articles lost in patient during surgery_

POST-TEST ANNOTATED ANSWER SHEET

No. 1 and No. 7 are true. (pp. 701 and 702)

12. To protect the patient's and the hospital's rights. (p. 701)

13. Refer to his doctor for clarification and withhold signing of the consent until the patient understands. (p. 702)

14. You do not need to persuade the patient, family, or guardian. Refer to the nurse and she will notify the physician. He will then determine what action to take. The final responsibility rests with the physician. (p. 702)

15. Any of these: Admission Agreement; Surgical Consent, Consent for Use of Experimental Drugs; Consent to Photograph; Autopsy Permit, etc. (p. 702)

16. Any of these: AMA; Release from Use of Siderails; Release of Body to Mortuary, etc. (p. 703)

17. Any person who has reached the age of 21 years or who has a valid marriage contract and is mentally competent. (p. 703)

18. Any of these: patient fall; patient burn; medication or treatment error; error in patient identification; broken thermometer; damaged or lost personal articles, etc. (p. 704)

PERFORMANCE TEST

1. Complete an Incident form from the following information.

At 3:45 A.M. Mrs. Mary Volk, 223^2, fractured hip, 87 years old, patient of Dr. G. Marshall, fell out of bed while trying to get up to the bathroom. Siderails were down, and the bed was in the low position. Patient had received her nembutal gr lss h.s.

2. Complete a Surgical Consent form for Mr. Victor Welk, 257^1, patient of Dr. S. First, for a right inguinal herniotomy. He is scheduled for surgery at 9:00 A.M. on Thursday, December 1.

3. Complete a Release of Siderails Form for Mr. V. Welk in question #2.

PERFORMANCE CHECKLIST

CONSENTS, RELEASES, INCIDENTS:

COMPLETION OF INCIDENT FORM

1. Obtain proper form.

2. Fill in preliminary information.

3. Wash hands.

4. Identify patient.

5. Explain procedure to patient.

6. Verify the patient's understanding of the form.

7. Complete history of incident as related by patient — the patient states that "   ".

8. Document report if possible, i.e., list all individuals familiar with incident.

9. Transmit form to appropriate departments.

COMPLETION OF CONSENT OR RELEASE FORM

1. Obtain proper form and necessary equipment.

2. Fill in all preliminary information.

3. Wash hands.

4. Identify patient, and explain procedure.

5. Permit patient to read form, clarify his understanding of the form.

6. Ask patient to sign the form.

7. Write in date and time the form is signed.

8. Witness the form as required.

9. Place the completed form with the patient's chart.

U
N
I
T
34

10. In the event that the patient will not sign, you sign the form, annotating the record appropriately.

11. In the event that the patient cannot write his name, obtain the signature of two witnesses.

12. In the event the patient is a minor, obtain parent's or guardian's signature.

COMPLETION OF CONSENT OR RELEASE FORM

1. Obtain proper form and necessary equipment.

2. Fill in all preliminary information.

3. Wash hands.

4. Identify patient, and explain procedure.

5. Permit patient to read form, clarify his understanding of the form.

6. Ask patient to sign form.

7. Write in date and time form is signed.

8. Witness form as required.

9. Place completed form with patient's chart.

10. In the event that patient cannot write his name but can make an "X" or "mark," obtain signatures of two witnesses.

11. In the event the patient is a minor, obtain parent's or guardian's signature.

Unit 35

POST-OPERATIVE
CARE OF A PATIENT

I. DIRECTIONS TO THE STUDENT

You are to proceed through this lesson using the workbook as your guide. In the skill laboratory, you will need to practice gathering the necessary equipment and preparing the bedside unit to receive the patient from the Recovery Room or from Surgery. Following your practice sessions and the completion of the lesson, you should arrange with your instructor to take the post-test for this lesson.

You will need the following items for your study and practice:

1. This workbook

2. A pen or pencil

3. Thermometer

4. Sphygmomanometer

5. Stethoscope

6. Cellu-wipes or tissues

7. Emesis basin

8. IV standard

9. Suction machine

10. Intake and output record

11. Drainage bottle and tubing, or disposable GU set

12. Extra linen as needed — gown, sheets, towel, wash cloth, etc.

13. Nurses' record

Please read the following paragraphs carefully. They will tell you exactly what you will be expected to know and how to provide safe post-operative care during the period immediately after surgery, and in the later period after recovery from anesthesia. If you feel that you have sufficient knowledge and skills to perform the post-test accurately and to take the written test with at least 80% accuracy with no further study of the lesson, discuss with your instructor the possibility of proceeding directly to the post-tests.

II. GENERAL PERFORMANCE OBJECTIVE FOR THIS LESSON

You will be able to assemble the required equipment and provide post-operative care to the unconscious or helpless patient recovering from anesthesia, or the patient who has fully recovered from anesthesia. You will do this to protect the patient's safety by the early detection and prevention (when possible) of post-operative discomforts and complications, and to promote his recovery and rehabilitation.

V. SPECIFIC OBJECTIVES

Upon completing this lesson you will be able to provide post-operative care to meet the following objectives:

1. Maintain open breathing for the unconscious or helpless patient through the use of an artificial airway, the proper positioning of the patient, and suctioning secretions from the mouth and throat.

2. Observe for signs of shock or hemorrhage by taking and recording the vital signs every 15 minutes during period immediately after surgery, by frequent inspection of the dressings for signs of unusual bleeding, and by checking any drainage or vomitus for the presence of blood.

3. Insure the safety of the patient by the use of siderails on the bed to prevent falling, by not leaving the unconscious or anesthetized patient alone, and by setting up post-op room completely and correctly.

4. Accurately record the intake and output from all sources as indicators of the patient's fluid and electrolyte balance, connect all tubes to suction or drainage as appropriate, and use care to keep the IV running in the vein.

5. Provide for the patient's comfort and relief of pain through careful handling, with frequent turning or change of position, avoiding unnecessary noise or confusion, and anchoring the drainage tubes. If pain persists, notify the team leader or the nurse in charge without delay.

6. Prevent respiratory complications by changing the patient's position at least every two hours, instructing him to breathe deeply and to cough, and supporting the operative site during coughing.

7. Observe and maintain an adequate urinary output by encouraging intake of sufficient fluids, checking for signs of urinary retention, and promoting the elimination of urine by encouraging voluntary voiding or the use of a catheter when ordered by the physician.

8. Reduce or relieve the discomforts related to the patient's gastrointestinal tract (i.e., nausea, vomiting, gas pains, and constipation) through appropriate medical and nursing measures.

9. Provide for the personal hygiene needs of the patient during the anesthesia recovery period by changing his gown and bed linen as needed, bathing his face and body of perspiration or secretions, and assisting with personal hygiene, usually for several days, giving particular attention to oral hygiene.

10. Provide passive exercise of the unconscious or helpless patient's arms and legs at least twice a day, encourage active exercise by the alert patient, and promote the goal of early ambulation.

III. VOCABULARY

By this time you have learned the meaning of most of the words used in the lesson, inasmuch as they were in the vocabularies of other lessons that you have studied. However, there are some which may be new to you. Study the words and their meanings carefully before proceeding further into the lesson.

1. Words related to post-operative complications:

apnea — stopped breathing, lack of respiration.
atelectasis — a diffuse blockage of tiny air sacs in the lungs due to bits or plugs of mucus, or possible result of a surgical opening into the chest cavity.

embolism — obstruction of a blood vessel by a foreign substance, i.e., air bubble, fat globule, purulent matter, blood clot.

embolus (emboli is plural) — a circulating embolism

evisceration — the separation of layers of an incisional wound with the exposure or protuberance of an organ of the body through the separation or opening.

hemorrhage — excessive flow of blood out of the blood vessels, an abnormal amount of bleeding.

hypoventilation — decreased or reduced column of air taken into the lungs.

shock — a clinical syndrome due to inadequate circulation, impending circulatory collapse, due to various causes.

thrombus — a blood clot that develops within a blood vessel, either attached to the vessel wall or lodged within the vessel. When it becomes dislodged and circulates in the blood system it is called a thrombotic embolus.

thrombophlebitis — an inflammation of a vein with a blood clot, especially in the legs.

2. Words related to the level of consciousness:

coma, comatose — state of being unconscious, unresponsive to stimuli.

conscious — state of being awake; responsive, alert.

disoriented — state of being confused, lack of response, or inappropriate response to stimuli.

semi-conscious (semi-comatose) — state of being able to respond to physiological stimuli, but reduced response to mental stimuli.

unconscious — state of being unaware, unresponsive to all stimuli.

3. Other words used in the lesson:

airway — the air passages of the body: the mouth, nose, larynx, pharynx, trachea, bronchi, and the lungs. Also, a plastic or metal tube inserted in the mouth and pharynx to insure clear air passage.

aseptic — a condition free of contamination or germs, sterile.

anesthesia — the absence of pain; drugs which block perception of pain. General anesthesia, such as induced by ether, produces unconsciousness. Local anesthesia, such as novocaine, blocks sensation of pain with no loss of consciousness.

cannula — a short hollow tube or pipe, usually made of plastic; often used instead of a metal needle on an IV.

cyanosis — bluish color of tissue resulting from lack of oxygen.

electrolyte balance — dissolved chemicals in such body fluids as blood and serum, capable of conducting an electrical charge; ionized particles in balance.

larynx — the voice box.

pharynx — the back of the throat (part of the air passages).

pulmonary — refers to the lungs and the function of breathing.

U
N
I
T
35

INTRODUCTION

The Importance of Post-Operative Nursing Care

The operation is over. The surgeon has used his knowledge, skills and talent to perform an operation designed to prolong the patient's life or to improve the quality of some aspect of that life. However, the very nature of the operation produces injury and stress to the patient's body. The anesthesia used during the surgery reduces the patient's ability to respond to the stimuli within himself and from the surrounding environment. This, then, is the state of the patient as he enters the post-operative period: his body has undergone a deliberate injury, and his response to stimuli has been reduced.

The patient has literally entrusted his life and welfare to the doctors and nurses during surgery and the post-operative phase of his illness. If something were to go wrong, the patient often could not even signal for help, much less take steps to correct the problem himself. The surgical injury and the reduced ability to respond to stimuli make the patient dependent upon the help and assistance of the nurse. The less the patient is able to respond, the more the nurse must be his eyes, ears, touch, judgment, and muscles, and his physiological watchdog.

In post-operative nursing, the *helping* and *caring* aspects of nursing become dramatically clear. The patient recovering from a spinal anesthesia is unable to turn himself, so the nurse turns him frequently. The unconscious patient is unable to control the secretions trickling down his throat, so the nurse controls them by positioning and by suctioning. In helping the patient, the nurse is guided by the doctor's orders for post-operative treatment and therapy, but the helping aspect of nursing is evident even as the nurse bathes perspiration from the patient's forehead, or adjusts the light so that it doesn't shine directly in his eyes.

The caring aspect of nursing is the feeling that is extended to the patient and experienced by him. It is the part of nursing that requires being with the patient, tending to his needs, heeding his responses, protecting him from dangers, and providing him with compassion, tenderness, concern, consideration, and respect. Through this caring aspect of nursing, we are able to nurse the patient, not just the disease.

The helplessness of the post-operative patient makes it essential that the nurse worker have the skills and knowledge to help maintain the life processes, provide for safety and comfort, and prevent complications. This lesson is designed to give you the *beginning skills* that you will need in order to provide post-operative care to patients under the direction of the doctor and the nurse.

A. In the post-operative period, the state of the patient is characterized by (1) *deliberate injury to body*, and (2) *reduced stimuli*.

B. The functions of nursing consist of the (1) *helping*, and (2) *caring* aspects.

C. The nurse is guided by the *doctor* in giving post-operative care to the patient.

ITEM 1.   WHERE POST-OPERATIVE CARE IS GIVEN

Regardless of the location in which post-operative care is given, the same meticulous and skillful nursing care is required. The surgical patient receives post-operative care in (a) the Recovery Room, sometimes called the PAR (Post-Anesthesia Room). (b) an Intensive Care Unit (ICU) or (c) his own room.

Many hospitals have Recovery Rooms to care for the patient from the time he has left the operating room until he has reacted or responded from the anesthesia. The recovery room is usually located near the operating rooms, staffed with skillful nurses, and supplied with equipment needed for most post-operative emergencies. Doctors or anesthetists from the operating room can be called when needed. The patient stays in the recovery room until he has reacted, or is able to respond to stimuli around him. It generally takes from 2 to 6 hours for the patient to react from general anesthesia and, if his condition is stable, he is then transferred to his room. Many recovery rooms are not open during the night hours when only emergency surgery is performed.

In recent years, Intensive Care Units have been established in many hospitals to provide highly specialized and complex nursing care in one central area. Some surgical patients are taken directly to the ICU following a complex and serious operation. The patient may remain there for several days if his condition continues to be unstable. As a beginning worker in nursing, you *should not* be assigned to work in the Recovery Room or an ICU until you have gained clinical experience.

Most of the post-operative care of the patient takes place in his own room. Before the use of Recovery Rooms became widespread, all patients were returned from the operating room directly to their rooms. The nursing staff on the unit stayed with the patient until he reacted from anesthesia, and continued his care through the recovery period until he was discharged from the hospital. (In hospitals that use Recovery Rooms, the patient will be reacted from the anesthesia before he is returned to his room.) However, you will need to check the patient frequently during the first 72 hours or so, and the patient will require more assistance for his personal needs during this early post-operative period.

D. As a beginning worker in nursing, you would provide post-operative care to the patient in _his room_

E. The patient is transferred from the Recovery Room to his own room when he has _responded_ _from anesthesia_

ITEM 2. PREPARING THE POST-OPERATIVE UNIT

In order to provide post-operative care to the patient, whether in his room or in the Recovery Room, certain equipment will be necessary. You should prepare the unit and collect the equipment before the patient arrives, so that observation and care of the patient can begin immediately. The patient's bed should be made up as a post-operative bed, as described in your lesson on Bedmaking. Even if the patient has reacted from the anesthesia, it is easier to transfer him onto the bed if the top bedding has been folded back. Many patients will experience some nausea and vomiting, or have some drainage, so the bed should be protected with a pad or towel at the head of the bed, and a plastic sheet, drawsheet, pad, or Chux to protect the middle portion of the bed. These pads can easily be changed if they become soiled.

On the bedside stand, you should place the following items: a package of *Cellu-Wipes*, or tissues, emesis basin, thermometer, sphygmomanometer, stethoscope, nursing records, and paper and pencil. Even the reacted patient should have his vital signs checked every 15 minutes for at least four times after arriving in his room. When the vital signs have been stable for some time, the doctor or the nurse may instruct that they be taken less frequently or discontinued. Most patients who have had major surgery will also have an IV running during the early post-operative period in order to supply the fluids that they are unable to take orally. An IV stand should be at the bedside to hold the bottle of fluids.

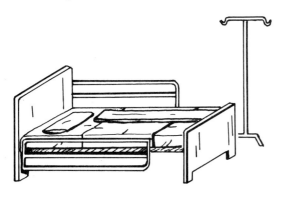
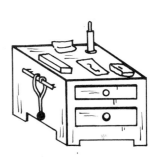

Other equipment may be needed at the bedside, depending upon the type of operation performed, or the patient's condition. The team leader, or the nurse in charge, will be able to tell you what may be needed. For instance, some patients will have a Levin tube that will be connected to a suction machine or wall suction outlet; some may have a urinary catheter which will need to be connected to a drainage set; some may need special traction or weights after orthopedic surgery; or, after tonsils have been removed, an ice pack to soothe the throat.

F. List seven items that should be placed in the patient's unit in order to provide post-operative care.

(1) _emesis bowl_   (3) _cellu wipes_   (5) _thermometer_   (7) _B/P equip_
(2) _paper pencil_   (4) _nursing record_   (6) _stethoscope_

U
N
I
T
35

G. The fully reacted patient who has arrived in his room from the Recovery room should have his vital signs checked every_____15_____minutes for at least_____four_____times.

ITEM 3.   PROCEDURE FOR PREPARING POST-OPERATIVE UNIT

In the skill laboratory, you should practice the procedure of collecting the required equipment and preparing the patient's bed so that post-operative care can be given to provide for his safety, reduce or prevent complications, and promote his recovery.

Important Steps	Key Points
1. Confer with your team leader or nurse in charge for special instructions.	The nurse may ask you to have special equipment or supplies at the bedside, based on her knowledge on the patient's condition and the type of surgical procedure being performed, e.g., a urine drainage set, throat or gastric suction machine, oxygen equipment or orthopedic appliances.
2. Collect the equipment and supplies needed and take them to the patient unit.	Use a utility cart to collect items and transport them to the unit. In preparing most post-operative units, you will need: Linen for the bed, including a rubber or plastic sheet and drawsheet; box of *Cellu-Wipes* or tissues; sphygmomanometer; stethoscope; nursing records; IV standard; and paper and pencil. A thermometer is usually in the patient unit; if not, be sure to take one with you.
3. Make the bed as a post-operative bed.	Follow the instructions given in the lesson on Bedmaking to prepare the post-operative bed. The top bedding should be folded to the side or the bottom of the bed, the rubber sheet and drawsheet used to protect the middle portion of the bed, and the pillow placed on the over-bed table or a chair. The bed should be equipped with siderails for safety.
4. Arrange the other items at the bedside.	Place the IV standard at the side or the foot of the bed. On the bedside stand, place the Cellu-Wipes, emesis basin, thermometer, sphygomanometer, stethoscope, and Intake and Output record. Arrange other special equipment, if needed.
5. Prepare for stretcher access to the bed.	Move furniture, such as chairs, out of the way so that there is a clear path at least 4 feet wide from the entrance of the room to the side of the bed to allow for the stretcher transporting the patient. It is often easier to transfer the patient from the stretcher to the bed if the bed is pulled out so that the head of the bed clears the front of the bedside stand.

ITEM 4.   CARDINAL RULES FOR POST-OPERATIVE CARE

1. *Maintain an open airway and adequate respiratory function.*

2. *Take vital signs until patient's condition is stable.*

3. *Record fluid intake and output.*

4. *Check the operative site for excessive drainage.*

5. *Provide for the patient's safety.*

6. *Provide for the patient's needs.*

Each of these cardinal rules will be explained in greater detail as we progress. The physiological needs of the surgical patient are of paramount importance. Once these needs are met, his psychological and social needs can be met. First things first; it does little good to help reduce the patient's anxiety about his job when he is hemorrhaging. Attend to the hemorrhage first, then the anxiety about the job.

ITEM 5.   MAINTAIN ADEQUATE RESPIRATORY FUNCTION

The patient must breathe and take in sufficient oxygen in order to live. Following surgery with anesthesia, the patient tends to have slow, shallow breathing. This is called hypoventilation, inasmuch as the volume of air in and out of the lungs is reduced. One result of hypoventilation is a reduction in the amount of oxygen available to the lungs. A dusky, bluish color to the fingernail beds is often the first indication of a lack of oxygen, and as it continues, the skin takes on a bluish tinge.

The patient's airway consists of the air passages in the head, the throat, and the chest. The parts of the airway are the nose, the pharynx, larynx, trachea, bronchi, and the lungs. The most common causes of obstruction of the airway are relaxation of the jaw and tongue so that the tongue falls back into the pharynx of the throat, and collection of secretions blocking the passage. The unconscious post-operative patient will usually have an airway inserted by the anesthetist to keep the tongue in place. An airway is shown in the sketch. Turning the patient's head to one side also keeps the tongue from falling back into the throat.

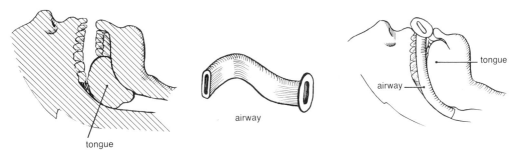

Tongue blocking pharynx.   Airway in place.

UNIT 35

Saliva, mucus, and other secretions often collect in the back of the unconscious patient's throat and interfere with breathing. Such secretions may be drawn into the lungs, where they cause irritation to the lung tissue and further interference with breathing. You can tell by the moist, rattling sounds of the patient's breathing whether secretions are obstructing his breathing. These should be suctioned from the mouth and throat as soon as possible. Again, the patient's head should be turned to one side, so that some of the secretions drain from the corner of the mouth.

To prevent other respiratory complications, the patient must be turned every two hours to relieve the pressure on the lungs so that all parts of the lung can expand with air. When the patient has reacted from the anesthesia, he should be encouraged to take at least five deep breaths, cough, and move his arms and legs every one to two hours. If the patient is unable to move himself, the nurse must give passive exercise.

H. Hypoventilation should be suspected when the patient (1) _Nail beds are blue_
skin dusty blue, and (2) _breathes shallow_

I. The unconscious patient should be turned every _two_ hours.

J. The common obstructions of the airway are (1) _accumulated_ and (2)
tongue falls back in throat. _Secretions_

K. Why is it advisable to turn the unconscious patient's head to one side?
So let the secretions drain & keep the
tongue from falling back in throat

ITEM 6. TAKE VITAL SIGNS UNTIL PATIENT'S CONDITION IS STABLE

The vital signs consist of the temperature, pulse, respiration, blood pressure, and the level of consciousness. In the post-operative patient, these are indicators of his physiological condition. A rise in temperature can be a sign of the body's response to injury, a sign of infection, or a sign of damage to part of the brain. The blood pressure reading and the pulse rate are indicators of the state of the circulatory system. Fluctuations in the blood pressure or the pulse may be the first signs of complications, such as shock or hemorrhage. The respiratory rate is a sign of the function and the ventilation of the lungs. The depth of respiration should also be noted in order to determine if there is hypoventilation. As the blood pressure rate decreases, the pulse and respiratory rates increase.

The level of consciousness should be recorded as part of the vital signs. Different levels of consciousness can be defined as unconscious, semi-conscious, disoriented, and awake (or conscious). The unconscious patient does not respond to stimuli and his reflexes are absent so that he is unable, for example, to swallow or to blink his eyes. General anesthesia produces unconsciousness and the patient should be observed constantly and should lie with his head turned to one side or have an airway in place until the swallowing reflex returns. The semi-conscious patient is able to respond to painful stimuli, move about restlessly, and swallow, but has difficulty comprehending or responding to oral stimuli (the spoken word). The disoriented patient may be able to respond to all stimuli, but is confused about persons, time, place, or events. The conscious (or awake) patient is able to respond to all stimuli with comprehension.

During the time the patient is recovering from anesthesia, the vital signs should be taken at least every 15 minutes and recorded. When the vital signs have been stable for one hour or longer, the doctor may order them taken at less frequent intervals. Stability of the vital signs is indicated by little or no change in the readings obtained from those of previous readings, and which are within the normal range for the patient. The normal range is determined by comparing the readings with those taken pre-operatively, or those recorded by the anesthetist during the operation.

L. Indicators of the patient's physiological condition may be obtained by (1) _temp_, (2) _pulse_, (3) _resp_, (4) _BP_, and (5) _level of consciousness_

M. Some changes in the function of the circulatory system are indicated by readings of (1) _pulse_, and (2) _respiration_

N. Stability of the vital signs means _little change from previous_ _readings & within normal range for patient_

ITEM 7. RECORD FLUID INTAKE AND OUTPUT

During surgery, the patient has lost blood and tissue fluid due to the nature of the surgical procedure. This loss is replaced either during surgery or in the early post-operative period in order to restore the body's fluid and electrolyte balance, and to promote the healing process. The doctor may order "Fluids orally as tolerated" for the patient who has had a spinal or a local type of anesthesia. Since the patient is conscious, he will ask for water while in the Recovery Room because his mouth is dry from the effects of the pre-operative medication. The water should be given in sips and small amounts in case his stomach has been upset by the surgery, medication, or anesthesia.

Intravenous fluids are given to many of the patients who are unconscious for several hours due to a general anesthesia, and to those patients who would have difficulty taking in enough oral fluids to replace the fluids lost in surgery. In taking care of the patient with an IV running, you should note whether the IV needle, or cannula, is in the vein and the arm carefully supported. Note also the rate of flow of the fluids, and whether the patient is to have another bottle of fluids to follow the current one. The rate of flow for the adult IV is 60 drops a minute, unless the doctor has specified a different rate. Blood transfusions may also be given post-operatively to replace blood lost during surgery. (If the surgeon expects a large blood loss, he may order a type and crossmatch [T and C] of a stated number of bottles of blood to be held in readiness for the patient should a blood transfusion be needed.) Except in unusual cases, the doctor will want to make sure that the patient's intake equals the amount of his output. During a 24-hour period, the average adult patient will put out 1200 ml. of urine, and lose another 800 to 1000 ml. of fluid through the skin and lungs. There is more rapid fluid loss from breathing when the airway is in place. If there is post-operative drainage from a Levin tube or the wound, additional fluid will be lost from the body. The patient's fluid intake should then be 2000 to 2200 ml. plus the amount lost as drainage.

The doctor's post-operative orders will state when the patient is allowed to take fluids orally and the type of diet to be given. If the patient has a gastrointestinal tube, or an IV connected, there may be an order for "Nothing by mouth (NPO)." The patient must not swallow fluids, but may relieve the parched mouth by rinsing it with water, or using a moistened cloth to sponge the lips.

It is very important that the kidneys continue to function and produce urine after surgery. Within 8 to 12 hours after surgery, the patient should void (discharge) urine. The kidneys should put out at least 30 ml. of urine an hour. If the patient has a catheter in place, check the drainage system at least every hour to see that the tubing is not kinked and that urine is draining through the tubing. If the patient is unable to void within 8 hours after surgery, be sure to report this to the nurse in charge at once.

All fluids taken in by the patient, whether orally or by IV, must be recorded on the Intake and Output record. All output, including urine, vomitus, and drainage, must be measured and recorded. The Intake and Output record provides one indication of the patient's fluid and electrolyte (chemical) balance to the doctor and the nurse. The nurse should always know about the patient's Intake and Output, regardless of whether this is a written order by the doctor or not. (*Note:* Some agencies may record the I and O on the nurse's notes. Follow your agency procedure.)

O. The amount of fluid lost through the lungs and skin, and that excreted as urine, total about ___2000-2200___ ml. a day for the adult.

P. The usual rate of flow for an IV is ___60___ drops per minute in the adult.

Q. You should report to the nurse if the patient has not voided in the ___8___ hour period following surgery.

ITEM 8. CHECK THE OPERATIVE SITE

When the patient is received from surgery or the Recovery Room, you should check the operative site as soon as possible. Look to see if the dressing over the wound is dry and in place so that it protects the wound. Some dressings may have a small amount of slightly bloody drainage on them, and it is important to check them frequently to see whether the bleeding continues or increases. Be sure to check the bed linen for signs of bleeding too. Cases have been known where the dressing appeared dry, but blood seeped under it and formed a pool beneath the dressing.

You should find out if the patient has tubes in place, and whether these are to remain clamped or connected to suction. The tubes should be secured to the bed in such a way that they do not pull on the patient, nor are they kinked or lying under the patient's body. The usual tubes are: the urinary catheter, which is attached to the urinary drainage tubing bottle; a Levin or other type of gastrointestinal tube attached to suction; oxygen in the form of a nasal tube; and various tubes or drains left in an incision to assist in the flow of drainage. (Commonly used drains would be catheters, Penrose, cigarette, etc.)

One word of caution: Do not change or reinforce a surgical dressing unless you are specifically instructed to do so by the doctor or the nurse in charge. Report to them about any bleeding or drainage which has soiled the dressing, because this may be a sign of complications.

R. The most common types of tubes the patient may have following surgery are (1) _Catheters_, (2) _N-S_____, and (3) _oxygen____.

S. _____ T __✗__ F If the patient's dressing is saturated with blood, you would apply a sterile dry dressing immediately.

ITEM 9. PROVIDE FOR THE PATIENT'S SAFETY

The pre-operative medication, the anesthesia, and the injury produced by the surgery all combine to reduce the patient's response to the stimuli in his environment. He is less aware of what is happening to him and what is occuring around him. He is dependent upon others to protect him from dangers at this time. The hospital and the nurse workers are legally responsible for protecting the patient and preventing harm to him. Assemble all needed equipment at the patient's bedside before he arrives from the operating room.

The patient who is not fully conscious, as well as the one who is under the influence of medication, needs protection from harm. These patients can respond to some stimuli, yet they are not fully awake or aware of dangers. They, as well as the unconscious patient, should have a nurse worker in constant attendance during the early post-operative period. This means that you must be in the room where you can readily see the patient and be at his side to help him within a second or so.

You should make it a habit to use siderails on the bed for the post-operative patient. Siderails help prevent the patient from falling out of bed, especially when he is not fully aware of his surroundings. If the patient is extremely restless, it may be helpful to attach a safety belt around his waist and to the mattress support of the bed. (The safety belt, or similar restraining device, should not be attached to the movable frame because raising the head or foot of the bed will squeeze the patient unduly.) In some Recovery Rooms, post-operative patients are kept on stretchers instead of being transferred into a bed. These stretchers should be equipped with siderails and safety belts to be used for the patient's security. Siderails also can be used to assist the patient in turning, by holding one siderail while turning self toward it.

Frequently changing the patient's position is another way of providing for his safety. You should know and use the procedures to immobilize or support parts of the body, and to reduce pressure areas in the post-operative positioning: (a) no head pillow is used for the unconscious patient or for 8 hours following a spinal anesthesia, and (b) the patient's head is turned to one side when in the supine position so that secretions can drain from the mouth, and the tongue cannot fall back into the throat to block the air passages.

One of the most important ways to provide for the patient's safety is to prevent the possibility of infection. The patient's resistance to infection is decreased due to surgery. You can reduce the possibility of infection by washing your hands before and after working with each patient, by maintaining sterility around the incisional wound, by turning the patient frequently to prevent respiratory infections, and by avoiding contact with patients when you yourself have a cold, sore throat, boils, or other type of infectious disease.

T. To reduce the possibility of danger or harm to the post-operative patient, you would take the following steps:

(1) _Siderails up_ (2) _Constant atten._ (3) _frequent change of position_ (4) _prevent infection_

U. Which of the following statements refers to measures providing for the patient's safety?

___1. Close observation of the patient to help maintain his respiratory and circulatory functions.

___2. When turning the patient who is receiving an IV, care is taken to prevent dislodging the IV needle from the vein.

___3. After assisting the patient to use the bed-pan for voiding, the nurse washes her hands before taking vital signs of patient.

___4. Every two hours, the nurse assists and encourages the reacted patient to breathe deeply, to cough, and to turn.

ITEM 10. PROVIDE FOR THE PATIENT'S NEEDS

As the patient begins to respond from the anesthesia, he needs reassurance from the nurse and orientation as to time, person, and place. You may need to repeat the reassurances several times, for although the patient reacts and seems to talk rationally, the medications and anesthesia reduce his ability to remember. He needs to be reassured that the operation is over, that he is doing well, that you are there to watch over him closely, that he is in the Recovery Room (or his own room), and even what day it is or the time of day.

When caring for the patient still under the effects of anesthesia, *Do not* slap the patient's face, yell at him or shake him in an effort to make him react or arouse him more quickly. The response you get from the patient is not a true awakening from anesthesia, but a defensive response by the patient to avoid pain or hurt. The patient's body needs time to break down the chemicals in the medications and anesthesia and to begin to excrete or get rid of them before he can emerge from their effects.

During the post-operative period, the patient will need your assistance for his personal hygiene. He should be encouraged to take care of many of his hygienic and personal needs as he gains strength in the days following surgery. On the day after surgery, the patient may be able to brush his teeth and wash his face and arms without becoming over-fatigued or uncomfortable. You will need to provide the supplies, water, towels, and to finish bathing him. During the patient's bath period, you should see that his joints are put through the range-of-motion exercises. When the patient is resting in bed, his body should be in good alignment, with supportive aids to maintain good position, and with protective aids to reduce and prevent formation of pressure areas.

It is common practice to get the patient out of bed hours after surgery, instead of keeping him in bed for prolonged periods, which may add to his discomfort and delay his recovery. These harmful effects were discussed in the lesson on Patient Movement and Ambulation. You should remain with the patient the first few times that he is out of bed. Assist him to dangle his feet at the side of the bed for a few minutes so that his circulatory system can adjust to his change of position. When he no longer feels dizzy or light-headed, assist him to stand, take a few steps and sit in a chair. In the post-operative orders, the patient's doctor will specify when the patient is to be ambulated, how often, for how long a period of time, or with any limitations.

The patient will suffer from various discomforts following surgery, the most common of which are pain, abdominal distention and "gas pains," nausea, vomiting, and constipation. He may also develop complications and must be observed closely for signs of these. The post-operative discomforts and complications are discussed in greater detail in the following items.

V. As the patient reacts from the anesthesia, you give _reassurance_ and _orientation_ by saying, for example, "The operation is over and I'm staying with you to take care of you now."

W. The patient is performing active _ROM_ of his arm and shoulder as he brushes his teeth the day after surgery.

X. In the days following his surgery, you will observe the patient closely for signs of _discomforts_ or _complication_

UNIT 35

ITEM 11. SHOCK AS A COMPLICATION

Every post-operative patient should be treated as though he might develop shock at any time. Shock is the body's response to inadequate circulation due to a variety of causes. In the post-operative patient, the stress of going to surgery, the anesthesia, the amount of blood loss (even when there is practically no blood loss), and the injury from the incision itself can lead to shock. Progressive and prolonged shock leads to death, so the faster the state of shock can be reversed, the better the patient's chances for a recovery. Unless circulation is restored, damage may occur in the brain, kidneys, or other organs due to the lack of blood and oxygen. With prompt and adequate treatment, the patient usually recovers from shock.

The most common cause of shock in the post-operative patient is the loss of blood. Other causes of shock may be: (a) faulty pumping of the heart, as in a myocardial infarction, or heart attack; (b) dilation of some blood vessels so that they become engorged and the blood does not move along rapidly enough to be part of the circulating volume; (c) an insult (injury) to the nervous system; (d) severe, strong emotional response such as extreme fear of pain; (e) infections which overwhelm the body's defenses, and (f) excessive blood loss from hemorrhage.

The signs of shock are related to the effects of the inadequate circulation. The symptoms are:

Skin: pale color, clammy to the touch.

Blood Pressure: progressive, consistent fall in pressure. This is the earliest change to signify shock.

Pulse: rapid (often over 120 beats per minute), thready, or feels quivery.

Respirations: very rapid and shallow, often grunting type as if hungry for air.

Cyanosis: blueness of fingernail beds or lips due to lack of oxygen; use inner lip for detection in a dark-skinned person.

Urine output: scanty or absent because of decreased circulation through the kidneys.

At the onset of shock, the patient may be anxious and apprehensive. As the state of shock progresses, he becomes listless, and finally becomes unconscious as the shock deepens. The early signs of impending shock are apprehension, a rapid and thready pulse, and air hunger. Profound shock is characterized by a change in the level of consciousness, profuse sweating, and very markedly low blood pressure.

Y. The body's response to _inadequate circulation_ is the condition known as shock.

Z. In the post-operative patient, the most usual cause of shock is _loss of blood_.

AA. A patient going into shock would have (1) _pale, clammy_ (2) _cyanosis_, and (3) _resp. rapid & shallow_ _skin_

BB. As you take the vital signs of the patient, you suspect he may be going into shock because he seems anxious, there is an increase in the _pulse_ and a decrease in the _BP_ in the last three recorded readings.

ITEM 12. THE TREATMENT OF SHOCK

The best treatment for shock is prevention and early recognition. Shock can be prevented by careful physiological and psychological preparation of the patient for surgery. Post-operatively, it can be prevented by replacing the blood and fluid loss, careful movement of the patient, judicious (careful) use of drugs that depress circulation or respiration, retaining body warmth with light covers and a warm room. (However *do not* apply external heat directly to the body because this dilates superficial blood vessels in the skin and further reduces deep circulation.) Keep patient in flat position, and provide for his sense of security through skillful care in a calm, quiet atmosphere. Early signs of shock are detected by carefully observing the patient and his vital signs.

If your observations indicate that the patient may be going into shock, you should *immediately* summon help and report the signs to the nurse so that the doctor can be notified. *Do not leave the room.* The team leader or the nurse in charge may instruct you to remain with the patient to calm and reassure him, or she may care for the patient and ask you to collect the supplies and equipment that will be needed.

You can help in the treatment of shock. Keep the patient warm by providing additional blankets and help put him in Trendelenburg (shock) position by mechanically elevating the foot of the bed or placing it on shock blocks. Exceptions: patients who are recovering from a spinal anesthesia or who have had brain surgery *must not* be placed in shock position, *but should be kept flat*. The doctor will order replacement of blood or fluids, so that if the patient does not have an IV running, you should have the equipment ready. He may also order the use of oxygen and various drugs to treat the shock. Close observation of the patient and his vital signs is essential until he has recovered from shock.

CC. When you observe signs of shock in your patient, what is the first thing you should do? *Immediately report it to the nurse, do not leave the room*

DD. Shock in the post-operative patient is best treated by *prevention* and *early detection*

EE. The treatment of shock by the nurse-doctor team, in which you also participate, consists of:

(1) *shock position* (2) *added warmth* (3) *replace blood or fluids*
(4) *oxygen* (5) *drugs* (6) *close observation*

ITEM 13. OTHER CIRCULATORY COMPLICATIONS

Hemorrhage can occur as a complication in the immediate post-operative period, and the loss of blood has been mentioned as one cause of shock. With external hemorrhage, the bleeding is visible. The other symptoms of hemorrhage are the same as shock since the volume of blood in circulation is reduced: pale color, anxiety or apprehension, rapid pulse, and lower blood pressure. In addition to taking the vital signs (BP then P), the dressings, drainage, and the bedding of the post-operative patient should be inspected frequently for signs of bleeding. Dark-brownish color of the blood in drainage or on dressings indicates that the bleeding occurred some time ago, while bright red blood is a sign of fresh bleeding. Report the color and the amount to the charge nurse and record on the patient's chart.

The treatment for hemorrhage is (a) to stop the bleeding, and (b) to treat the shock. If your patient starts to hemorrhage, you should call for help immediately, notify the nurse in charge and the doctor, attempt to staunch (or stop) the bleeding if possible (some patients may have to return to surgery so that the doctor can stop internal bleeding), and treat the shock. Place the patient in a flat position or a shock position, provide additional blankets if necessary, and collect the supplies and equipment needed to replace the blood loss with IV's or transfusion.

Another complication is that long word "thrombophlebitis" (thrombo = blood clot, phleb = vein, = itis = inflammation). It is an inflammation of the vein and commonly occurs in the leg, which has a sluggish blood flow that leads to the formation of a clot. The condition may be caused by the patient's prolonged inactivity, especially of his legs, or pressure caused by a pillow under the knees, or a tight strap around the arm or leg that restricts venous circulation. The symptoms are pain, heat, redness, and swelling around the affected area of the leg. The treatment given is complete bed rest, elevation of the limb, warm wet packs applied to the area, and drugs as ordered by the doctor. Thrombophlebitis is not as common a complication today since post-operative patients are encouraged to move and ambulate early.

The most dreaded consequence of thrombophlebitis is a possibility that the blood clot may become dislodged from the vein and travel through the bloodstream to the heart and the lungs. This is called a cardiac or pulmonary embolism, which at its best produces pain and an extended period of illness, but at its worst causes sudden collapse and death. The symptoms are severe chest pain, cough, and difficulty in breathing. Because of the danger and possible tragedy from pulmonary embolism, all efforts should be made to prevent thrombophlebitis and embolism in the bloodstream. Preventive measures include exercise of the legs, wrapping them with elastic bandages, and slight elevation of the foot of the bed to improve venous return of blood. Because of the danger of dislodging possible clots, one good rule to remember is: *Avoid rubbing or massage of legs, even as a comfort measure.*

FF.   Mr. Smith had an operation on his stomach three hours ago. Which of the following statements would lead you to suspect that he may be hemorrhaging? More than one answer may be correct.

     ____ (1)   You notice more dark, reddish-brown drainage on his abdominal dressing.

     ____ (2)   He has started moving restlessly from side to side, his eyes seem to roll around, and he is moaning.

     ____ (3)   In the last few minutes, the Levin tube has filled with bright red drainage.

     ____ (4)   His IV fluids have slowed down to a rate of 20 drops per minute.

     ____ (5)   His pulse is now 116 beats per minute, but had been around 60 to 80 in surgery.

GG.   The day after surgery, Mr. Smith asked you to put a pillow under his knees to ease the strain on his abdomen, and also wanted you to rub his legs because they seemed sore. What would you do and why? *Would not — danger of thrombus + emboli explain better to exercise*

HH.   What measures can you take to prevent thrombophlebitis from becoming a complication for Mr. Smith? *encourage movement + exercise of the legs*

ITEM 14.   RESPIRATORY COMPLICATIONS

The most common post-operative complications are respiratory problems, and these occur more often than all the others combined. Hypoventilation is the underlying factor in all respiratory complications. In hypoventilation, the breathing is slow and shallow so that a smaller amount of air is taken into the lungs. Portions of the lungs do not receive enough air to expand all of the air sacs so that the scene is set for complications to develop. The treatment of hypoventilation consists of nursing measures that increase the respiratory function: deep breathing, coughing to clear mucus from the passages, and frequent turning to relieve pressure on the lungs and to allow lung expansion. Without treatment, hypoventilation may progress so that there is cyanosis (from decreased oxygen and increase of carbon dioxide) which lowers the heart output, shock, and apnea (or cessation of respiration).

Post-operative or hypostatic, pneumonia is a common complication of hypoventilation. Air sacs in the lungs which are not expanded with air become filled with fluid or they collapse. They become a fertile field for the growth of viruses and germs which cause inflammation of the lung or pneumonia. Decreased respiratory function and the possibility of infection occur when the air sacs are plugged with bits of mucus in a condition called atelectasis. The treatment of both pneumonia and atelectasis includes ventilating the lungs and administering antibiotics or other drugs.

II.   The underlying cause for all respiratory complications is *Hypoventilation*

JJ.   To increase the post-operative patient's respiratory function, you should assist and encourage him to (1) *breathe deep* (2) *cough* and (3) *turn frequently*

KK.   Two complications that result from decreased respiratory functions are (1) *pneumonia* and (2) *atelectasia*

ITEM 15. WOUND COMPLICATIONS

The two types of wound complications are infections and the breaking open of the incision. During recent years, some organisms have emerged that are resistant to the action of various antibiotics. It is still very important to prevent wound infections because the use of antibiotics may prove ineffective in treating the infection. Prevention of infections of the wound depends on careful handwashing, scrupulous cleaning of equipment, the use of sterile supplies, and the use of aseptic techniques by the nurse.

The first sign of wound infection is increased pain in the incision. In normal recovery, pain decreases each day. The incision shows signs of infection by becoming reddened, warm, swollen, and in draining pus-like material. If a patient develops a wound infection, it is important to prevent the spread of the infection to others. The treatment prescribed by the doctor may include antibiotics to fight the infection, drainage of the pus, and often, application of wet or dry heat.

Wound separation, where the edges of the incision break apart, may occur in some patients during the sixth to eighth day after surgery. The causes of wound separation are malnutrition (which interferes with the normal healing process), defective suturing, and excessive strain on the wound from retching, coughing spasms, etc. When the wound separates completely so that body organs (viscera) are exposed, the condition is called evisceration. Usually the patient will feel that something has "broken loose," or "given way." You should have the patient stay at complete bed rest, inspect the dressing for pinkish drainage, look to see if the wound has separated, relieve strain on the wound, and reassure the patient by saying that you would like the doctor to check his dressing. The nurse in charge and the doctor should be notified immediately. If there is evisceration of the wound, the nurse will cover the wound with a sterile dressing moistened with sterile saline solution to protect the exposed organ.

LL. Antibiotics have been so miraculous in curing so many infections; why is it necessary to go to all the trouble of cleaning and sterilizing equipment and using aseptic technique to prevent infections?
Many organism may be resistant to antibodies

MM. Wound infections produce inflammation; the symptoms of inflammation are:

(1) _pain_   (2) _redness_   (3) _heat_
(4) _swollen_   (5) _drainage of pus_

NN. Evisceration means the exposure of _an organ_

ITEM 16. DISCOMFORTS FOLLOWING SURGERY

Most post-operative patients experience some type of discomfort following surgery. The common discomforts are pain, nausea and vomiting, abdominal distention with "gas pains," and constipation. Although the discomforts are less serious than the complications of surgery, the patient may feel miserable unless they are promptly and effectively relieved.

Pain. A certain amount of pain is expected after surgery and the most severe pain occurs during the first 48 hours. It will normally decrease with each passing day. The doctor's orders for post-operative care prescribe the medication to be given for pain. However, there are things you can do to help relieve the pain. The patient should be made comfortable by assisting him to turn or change his position, by giving a backrub, etc. When a patient complains of pain, you should try to find out what kind of pain and the probable cause. If it is pain in the operative site, he should have his medication promptly because minutes seem like hours if he has to wait. Often a lesser amount of medication will be needed if given promptly. If pain persists over a period of time, a larger dose usually will be needed. Often you will find that the patient has less pain if he can talk about his worries and anxieties. The patient may resist turning, doing his exercises, or getting up during the first few days when pain is severe. You should discuss with the team leader the best time for assisting the patient with these activities in relation to his medication for pain.

Nausea and Vomiting. Vomiting is less a post-operative problem today than it was some years ago when ether was the main agent used in general anesthesia. Ether is still used but not to the extent it was in the past. Although the patient may not have vomiting, most patients will have some nausea and lack of appetite after surgery.

One of the goals for the post-operative patient is to regain the normal function of his gastrointestinal tract as soon as possible. Most patients will begin to take food and fluids within a short time after recovering from the anesthesia. You can help to overcome nausea and vomiting by the following actions: begin by giving the patient small sips of liquid. Tap water (not ice water), tea, or ginger ale are tolerated best, although small children may want only milk. If the patient seems nauseated, suggest that he take several deep breaths through his mouth until the feeling passes. Abrupt movements should be avoided. If the fluids are retained, the patient may take more. When his meal tray arrives, he should be encouraged to taste the food even if he does not have an appetite. If he is nauseated, the sight of a tray of food may lead to vomiting, and therefore it would be better to ask him in advance if he would like to try one or two items from the tray, and then take only those in to him.

Abdominal Distention and Flatus. The distention of the abdomen with flatus occurs as a result of a hypoactive bowel. Medications, anesthesia, handling of the bowel in some types of surgery, inactivity following surgery, and change in diet habits all contribute to the hypoactive bowel.

The accumulation of swallowed air and the flatus cause the patient's abdomen to become swollen and painful. Narcotics tend to enhance distention by decreasing bowel activity. The doctor usually prescribes the use of a rectal tube, enema, Harris flush, or medication to stimulate the passage of flatus to relieve the distention. You can help relieve the discomforts of distention by assisting the patient to turn frequently, or to get up if he is allowed to do so. Iced liquids seem to aggravate the flatus, but hot liquids and some solid food help to reduce it. When the rectal tube is used, remember to remove it after 30 minutes, then clean it; it can be reinserted in an hour or so if the patient continues to be uncomfortable.

Constipation. When the surgical procedure has been a minor one, the patient will probably experience no change in his bowel habits. However, some patients will not have a normal bowel movement until the third or fourth day after surgery, due to decreased intake of food and fluids, less movement and exercise, and because of the hypoactive bowel. Narcotics and other medications, anesthesia, and surgery all contribute to decreased activity of the bowel.

You can help the patient who is troubled by constipation by encouraging him to eat a diet with normal amounts of roughage, to drink a large amount of fluids, to get some form of exercise, and to walk about if able. Provide privacy and time when he is attempting to move his bowels. An enema or a suppository may be given when ordered by the doctor.

Other Discomforts. Less frequently, the patient may develop (1) *parotitis*, (2) *urinary retention*, or (3) *hiccups* (singultus) during the post-operative period, and these can be just as distressing as the problems already discussed.

Parotitis is an inflammation of one or more of the salivary glands and is seen in patients who have not eaten or taken fluids orally for a period of time, or who have not had good mouth care frequently and have thus lacked stimulation of the salivary gland. Prevention is accomplished by frequent mouth care.

Urinary retention is the inability to void or to empty the bladder when voiding does occur. Small, frequent voidings are often a sign of overflow from a full and distended bladder. To assist the patient to empty his bladder, position, privacy, a high fluid intake, and reassurance are all important.

Having the patient breathe into a paper bag will often relieve hiccups, but persistent hiccups require more vigorous treatment prescribed by the doctor.

OO. Almost without exception, the post-operative patient will experience the discomfort of _pain_.

PP. The depressing action of drugs and anesthesia given the patient causes hypoactivity of the bowel and contributes to the discomforts of _abd distention_ and _constipation_.

QQ. The patient had surgery about ten hours ago and is allowed to take fluids and diet as tolerated, but continues to have moderate nausea. Some actions you might take to reduce the patient's nausea are:

(1) _sips of fluids_ (2) _preferred liquids_ (3) _deep breaths thru_

(4) _rest quietly_ (5) _after only food mouth_

he thinks he can eat

ITEM 17. CONCLUSION OF THE LESSON

You have now completed the lesson on post-operative care of the surgical patient. After sufficient practice in the skill laboratory, you should be able to collect the necessary equipment and prepare the patient's unit for his arrival following surgery so that there is no delay in giving him care. Your responsibility for the patient is based on the cardinal rules of post-operative care, knowledge of ways to identify and prevent complications, and ways to reduce the patient's discomforts through nursing measures.

You should now make an appointment with your instructor and arrange to take the post-test. After that, you should be able to use your beginning skills to provide safe and effective nursing care to the post-op patient in the clinical area.

IV. ADDITIONAL INFORMATION FOR ENRICHMENT

Post-operative care of the patient is a rich and rewarding field of study. It is complicated by the wide variety of special needs, precautions, and procedures that are used depending on the type of surgery performed and the condition of the patient. Those of you who are interested may wish to read and learn more about the nursing care of the patient after surgery has disrupted the function of a particular organ or system of the body. For instance, you may wish to investigate the special nursing care requirements of the patient following a kidney transplant, a knee operation for torn cartilages, removal of a brain tumor, or the amputation of a limb or breast. In each case, the surgery has interfered with the function of a body part or a system, and the post-operative emphasis is on assisting the patient to regain, maintain, or adapt to a change in this function. The lesson you have just completed provides the basic framework for *all* post-op care, but it has not been possible to cover all the special variations.

As you take care of post-op patients in the clinical setting, you may want to read more about their particular needs. Textbooks on surgical nursing are quite detailed concerning the nursing care, and articles in various journals provide sources of up-to-date information. To start you on your reading, you may want to select a few articles listed below, most of which are in the *American Journal of Nursing.*

1. Transplants of organs:

Bois, Marna, *et al.*, "The Patient with a Kidney Transplant," *American Journal of Nursing,* 68:1238-1247, June 1968.

Taylor, Karleen, Nancy Commons, and Mary Sue Jacks, "Liver Transplant," *American Journal of Nursing,* 68:1895-1899, Sept. 1969.

Topor, Michele, "Nusing and Renal Transplant Patient," *Nursing Clinics of North America.*

2. Post-operative discomforts and complications:

Gardner, Arlene M., "Responsiveness as a Measure of Consciousness," *American Journal of Nursing,* 68:1034-1038, May 1968.

3. Nursing care related to heart and blood vessel (cardiovascular) surgery:

Betson, Carol, Patricia Valoon, and Cynthia Soika, "Cardiac Surgery in Neonates: A Chance for Life," *American Journal of Nursing,* 69:69-73, Jan. 1969.

Breslau, Roger, "Intensive Care Following Vascular Surgery," *American Journal of Nursing.* 68:1670-1676 Aug. 1968.

Coleman, Doris, "Surgical Alleviation of Coronary Artery Disease," *American Journal of Nursing,* 68:763-766, April 1968.

Hunn, Virginia K., "Cardiac Pacemakers," *American Journal of Nursing,* 69:749-754, April 1969.

4. Nursing care related to head and neck surgery:

Dison, Norma, "A Mother's View of Tonsillectomy," *American Journal of Nursing,* 68:1024-1027, May 1969.

Pitorak, Elizabeth F., "Laryngectomy," *American Journal of Nursing,* 68:787-791, April 1968.

5. Nursing care related to surgery of other systems and cancer:

Boegli, Emily, and Mary Steele, "Scoliosis: Spinal Instrumentation and Fusion," *American Journal of Nursing,* 68:2399-2403, Nov. 1968.

Svoboda, Emma, "Wilms' Tumor and Neuroblastoma: The Child Under Treatment," *American Journal of Nursing,* 68:532-535, Mar. 1968.

Seaman, Florence W., "Nursing Care of Glaucoma Patients," *Nursing Clinics of North America,* Sept. 1970, pp. 489-496.

Formation of Thrombus and Embolus

You may be interested in learning how the blood forms a thrombus within the blood vessel. Without going into the complex clotting mechanisms of blood, we can consider the physical conditions which are involved.

The causes of blood clotting within blood vessels are: (1) a roughened surface of the vessel, or (b) the slow movement of blood through the vessels. The slow movement of blood allows the clotting factors which are always being formed to concentrate in one area rather than being dispersed in the blood flow. Once the clotting begins, the clot tends to promote further clotting, so that it grows in size.

Some elements of the circulatory system need to be considered. The blood circulation is a closed system — that is, there are no normal openings between the system and the outside of the body. The heart pumps blood from its chambers by contracting, and the force increases pressure that speeds the blood along through the vessels. The heart rests for a fraction of a second, then pumps again to send out more blood under pressure. This second contraction, rest, contraction action causes the beat of the pulse that you can feel in various parts of the body. The action can be compared to a roller coaster. The cars approach the starting point (the heart); the first car fills with people (picks up oxygen); it is given a push onto the course (contraction of the heart); it speeds down the declines, swoops around the curves, labors up the inclines (blood circulates through the body), and then it returns to the starting place while other cars follow it around the course. The process is then repeated.

Now let's see what happens to the roller coaster car when the track near one of the curves is slightly larger than the wheels of the car (roughened surface of the vessel). The car slows down and unless it had sufficient speed to begin with, it will stop, causing the cars behind it to slow and stop (formation of a clot). Or the car runs out of energy or power and goes slowly until it comes to an incline, then travels even more slowly or stops. Cars following it are slowed, stopped, and unable to pass (formation of a clot). The formation of a blood clot in a vessel is shown in the following figure.

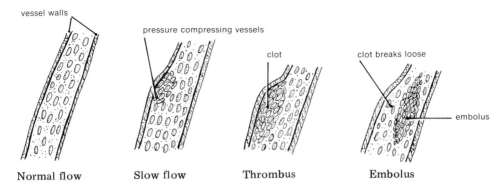

vessel walls

pressure compressing vessels

clot

clot breaks loose

embolus

Normal flow   Slow flow   Thrombus   Embolus

The immobility of the surgical patient slows the rate of his blood flow. This sluggish flow of blood is further aggravated by bed rest and the former practice of putting pillows under the knees. Blood flowing slowly through the legs will begin the clotting process within a matter of a few hours.

Clots (thrombi) have been known to grow in size and length until they are the length of the leg itself. When a portion of the clot breaks loose from the wall of the vessel, it becomes an embolus and circulates until it reaches a vessel too small to pass through. If that vessel is a vital one, such as those in the lungs, brain, or heart, sudden death of tissues occurs. There are certain drugs available for treatment which interfere with and retard the clotting process when thrombus or embolus formation is suspected.

WORKBOOK ANSWER SHEET

Introduction	P. 714	A.	(1) deliberate injury to body
			(2) reduced response to stimuli (may be transposed)
		B.	(1) helping
			(2) caring (may be transposed)
		C.	doctor's orders
Item #1	P. 714	D.	his own unit or room
		E.	reacted
Item #2	P. 715	F.	listed in any order: Cellu-Wipes or tissues, emesis basin, thermometer, stethoscope, sphygmomanometer, Intake and Output record, and IV standard.
		G.	every 15 minutes; four
Item #5	P. 717	H.	(1) breathes shallowly
			(2) has bluish tinge to nails or skin (may be transposed)
	P. 717	I.	two
	P. 717	J.	(1) accumulated secretions
			(2) tongue falling back in throat (may be transposed)
		K.	to help secretions drain and keep tongue from falling back into the throat.
Item #6	P. 718	L.	(1) blood pressure
			(2) temperature
			(3) respirations
			(4) pulse
			(5) level of consciousness (any order)
		M.	(1) blood pressure
			(2) pulse (any order)
	P. 718	N.	little change from previous readings and within normal range for the patient.
Item #7	P. 719	O.	2000 to 2200
		P.	60 drops
	P. 719	Q.	8 hour
Item #8	P. 720	R.	(1) urine catheter
			(2) Levin or naso-gastric tube
			(3) oxygen (any order)
		S.	False

Item #9   P. 720   T. (1) constant attention until fully conscious

                           (2) keep siderails up

                           (3) frequent change of position

                           (4) prevent infections

                       U. All four answers are correct

Item #10   P. 721   V. reassurance; orientation

                       W. range-of-motion

                       X. discomforts; complications

Item #11   P. 722   Y. inadequate blood circulation

                       Z. blood loss

            P. 722   AA. (1) rapid, thready pulse

                           (2) apprehension

                           (3) air hunger (any order)

                       BB. pulse rate; blood pressure

Item #12   P. 722   CC. summon help

                       DD. prevention; early detection (any order)

            Pp. 722 and 723   EE. (1) added warmth (any order)

                               (2) shock position

                               (3) replacement of blood or fluids

                               (4) oxygen

                               (5) drugs

                               (6) close observation of patient

Item #13   P. 723   FF. answers (3) and (5)

            P. 724   GG. I would not use a pillow under his knees or rub his legs because of the danger of thrombus and emboli. I would explain that it would be better to exercise his legs, change his position.

            P. 724   HH. Encourage movement and exercise, especially of the legs.

Item #14   P. 724   II. Hypoventilation

            P. 724   JJ. (1) breathe deeply

                           (2) cough

                           (3) turn frequently (any order)

                       KK. (1) pneumonia

                           (2) atelectasis   (any order)

U
N
I
T
35

Item #15   P. 725   LL. Many organisms have become resistant to anti-biotics.

MM. (1) pain

(2) redness

(3) heat

(4) swelling

(5) drainage of pus (any order)

NN. an organ

Item #16   P. 725   OO. pain

P. 726   PP. abdominal distention; constipation (any order)

QQ. (1) give sips of fluid

(2) give preferred liquids if allowed

(3) have patient take deep breaths through his mouth

(4) have patient rest quietly

(5) offer only the food he thinks he could eat. (any order)

POST-TEST

Matching Test

Select a word from List I which most closely means the same as the phrase in List II. Not all of the words in List I will be used. Place the letter from List I in the space provided.

List I   List II

A. unconscious   _F_ 1. reduced amount of air inhaled into the lungs.

B. thrombus   _D_ 2. a device to keep the tongue from falling back into the throat.

C. cannula
                        _J_ 3. a clot circulating within the blood vessels.
D. airway
                        _G_ 4. the bluish-tinged color of the skin and nails.
E. atelectasis
                        _I_ 5. inadequate circulation of blood.
F. hypoventilation
                        _B_ 6. a blood clot formed in the inner wall of a blood vessel.
G. cyanosis
                        _A_ 7. unresponsive to all stimuli.
H. antisepsis
                        _L_ 8. state of being unaware of pain.
I. shock
                        _E_ 9. blockage of air sacs in the lungs with mucus.
J. embolus
                        _M_ 10. excessive amount of bleeding.
K. apnea

L. anesthesia

M. hemorrhage

Multiple Choice Test

For each of the following situations, you are to select the one best answer to the question. Place a check mark in the space provided for the answer that you select.

Your patient, Mr. Blake, has gone to surgery to have an operation for a bleeding duodenal ulcer. Your team leader has assigned you to prepare Mr. Blake's unit for his return and has mentioned that he will probably have a Levin tube in place. In setting up his unit and bed for post-operative care you would provide:

11. ___ a.   an Output record to keep track of all drainage from the Levin tube.

___ b.   extra blankets and hot water bottles to conserve his body heat in case of shock.

___ c.   an extra airway you could insert to keep his tongue from blocking the air passages.

___ d.   a suction machine to withdraw drainage from the stomach or upper bowel.

After the operation, Mr. Blake is taken to the recovery room. He has had a general anesthesia and while unconscious, he would:

12. ___ a.   need the nurse's assistance to cough.

___ b.   be unaware of any stimuli.

___ c.   react to stimuli, but feel no pain.

___ d.   be unable to swallow salivary secretions.

The nurses in the recovery room have started their post-op care of Mr. Blake. The *first* observations they would make would be:

13. ___ a. see that he is breathing.

___ b. take the blood pressure and pulse.

___ c. observe the level of consciousness.

___ d. inspect the dressings for bleeding.

The recovery room nurse noticed that Mr. Blake's vital signs at the end of the operation were: B.P. 124/80, P. 84, and R. 16. Now, a half hour later, the vital signs are B.P. 118/80, P. 92, and R. 10. From these readings, the nurse would suspect that Mr. Blake may be:

14. ___ a. bleeding internally.

___ b. in early stage of shock.

___ c. developing a thrombus.

___ d. under-ventilating his lungs.

As part of Mr. Blake's care in the Recovery Room, the nurse has taken his vital signs every 15 minutes, checked the dressing which has remained dry, and noted the dark, greenish-brown drainage from the Levin tube. Now, Mr. Blake has become more restless, moving his arms, and moaning. As he groggily opened his eyes several times and started to spit out the airway in his mouth, the nurse would know that:

15. ___ a. she should remind him to leave the airway in place.

___ b. he is restless because of pain and should have medication.

___ c. he is beginning to react from the anesthesia.

___ d. his restlessness is a symptom of impending shock.

Mr. Blake is now waking up, and the nurse hastens to reassure him by saying, "Your operation is over, and you are in the Recovery Room. I'm Miss Jones and I'm taking care of you." In addition, Miss Jones would also ask him:

16. ___ a. to keep his head turned to one side so secretions would drain out of his mouth.

___ b. to take several deep breaths, cough, and move his legs in the exercises.

___ c. whether he is thirsty, and what type of fluid he would prefer to drink.

___ d. to lie quietly so that the Levin tube and the dressing on the incision would not be disturbed.

The nurse helps turn Mr. Blake to his side and he dozes off. The reason the nurse turned him was:

17. ___ a. to help make him more comfortable.

___ b. to relieve pressure areas on his back.

___ c. to promote the expansion of the lungs.

___ d. all of the above.

A short time later, Mr. Blake complained of pain and was given medication for it, because he had fully reacted from the anesthesia and his vital signs were quite stable. Stable vital signs indicate that:

18. ___ a. there was no change from the previous reading.

___ b. there were no post-op complications or discomforts.

___ c. the readings were within the patient's normal range.

___ d. there is rapid recovery from the general anesthesia.

You have been notified that Mr. Blake is being transferred from the Recovery Room to his own unit. When he arrives, you notice that he is very relaxed from the medication and that he has an IV still running in one arm. As you help settle him in his bed, you would be careful to:

19. ___ a. avoid dislodging the IV needle from the vein.

___ b. elevate the knees of the bed to prevent strain on abdominal muscles.

___ c. raise the siderails before leaving the bedside.

___ d. take his vital signs every 15 minutes for one hour.

___ e. all except b.

___ f. all except c.

Now that Mr. Blake is back in his room, it is important that you:

20. ___ a. check his condition frequently.

___ b. stay with him constantly until the IV is completed.

___ c. help him to turn, cough, and breathe deeply every 4 hours.

___ d. massage his back and legs as a comfort measure.

It is now nearly 8 hours since Mr. Blake had his surgery. You offer him a urinal and ask him to void. The reason for doing this:

21. ___ a. you need to write down the amount as output on the Intake and Output Record.

___ b. distention of his bladder with urine causes him additional discomfort and pain.

___ c. you want to make sure his kidneys are putting out urine following the surgery.

___ d. the doctor needs to know how long to keep him on IV fluids.

Since Mr. Blake returned to his room, you have assisted him to turn and encouraged him to breathe deeply, to cough, and to move his legs at least every 2 hours. By coughing, Mr. Blake will be less likely to develop the post-op complication of:

22. ___ a. embolus.

___ b. pneumonia.

___ c. shock.

___ d. hemorrhage.

By moving his legs every 2 hours, he is less likely to develop the complication of:

23. ___ a. pain.

___ b. shock.

___ c. thrombus.

___ d. hypoventilation.

The second day after surgery, the doctor removes Mr. Blake's Levin tube and leaves an order for fluids as tolerated and a liquid diet. Mr. Blake is eager to try taking fluids. What would you recommend that he do?

24. ___ a. Wait until his liquid diet arrives at the next meal time.

___ b. Go ahead and drink all the water he wants.

___ c. Take at least 2000 ml. of fluids daily.

___ d. Start with small sips at first to see if it is retained.

Later that day Mr. Blake complained of gas pains in his abdomen. The most probable reason for the gas pains would be:

25. ___ a. his bowel is hypoactive following surgery.

___ b. the Levin tube was removed too soon.

___ c. he has not had enough solid foods.

___ d. his fluid intake has been too high.

You can help relieve Mr. Blake's gas pains by which of the following nursing measures?

26. ___ a. Providing a paper bag for him to breathe in.

___ b. Assisting him to turn or to get up and walk about.

___ c. Giving him only ice-cold fluids to drink.

___ d. Having him breathe deeply and pant through his mouth.

On his third post-operative day, Mr. Blake stated that he did not feel well; that he had a lot more pain in his incision. You call the team leader, and both of you inspect his incision. You notice that the area around the lower end of the incision is very red. From the symptoms, you would suspect that Mr. Blake had developed:

27. ___ a. an embolus.

___ b. strained muscles.

___ c. an evisceration.

___ d. a wound infection.

Suppose that Mr. Blake had been on complete bed rest for several days after surgery, that he had not moved his legs, and that he had kept a pillow under his knees. If he then complained of soreness and pain in one leg, what probably has happened?

28. ___ a. He has cramping in his leg muscles due to lack of exercise.

___ b. He has become weak due to the prolonged bed rest.

___ c. He has an inflammation and blood clot in a leg vein.

___ d. He has developed a contracture from flexion of the knees.

Mr. Smith, who is in the room next to Mr. Blake, went to surgery today and has just returned to his room from the Recovery Room. He had a spinal anesthesia for his operation less than 4 hours ago. If he were to develop symptoms of shock, what should you *avoid* doing when helping to treat the shock?

29. ___ a. Provide warmth to his body with extra blankets.

___ b. Lower the head of his bed in the shock, or Trendelenburg, position.

___ c. Remain with the patient at all times and give reassurance.

___ d. Take and record the vital signs until they have stabilized.

One of the doctor's orders for Mr. Smith post-operatively was "Diet as tolerated." Mr. Smith began taking some liquids by mouth in the Recovery Room, but now is experiencing a great deal of nausea. You have suggested that he do all but one of the following until the nauseated feeling passes. Which one does not apply?

30. ___ a. Breathe deeply through his mouth several times.

___ b. Cough several times and turn frequently.

___ c. Take small sips of any liquid he chooses.

___ d. Lie quietly in one position or on right side.

POST-TEST ANNOTATED ANSWER SHEET

1. F   (p. 713)

2. D   (p. 713)

3. J.   (p. 713)

4. G   (p. 713)

5. I   (p. 713)

6. B   (p. 713)

7. A   (p. 713)

8. L   (p. 713)

9. E   (p. 712)

10. M   (p. 713)

11. d   (p. 715)

12. b   (p. 714)

13. a   (p. 716)

14. d   (p. 717)

15. c   (p. 717)

16. b   (p. 717)

17. d   (p. 720)

18. c   (p. 718)

19. e   (p. 717, 720 and 718)

20. a   (p. 715)

21. c   (p. 719)

22. b   (p. 724)

23. c   (p. 724)

24. d   (p. 726)

25. a   (p. 726)

26. b   (p. 726)

27. d   (p. 725)

28. c   (p. 723)

29. b   (p. 723)

30. b   (p. 725)

PERFORMANCE TEST

In the skill laboratory your instructor will ask you to perform the following procedure without reference to other resource material.

Given an adult patient returning from surgery on his abdomen, collect the equipment needed, and prepare the patient's unit for his arrival in such a way that you would be able to begin his post-operative care safely and without delay. For the purpose of this exercise, the patient will have an IV running and will have a urinary catheter in place.

Record the following notes on the nurses' notes that you have written on scratch paper during the immediate recovery of Mr. Bruce Lemo, 213^2, Dr. G. Marshall, Choleuptectomy.

From OR 3:10 P.M.	144/94 98-22 color pink, beginning to respond. Cath. attached, IV running, 500 cc absorbed.
3:30	Dr. Marshall 90/60 120-30 Restless, pale, clammy Shock blocks IV speeded
3:45	emesis 200 cc bile 110/68 100-26 color improved, pink tone. Demerol 50 mgn. Im. RT hip — J. Reed, RN Responding to questions DSG dry
4:00	120/80 88-22 quiet, color good, pain relieved
4:15	120/80 88-22 IV completed — 1000 cc 5/0 DW added.

PERFORMANCE CHECKLIST

POST-OPERATIVE CARE

PREPARATION OF PATIENT UNIT FOR POST-OPERATIVE CARE

1. Obtain instructions for securing special equipment (type of equipment is dependent on patient's condition and surgery procedure performed).

2. Collect appropriate equipment, including at least following items:

   A. Linens

   B. Tissues

   C. Sphygmomanometer

   D. Stethoscope

   E. Intake/Output record

   F. IV standard

   G. Airway

   H. Paper and pencil

3. Prepare post-operative bed (refer to bed making unit if necessary).

4. Arrange equipment appropriately.

5. Ensure that bed was accessible by stretcher.

6. Maintain respiratory functions.

7. Take vital signs as directed.

8. Observe and record Fluid Intake and Output.

9. Check operative site.

10. Maintain IV (if appropriate).

11. Provide for patient's safety.

NOTES

Unit 36

ISOLATION TECHNIQUE

Direct, Reverse, and Terminal Disinfection

I. DIRECTIONS TO THE STUDENT

Study the entire unit, write the post-test, and be ready to demonstrate your proficiency in handling direct isolation technique, reverse isolation technique, and terminal disinfection for your instructor.

II. GENERAL PERFORMANCE OBJECTIVE

Upon completion of this lesson, you will correctly employ isolation technique to protect yourself and others when caring for a patient in an isolation unit. You will be able to use reverse isolation technique to protect the patient who is suffering from a denuded skin area (e.g., after a burn) or a weakened condition such as leukemia or post-organ transplant, from infecting himself. You will know the principles and practices of terminally disinfecting a unit occupied by a patient who has a communicable disease.

III. SPECIFIC PERFORMANCE OBJECTIVES

When you have finished this unit, you will be able correctly to do the following:

1. Prepare a unit for isolation of a patient who has a communicable disease or who needs protection from infection.

2. Use proper technique to put on and remove a gown worn in an isolation unit.

3. Put on a mask and tell your instructor how to change it to retain safe isolation technique practice.

4. Put on and remove rubber gloves using proper technique.

5. Care for contaminated dishes, linen, and dispose of waste.

6. Collect specimens and transfer them to designated places using proper protection.

IV. VOCABULARY

Common Communicable Diseases Needing Isolation Technique

anthrax—bacterial infection of skin; can be transmitted from hair of infected animals.
bacteria—microorganisms, one-celled, disease-producing germs. This large group of bacteria vary in size and shape: rod-shaped, spiral-shaped and round. Some are capsulated (e.g., tb) in a waxy coat and are very difficult to kill.
blastomycosis—fungus disease of skin; can be transmitted in dirt and dust.
chickenpox—systemic virus infection which affects the skin; can be transmitted through direct or indirect contact with an infected person.

cholera—bacterial infection of entire body; transmission is through direct or indirect contact with infected food or person.

coccidioidomycosis (valley fever)— systemic fungus infection; transmitted by water or from inhaled dust.

common cold—virus infection of respiratory tract; transmitted by direct or indirect contact with infected person.

conjunctivitis—bacterial infection of the eyes; transmitted by direct or indirect contact with an infected person.

diarrhea of newborn—bacterial infection of g.i. tract; transmitted by direct or indirect contact (can be fatal to a newborn or infant).

diphtheria—bacterial infection causing a membrane to form on any mucous surface, most frequently in the throat, which can be fatal. Everyone should be immunized (protected from the disease by inoculation with antitoxin). It is transmitted by direct and indirect contact.

dysentery—bacterial infection of g.i. tract; transmitted by direct or indirect contact.

fungi—this disease-producing group is a type of plant (mildew, mold, mushrooms, and toadstools are non-disease-producing fungi). Athlete's foot, ringworm, and histoplasmosis are examples of disease-producing fungi.

gonorrhea—bacterial disease of the genitourinary tract; usually transmitted via sexual intercourse (commonly called venereal disease or VD).

granuloma inguinale—bacterial infection of genital skin area and mucous membrane; transmitted by direct contact.

hepatitis, infectious—virus infection of body with invasion (involvement) of the liver; transmitted via direct or indirect contact.

histoplasmosis—systemic fungus infection; transmitted by indirect contact.

leprosy (Hansen's disease)—bacterial infection of skin and nerves; transmitted by direct and indirect contact. Not as contagious as once believed.

measles—systemic virus infection; transmitted via direct or indirect contact.

meningitis (meningococcal)—bacterial infection involving the neurological system; transmitted through direct or indirect contact.

mononucleosis—systemic disease with glandular involvement of unknown cause.

mumps—viral infection of the parotid glands; transmitted via direct or indirect contact.

plague—systemic bacterial infection carried by rats and fleas; transmitted by direct or indirect contact.

pneumonias (pneumonitis)—bacterial or viral, involve the lungs; transmitted from respiratory tract and indirect contact.

poliomyelitis—virus infection involving the nerves and muscles; transmitted by direct or indirect contact; can be prevented by immunization, e.g., Salk or Sabin vaccine.

Q fever—systemic rickettsia infection transmitted through air and indirect contact.

rabies—virus infection involving the nervous system and body; transmitted via saliva of infected dog or animal bite.

rickettsiae—microorganisms which are in size between viruses and bacteria. Examples of disease caused by this are Q fever, Rocky Mountain spotted fever, and typhus.

rubella (German measles)—virus infection of body characterized by skin rash; transmitted through direct or indirect contact.

salmonella—bacterial infection of digestive tract; transmitted chiefly via indirect contact through ingestion of contaminated food and fluids.

smallpox—virus infection of the skin; transmitted by direct or indirect contact.

staphylococcus—bacterial infection of the skin in the form of boils, abscesses, carbuncles, rashes, furuncles, pimples, styes, impetigo; or it may involve the body system; transmitted by direct or indirect contact, or a bacterial infection involving the digestive tract; transmitted by contaminated food.

streptococcus—bacterial infection; may cause strep throat, scarlet fever, erysipelas or puerperal infection; transmitted through direct or indirect contact.

syphilis—spirochete infection which may involve any part of body; transmitted via direct contact (sexual intercourse).

tuberculosis (tbc)—bacterial infection which may involve any part of the body, but usually lung tbc; transmitted by direct or indirect contact.

typhoid—bacterial infection of body; transmitted by direct or indirect contact; can be prevented by immunization.

viruses—these are minute (very small) microorganisms. Some may be filtered and can be studied; others are non-filterable. There are many different kinds and strains.

General Vocabulary

aerobic—requiring the presence of oxygen to live.

anaerobic—life can continue without free oxygen.

aseptic—free from all germ-producing organisms.

asepsis—condition free from germs; sterile.

autoclave—mechanical equipment used to render sterile by steam under pressure.

bacteriostatic—arrest (stop or inhibit) bacterial growth.

bactericidal—solution which destroys bacteria.

burns—injury to skin from chemical or thermal (heat) sources; may require reverse isolation technique to protect the patient.

carrier—one who carries disease germs (usually not currently ill from the disease); e.g., Typhoid Mary was a carrier of the typhoid germ and she infected others who came in contact with food she handled.

communicable—an illness that may be transferred directly or indirectly from one person to another.

contaminate—to render unclean or unsterile.

denude—removal of a protective layer, e.g., as in a 3rd degree burn.

direct contact—communication of a healthy person with a contagious person (one who has a communicable disease) through *touching* an infected part.

genital—pertaining to organs of reproduction.

genitourinary—pertaining to organs of reproduction and urinary excretion.

germicide—a solution that kills germs, but not resistant spores.

g.i. tract—pertaining to organs of stomach, intestines and mouth.

immunity—state of being resistant to disease; immunity may be brought about by medical practice, e.g., vaccinations or immunizations.

indirect contact—spread of a contagious disease through some medium other than directly touching the person, e.g., sputum, dressings, clothing.

isolation—to separate, set apart from others; method utilized for controlling spread of communicable or infectious disease.

microorganism—minute (small) living body not visible to the naked eye.

reverse isolation—type of isolation technique used for patients suffering from burns or conditions in which the protective mechanisms of the body are defective or inadequate. The patient is protected through use of sterile sheets and other isolation techniques from the worker and other patients.

venereal disease—a disease usually acquired as a result of sexual intercourse with an individual who is infected (e.g.,gonorrhea, syphilis, chancroid, Vincent's infection of the genitals, venereal lymphogranuloma).

V. INTRODUCTION

The prevention of the spread of infections and communicable diseases in hospitals and other health agencies presents one of the most common problems health workers must face. The National Communicable Disease Center in Atlanta, Georgia, states that *"handwashing before and after contact with each patient is the single most important means of preventing the spread of infection."*

However, there are certain added precautions which must be taken in the case of certain communicable diseases. Federal, state, and local public health agencies set forth specific regulations defining which diseases must be reported, isolated, to what extent, where, and for how long. All health agencies are legally required to carry out these regulations.

UNIT 36

Preventing the spread of infections can be accomplished by controlling one or more of these elements:

1. The source of the infecting organism (patients, visitors, and inanimate carriers of the disease).

2. The route of transmission of the organism (via contact with an inanimate object like a pen or pencil, or via vehicle which could be airborne, or vector-borne, i.e., carried by an insect).

3. A susceptible host (an individual with an illness: the very young or very old, or one who has been exposed to a disease or infection). Susceptibility to the disease is also based on the strength and size of the infecting dose, the organism's ability to survive in the environment in which it finds itself (light versus darkness; with oxygen versus without oxygen) and its ability to resist various disinfection methods.

Microorganisms are transmitted by four general routes:

1. **Contact**

   A. *Direct*—actual touching of a person with a communicable disease, or an infected animal, by a susceptible person. Kissing and sexual intercourse are two common means of direct transmission.

   B. *Indirect*—touching of contaminated objects used by an infected person (e.g., soiled clothing, bed linen, surgical instruments, dressings, handkerchiefs, or toys) and then touching your mouth, nose, or food and transferring those microorganisms to yourself.

   C. *Droplet spread*— a spray of mist ejected from the nose or mouth when coughing, sneezing, or talking. These droplets do not usually travel more than three feet. Most hospital regulations require a distance of at least six feet between the beds as well as the use of proper screening methods.

2. **Vehicle**

   Transmission of disease through contaminated food, water, drugs, or blood.

3. **Airborne**

   Evaporated droplets of an infectious agent or those which lodge in dust can remain infectious in the air and may be inhaled or digested by a susceptible host.

4. **Vector borne**

   Disease organisms carried by an animal, usually an insect or tick (e.g., malaria, transmitted by the mosquito).

   Reservoirs (containers) of infection include: man, animals, plants, soil, or objects used in daily living. Man is the most common harborer of infection or disease.
   Communicable diseases can be controlled by one or more of the following methods:

1. **Isolation**

   The patient who has the communicable disease is separated from others, either in a private room or a cubicle in a ward area. Everything inside the isolation unit, except designated clean areas, is considered contaminated.

2. **Disinfection**

   Attempt is made to kill pathogenic microorganisms either through chemical or physical means applied directly. Agents used to destroy microorganisms include:

   A. Steam under pressure (best method) as by autoclave.

   B. Boiling (212°F. for 20 minutes) kills most bacteria.

C. Dry heat as in an oven (320°F. for one hour).

D. Open flame or fire.

E. Direct sunlight for 6 to 8 hours.

F. Drying prevents growth and kills some bacteria (because moisture is needed to sustain life).

G. Cold temperature retards growth but is not a reliable method of destroying bacteria.

H. Chemicals may be used to inhibit or destroy bacteria (antiseptics, bacteriostatics, germicides, antibiotics, and ethylene oxide gas sterilization).

Concurrent disinfection—continuous process of disinfection throughout the hospitalization period.

Terminal disinfection—destruction of infectious material when the disease is over (after recovery, discharge, or death).

ITEM 1. SETTING UP A UNIT

Use a cubicle or private room with running water. A signed marked ISOLATION or similar designation used in your agency should be placed on the outside door, or at the entrance to the cubicle. If a cubicle or private room is not available, a selected area of the room can be established as an isolation zone. Screen this area; identify it by hanging a sign ISOLATION on the outside of the screens. Acquaint other workers with the limits of the isolation area. Collect these items, properly place them in the patient's unit:

For Patient Use

1. Thermometer and holder

2. Paper bags and wipes

3. Toilet tissue

4. Paper towels

5. Bath basin and soap in holder

6. Emesis basin, water glass, toothbrush, and dentifrice

7. Razor, shaving cream, and mirror (if patient is a man)

8. Bedpan and/or urinal

9. Wastebasket lined with plastic bag

10. Food tray with silverware unless plastic disposable tableware is used. Salt may be included if allowed on the patient's diet.

11. Plastic covering for pillow and mattress

12. Linens

13. Other special equipment designated by the charge nurse as needed

For Health Worker Use

1. Extra bedside stand to hold rubber gloves, masks, and gowns unless a special cabinet is provided for that purpose.

2. IV standard on which to hang the gown (check with your agency; "Discard Gown Method" may be used and you may have to put on a new gown every time you enter a different room).

3. If running water and sink are not available, provide a means to pour 70% alcohol over hands or use alcohol pledgets to clean hands.

4. Hamper for soiled linen.

5. *Floors are contaminated.* (Nothing must be used after it is dropped on the floor.)

6. Laundry bag and holder

7. Containers for soiled syringes, gloves, needles, and instruments

UNIT 36

Note: An interesting report appeared in the Hospital Tribune, dated Monday, April 9, 1971, concerning Walter Reed Medical Center's development of a jet lavage: "a machine which when used for 90 seconds has proven more effective than the traditional 10 minute scrub." Undoubtedly you will be hearing more about this development in the future. In the meantime, we will have to use the present prescribed techniques for handwashing.

After you have assembled the supplies and equipment, proceed with the following series of steps:

ITEM 2. PUTTING ON A FACE MASK

Important Steps	Key Points
1. Take mask from container.	Masks may be made of cloth or one of a variety of disposable materials. Handle the mask as little as possible because it will be coming in contact with your face and you will be breathing through it. *Note:* The National Communicable Disease Center recommends the use of high-efficiency disposable masks.
2. Put on mask. 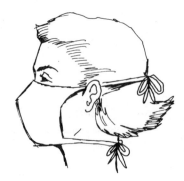	Unfold mask and place it over your *nose* and *mouth.* Tie the mask with top strings at back of head; be sure the strings pass over your ears. (If you wear glasses, the mask should fit snugly over your nose and under the bottom edge of your glasses. This will prevent your glasses from steaming.) Tie lower strings of mask at back of your head at the neckline. Be sure to fasten ties securely; if not tied securely over chin, they may work themselves loose during movement.
3. Wash hands and remove mask.	Remove mask by untying lower strings first, then upper strings. Take care not to let strings or mask drop on your gown. Discard mask in appropriate container. Proceed to untie waistband of gown and follow above gown procedure. *Note:* A mask should never be reused. Therefore, *do not* slide the mask off your nose and mouth down around your neck. Always discard your mask when finished with the procedure. Start with a clean mask each time.
4. Change mask.	Your mask will become moist as you breathe through it over a period of time. Change your mask whenever it becomes moist. Germs can grow in a wet environment. (Mask becomes moist in about 20 minutes.)
5. Rewash your hands before putting on another mask.	

ITEM 3. PUTTING ON AN ISOLATION GOWN

Important Steps	Key Points
1. Remove rings and wristwatch. 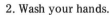	Rings and wristwatch may harbor micro-organisms which could be carried to others outside the isolation unit. If your watch is needed for the TPR, remove it and place it on a clean paper towel at the patient's bedside. (Take paper towel from dispenser in patient's room.)
2. Wash your hands. 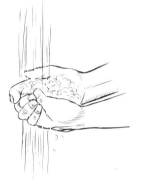	Refer to unit on handwashing. Use a liquid anti-microbial soap.
3. Select a clean gown. 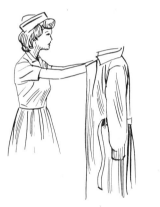	Hold gown at neck opening and let the gown unfold downward (gowns are usually folded in thirds for neat storage). The open part at the back should face you. The gown will be full length so it will cover your entire uniform to prevent contamination of your uniform while working in the isolation unit. *Note:* The National Communicable Disease Center in Atlanta, Georgia, recommends the use of the "individual gown technique." That is, use the gown only once and then discard.
4. Put your arms through gown sleeves.	Touch only the *inside* of the gown. Holding the inside of the gown, slip one arm at a time into the sleeve. Pull the gown on as far as possible.
5. Work inside sleeves of gown. 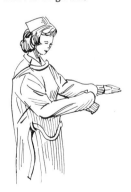	Work carefully to avoid contaminating your hands. Grab the opposite sleeve with your gown-covered hand (see opposite diagram); gently pull sleeve up on your arm and shoulder. When this procedure is completed, go on with the other sleeve in the same manner, always working from the inside of the gown.
6. Adjust gown on shoulders.	Place your fingers *inside* the neckband (at the back), and adjust the gown so that it fits comfortably on your shoulders. Remember to work

U
N
I
T
36

Important Steps	Key Points
	with the *inside* of the gown: keep your hands clean. If you touch the outside of the gown, or your hair, you must repeat the *handwashing procedure.*
7. Tie neck tapes (ties).	Handle the ties carefully. Keep your hands clean. Do not touch your hair.
8. Draw edges of gown together. 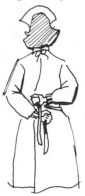	The open part of your gown is at your back. Bring the right side of gown over the left side of the gown. Adjust the gown so that it fits snugly (if you are left-handed, you would proceed from the left; putting the right side over the left, then adjust snugly).
9. Tie waist belt. 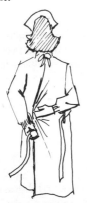	Grasp waist belt, at the far (distal) ends, draw together at your back, and tie snugly.

You are now ready to give nursing care unless you need a mask or rubber gloves. If they are required, proceed in the manner prescribed later in the lesson. You are now ready to leave an isolation room—follow this procedure.

ITEM 4.   REMOVING AN ISOLATION GOWN

Important Steps	Key Points
1. Untie waist belt.	Pull sleeves up above wrists.
2. Wash your hands.	
3. Untie neck ties.	Take care not to contaminate your hands by touching your hair or the *outside* of the gown. Remember, it is contaminated. If you do, you must *rewash* your hands.
4. Remove first sleeve of gown.	Place forefinger *under cuff* of sleeve and pull sleeve down over hand, without touching the outside of the gown.

Important Steps	Key Points
5. Remove other sleeve.	With hand inside first sleeve, i.e., working with your gown-covered hand, draw second sleeve down over your hand.
6. Slip out of gown.	Discard it carefully in the soiled linen hamper in the patient's room. Remember, the National Communicable Disease Center recommends one-time gown usage.
7. Wash your hands.	Wash according to procedure; dry thoroughly. Turn off faucets with towel and discard towel in the designated place. *Avoid touching* anything in the room as you leave. (If you used your wristwatch during the procedure, retrieve it at this time and put it on. Open door with paper towel. Discard paper towel. Handle towel from the top side only. Remember — the underside is contaminated.)
8. Record nursing tasks accomplished.	Record appropriate information on patient's chart. Report any unusual signs or symptoms to your team leader. Charting example:
	Placed in Isolation per order. Explained procedure. Appears to take news very well, is cooperative. B. Bee, SN

For some infectious cases you may be required to wear a mask (see sample chart, page 763). If so, follow the next procedure. *You will put the mask on before washing your hands and putting on a gown, if it is used.* Masks are usually worn in caring for patients who have an airborne disease, draining skin lesions, or who are on Reverse Isolation Technique.

ITEM 5. PUTTING ON STERILE OR NON-STERILE SINGLE-USE GLOVES

In some infectious cases, you may be required to wear rubber gloves for your protection. (Check the sample chart on page 763). Gloves may be used in cases where you will be handling soiled dressings. Check your agency procedure for the specific cases in which you will use rubber gloves.

Important Steps	Key Points
1. Obtain and unfold glove wrapper.	Lay glove wrapper on flat, clean surface and unfold. (Of course, your hands will have been washed before you put the gloves on. Gloves may be put on inside or outside the room. Check your agency procedure.)
2. Remove powder packet from wrapper (if there is one).	Some gloves are pre-powdered. Remove powder packet, tear open, and carefully powder your hands. It will make it easier to slip hand into the glove. Discard powder packet in wastebasket. Take care not to spread powder around the room.

UNIT 36

Important Steps	Key Points

3. Remove glove from wrapper.

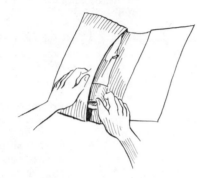

Grasp the folded edge of the left cuff-tip with your right hand. In other words, you are touching the inside of the glove with your clean hand. Keep your fingers straight while pulling the glove on the hand.

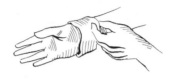

4. Put on second glove.

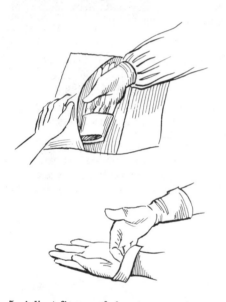

Grasp the folded edge of the cuff-top of the right glove with your left hand. In other words, you are touching the *inside* of the glove with your clean hand. Be sure to keep the fingers of your left hand off the outside of the glove and your skin. Pull glove on hand. With gloved right hand, slip fingers *under* the folded cuff of the left glove (sterile surface to sterile surface). Pull up over your hand and cuff to your gown. (Reverse these last two steps if you are left-handed.) Adjust gloves over gown cuff. Be careful to avoid touching your skin with the gloved hand—you will contaminate it and need to start at the beginning of the procedure with a new pair of gloves.

5. Adjust fingers of gloves.

When both gloves are in place, you can adjust the fingers of the gloves just as you would regular gloves you wear for dress or cold weather.

ITEM 6. REMOVING STERILE OR NON-STERILE SINGLE-USE GLOVES

Gloves will be removed before your gown is removed, if you are wearing one.

Important Steps	Key Points

1. Remove right-hand glove.

With your left hand, pull right glove off with cuff, taking care not to touch your skin with the contaminated glove. Dispose of gloves in designated container.

2. Remove left-hand glove.

Place fingers of your right hand *inside* the cuff of left glove. Pull glove down over and off your hand. Discard in designated container. (Reverse last two steps if you are left-handed.)

Important Steps	Key Points
3. Wash your hands. 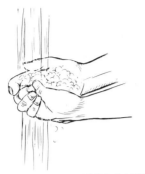	Wash them before removing mask. Untie waist belt if you are wearing a gown, and then wash your hands. Follow gown removal procedure.

ITEM 7.   SERVING DIET TRAY TO PATIENT IN ISOLATION

Important Steps	Key Points
1. Take tray to isolation door. *(Note:* Check agency procedure for conditions which require tray isolation.)	Transfer dishes sent from the cafeteria to the tray which is kept inside the patient's room. Take care not to touch the patient's tray with your hands—it is contaminated. You may do this unassisted or you may have help. Hold tray in your arm as you transfer dishes to patient's tray.
2. Return clean tray.	Take it back to the cafeteria or to the unit diet kitchen.

3. Serve patient's tray.	Unless your agency regulations state otherwise, you do not need to put on a gown if you are careful to touch nothing in the patient's room with your uniform. Identify the patient; compare the identification band with the name card on the diet tray.
	    Note: If you will be assisting the patient to eat, you will need to gown.
	    Place tray on patient's overbed table. Be sure your uniform touches nothing in the patient's room; otherwise you should put on a gown. Assist in cutting foods, pouring milk or coffee. Adjust bed to semi-Fowler's position if permitted. Move overbed tray close to the patient.

4. Wash your hands.	Wash according to procedure and leave room.

ITEM 8.   REMOVING THE DIET TRAY

(For patients who are on tray precautions—check your agency Isolation Procedure Manual.) When the patient has finished his meal, return to his room. *Wash your hands.*

Important Steps	Key Points
1. Remove dishes from tray.	Usually take one at a time. If disposable dishes are used, empty liquid contents in the patient's toilet and also any soft foods. Flush toilet. Solid foods such as gristle or bones should be disposed of in waterproof bags provided for that purpose. *Do not* throw in toilet. This

Important Steps	Key Points
	would stop up the sewer lines. *Disposable dishes* are then placed in the designated containers or wastebasket in the patient's room. If the dishes and utensils are *reusable*, the liquids and solids are disposed of in the above manner. The dishes are then placed in designated bags.
2. Remove dishes from isolation room (use double-bagging technique).	You will need a "clean person" on the outside of the room to assist you with this step. Place your carefully wrapped dishes *inside* a clean wrapper which is being held by the "clean person" outside the door. (Double-bagged = wrapped in one bag of paper, plastic or linen inside room. Then insert into second clean bag outside room.) He will close and secure the edges of the bag with masking tape. Label package with patient's name and identify package with isolation label.
3. Return articles to Processing Department (or Diet Kitchen).	Return labeled double-bagged package to the processing room or Diet Kitchen for sterilization. Sterilization may be done either in the Dietary Department or the Central Supply; check for your agency's procedure.

ITEM 9. GENERAL INFORMATION ABOUT USE OF BEDPANS AND URINALS IN ISOLATION

In addition to usual procedure, you *must follow* these suggestions:

Important Steps	Key Points
1. Provide assistance when needed.	
2. Remember to *wear gown and mask if designated by your procedure manual.*	
3. Contents of bedpan and urinal are flushed down the toilet unless obtained for a specimen.	Public Health Department Regulations prescribe that the sewage system used in most hospitals and extended care facilities (ECF) are constructed to take isolation liquids and excretions.
4. Rinse bedpan or urinal after *each* use.	Dry and return to storage. *Note:* If excretions must be emptied in the utility room, transport the bedpan or urinal covered through the hallways. Avoid touching anything with your "contaminated hands" and equipment. Use foot pedal to flush the "hopper" (multipurpose sink) frequently used in the central utility room.
5. Wash your hands.	

ITEM 10. COLLECTION OF SPECIMENS IN ISOLATION

Important Steps	Key Points
1. Secure appropriate container (urine, sputum, etc.).	Obtain from storage room. Follow procedures in units on bowel and urine elimination and sputum collection.
2. Label container.	(See agency specifications regarding name, etc.)
3. Collect specimen.	Obtain in the usual manner. See previous units on specimen collection.
4. Place specimen in container.	Transfer specimen from utensil (bedpan, urinal, etc.) to the specimen container.
5. Place specimen container in clean water-proof bag.	Bag should be held by someone *clean* on the outside of the room. Take care not to touch the exterior of the bag. If you touch the bag, you will contaminate it and will need to discard the bag and start over. The *clean* person on the outside of the room will carefully close and secure the opening with masking tape and attach the requisition to the bag.
6. Take to designated department.	*Transport* promptly to the designated department.
7. Record activity on nurses' notes.	Enter time collected, specimen, sent to lab, X-ray, etc.

ITEM 11. SIGNING A DOCUMENT

Note: This procedure would be carried out only for patients who have smallpox.

Important Steps	Key Points
1. Place clean paper towel on overbed table.	
2. Place the document on the paper towel.	
3. Place another paper towel with edge close to the line provided for the patient's signature.	The patient's hand will be resting on the paper towel.
4. When signature is completed, remove document from room.	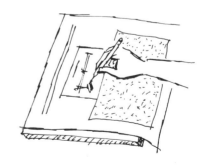
5. Wash the pen with soap and water, or a specified germicidal solution (if it is to be removed from the room; otherwise, place it in patient's bedside stand).	
6. Wash your hands.	Wash them before leaving the patient's room.
7. Record action on nurses' notes.	Designate the time and type of document that was signed.

ITEM 12. DISPOSAL OF WASTE MATERIALS: DOUBLE-BAG
          TECHNIQUE

Important Steps	Key Points
1. Empty the wastebasket.	Collect all used dressings, dishes, utensils, etc., in the designated disposable bags (waxed brown paper or plastic).
2. Seal bags securely.	Seal with string, tape, or whatever method is used in your agency.
3. Place soiled bag or bags of materials in *clean* plastic bag held by someone at the entrance of the room. 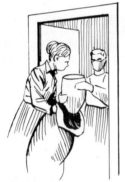	*Note:* This same method of transfer at the entrance of the isolation unit may be used for linens, specimens, waste products to be burned (paper, dressings, etc.). The *clean person* on the outside of the room places his hands under the cuff of the bag to protect himself from being touched by the *contaminated* articles.
4. The articles are carefully placed inside the plastic or linen bag.	Secure bag. The *clean person* then carefully secures the bag with tape, safety pin, or tie, labels it *Isolation*, and takes it to area for disposal: laundry chute, trash chute, etc. Isolation linens are frequently color-coded with a yellow marker.

ITEM 13. REMOVAL OF LINENS

Important Steps	Key Points
1. Place linen in hamper.	A laundry hamper with a heavy cloth bag is usually provided in the *clean area* of the patient's room for collection of soiled linens.
2. Remove linens from isolation room.	The filled laundry bag in patient's room is placed in a pre-labeled clean bag handled by the clean person *outside* the room. Send soiled linens to the laundry room. Follow remainder of procedure for removal of waste materials from the isolation room (Item 12).

ITEM 14. TAKING TPR AND BP

Important Steps	Key Points
1. Leave thermometer and sphygmomanometer in the isolation room until the patient is discharged or removed from isolation.	

Important Steps	Key Points
2. Wear gown and/or mask if indicated.	
3. Follow regular procedure for taking TPR and BP.	
4. Wash your hands after taking TPR and BP.	
5. Record.	Record observations promptly on clean paper in the clean area of the unit. Transfer to patient's chart at earliest opportunity.

ITEM 15.   TRANSPORTING PATIENT OUT OF UNIT

Important Steps	Key Points
1. Notify unit to which patient is being transferred.	
2. Place clean sheet over wheelchair or stretcher.	If patient goes in a wheelchair, place a clean sheet over the chair and wrap it around the patient after he is seated for warmth and to protect the patient's modesty. If patient goes on a stretcher, place clean sheet or cotton blanket on the stretcher. Place patient on it.
3. Place blanket on or around patient.	This provides warmth and privacy.
4. Place mask on patient.	*Note:* Masks are *always* worn by patients with respiratory diseases or those patients who are on strict isolation precautions when being transported in the hallways. (Check your agency procedure.)
5. Transport patient to designated area.	Remember to use proper body alignment, balance and movement for both you and your patient.
6. Return patient to his room.	Strip the linen from the stretcher or wheelchair. Dispose of it in the patient's linen hamper.
7. Return used wheelchair or stretcher for cleansing.	

ITEM 16.   TRANSFERRING ISOLATION PATIENT TO ANOTHER HOSPITAL OR UNIT

Important Steps	Key Points
1. Collect belongings and take them with patient.	Remember to take all personal belongings: dentures, glasses, clothing, toilet articles, etc.
2. Place mask on patient, if indicated.	
3. Prepare wheelchair or stretcher as needed.	See Item 15.
4. Accompany patient to new unit, and settle and orient patient in new room.	Introduce new personnel. Remember your admission procedure. If you have forgotten, review that unit.

U
N
I
T
36

Important Steps	Key Points
5. Provide for *terminal disinfection* of room from which the patient came, as well as for the transporting equipment.	Transportation equipment is either washed with designated germicidal solution by unit personnel as soon as patient has been returned to his room or is sent to the central processing area in your agency for terminal cleaning. *Note:* After cleaning, stretcher should be made up with a clean sheet and made ready for use by the next patient. Wash hands.
6. Record transfer on nurses' notes.	

ITEM 17. TERMINAL DISINFECTION

This procedure is done to clean the room, supplies and utensils when a patient is discharged, expires, or is removed from isolation. Because this room has more than the usual number of germs in it, *special precautions* must be taken during the final cleaning process before admitting a new patient.

You will need assistance with this procedure. Your co-worker can remain "clean" outside the room, ready to receive your supplies and equipment in the appropriate receptacles.

Important Steps	Key Points
1. Gown (mask and gloves if required by agency procedure).	Usually at least a gown is required to protect your clothing while you are working in the contaminated room. You will be assisted by a clean person who remains outside the isolation room to receive the specially prepared contaminated equipment.
2. Prepare utensils and supplies for removal from isolation room.	Articles which can be sterilized in the autoclave are placed in a special bag and handed to your clean assistant outside of the room. You will place your carefully wrapped contaminated articles inside a clean bag held by your outside assistant. Take care to touch only the inside of the bag he is holding. Your clean assistant will label the bag "Isolation" with patient's name, room number, and contents. *Note:* All linens, clean dressings, metal or glass articles except thermometers can be handled in this way. (Follow agency disposal procedure.)
3. Prepare basin with agency's germicidal solution.	*Note: Delicate instruments,* e.g., sphygmomanometers, otoscopes, scissors, thermometers, and *plastic articles* must be wiped off with a cold germicidal solution. (They would be melted or destroyed by the high temperature autoclave sterilization.) Use your agency's germicidal solution. If your agency uses disposable thermometers, dispose of them in the trash using special glass handling precautions established by your agency. *Note: Aerosol cans* cannot be autoclaved or burned—they would explode. Therefore, they, too, must be wiped off with a cold germicidal solution and sent home with patient. If aerosol

Important Steps	Key Points
	can is completely empty, it can be discarded in trash according to agency procedure. Examples of aerosol cans are containers for deodorant, hair spray, shave cream, spray cologne.
4. Wash gown standard (if portable) with germicidal solution.	When wiped clean, roll the standard from the room. The "clean" assistant will take it to the storage area.
5. Wipe instruments with germicidal solution.	Give them to your "clean" assistant to return to the central processing area for further decontamination. Follow double-bagging and labeling procedure.
6. Remove all burnable supplies.	Burnable items such as paper, dressings, and cotton can easily be burned. You have been placing them in waterproof bags in the waste containers in the patient's room as you have been working with the patient. Be sure the package is sealed and labeled "Isolation" before sending for incineration.
7. Remove the bags.	Seal the tops carefully by folding them down several times. Place in a clean bag held by your "clean" assistant outside the room. Be sure to drop your bags into the center of the clean bag, taking care not to touch the outside of the clean bag—you would contaminate it. Your "clean" assistant will close the clean bag by rolling the top edge downward. He will fasten it securely with tape, to be taken later to the trash collection area for transfer to the incinerator. From there it will be sent to the incinerator for burning.
8. Remove other used items.	Items such as needles and syringes must be specially disposed of. Follow your agency procedure.
9. Remove all other unused supplies or equipment.	Place items which can be autoclaved in a bag for sterilizing. Hand it to your assistant to double-bag, secure top and label for identification: isolation, patient's name, room number, and list of articles in package. Articles which cannot be autoclaved should be scrubbed thoroughly with your agency's disinfectant solution, taken out of the room and sent back to the Central Processing Room for further decontamination and storage.
10. Remove bedding and all other soiled linen.	Place soiled linens in laundry bag in the hamper. *Wash your hands.* Remove your gown and place it in the linen hamper. Carefully close the top of the bag securely by pinning or taping. Without touching your uniform, place in clean bag held by "clean" assistant who will close and label the bag securely for transportation to the laundry room.
11. Notify the Housekeeping Department that terminal cleaning is required.	Be sure to notify them that it was an isolation room. They also must take special precautions.

UNIT
36

Important Steps	Key Points
12. Make a closed bed and set up unit ready for new admission.	As soon as the housekeeping personnel have finished cleaning the unit, you can prepare the room for the next procedure. *Note:* This step may also be done by the housekeeping personnel. Check your agency procedure.

ITEM 18.   REVERSE ISOLATION TECHNIQUE

Reverse isolation technique, sometimes called protective isolation, follows the regular isolation technique in many respects. The difference is the purpose. In *regular isolation* technique the patient has a communicable disease, and an attempt is made to *protect the health worker* and others from the disease process. In *reverse isolation* technique the *patient is being protected* from the health worker and others of the health facility.

Persons with extensive burns in which the skin is denuded, patients with open lesions, and those who have very low resistance to infection because of a low white blood count or poor kidney function, benefit from reverse isolation technique. This technique is similar to that of surgical asepsis where all things are kept sterile. In other words, for patients who have low resistance to infection, we must take extra precautions. We set up as near sterile (free from pathogenic organisms) environment for him as possible.

Note: If the burn becomes infected, you would observe the Strict Isolation procedure.

Set up the unit the same as for regular isolation technique. Follow the items listed under general reminders on the next page.

Follow the Items 1 through 10 procedures for disposal of waste and soiled linen; however, food trays need not be included since the patient has no contagious disease, but is being protected from others.

In reverse isolation technique the health worker always wears a gown, gloves in some cases, and *always* a mask. The health facility will advise about each specific case as to the need for gloves.

Terminal disinfection is not needed upon discharge of this patient because the room will not need fumigation as in a contagious disease. The regular hospital facility terminal cleaning of a unit may be followed.

Summary:

1. The patient in a reverse isolation unit is being protected from *you* and others.

2. The patient is in a debilitated state and must be protected from any possible respiratory infection or other microorganism that may be brought *to* him.

3. Reverse isolation care is similar to that of surgical asepsis:
   — Hands must be washed carefully and frequently.
   — Gown, mask and sometimes gloves must be worn during care.
   — Use sterile equipment for care of the patient.
   — Restrict visitors and require that each wear a gown and mask (follow your agency procedure).
   — Limit trips in and out of the room. Plan in advance what equipment must be taken into the room.

ITEM 19.   GENERAL ISOLATION REMINDERS

1. Floors are contaminated. Anything dropped on the floor is contaminated and must be discarded or cleaned carefully before reuse.

2. Patients with communicable diseases should be grouped according to the epidemiology of transmission:

   A. Contact through respiratory spread.

   B. Gastrointestinal tract.

   C. Direct contact with wound or skin infection.

3. Keep dust down. Sweeping compounds or wet-mops with disinfectants are used.

4. Protect the patient from drafts.

5. Establish contaminated and clean zones. The clean areas should include those used by the health worker. Items like telephones should not be used by the patient outside the unit. There should be a "clean" area in the isolation unit where no contaminated articles are permitted. In other words, items not in the clean area are considered contaminated.

6. Anything that is brought into the isolation area must not be removed except in proper containers, then placed in an outside clean container and labeled *isolation.*

7. Never rub your eyes or nose, or put your hands near your mouth when you are taking care of a patient in an isolation unit.

8. Never shake linen when you are removing it or placing it on the bed.

9. Wash your hands often. Refer to unit "Handwashing Technique for Medical Asepsis."

10. Use clean squares of paper or tissue to touch contaminated articles.

11. Paper towels or clean squares of paper provide a clean area on which to place articles within a unit.

12. Keep water pitcher and glass in room. Ice and fresh water are brought to the door and transferred. (Use same technique for food.)

13. Faucets should be turned off and on with a paper towel.

14. Nursing procedures are carried out for these patients, the same as for any patient. However, you have also learned some additional safety precautions (masking, gloving, gowning, and disposal techniques).

15. Inform charge nurse of skin lesions, sore throat, or other evidence of your lowered resistance to infection or disease. (She may reassign you to protect you and the patient.)

VI. ADDITIONAL INFORMATION FOR ENRICHMENT

The health worker may further protect himself from communicable diseases by:

1. Taking a shower daily and shampooing hair as needed (at least once a week).

2. Establishing regular sleeping patterns and sleeping at least 8 hours each night. (Sleep cannot be stored like money in the bank; sleep is required daily for good body resistance to infection and for high performance.)

3. Eating a sensible, well-balanced diet. Avoid crash diets. Use fresh fruits and vegetables for necessary minerals and vitamins. Eat protein foods.

4. Drinking plenty of fluids. Two-thirds of the body is water, and because fluid is lost daily by perspiration and elimination, it must be replaced. Drink 6 to 8 glasses of water daily.

UNIT
36

5. Developing good habits of elimination. (Do not deny the body urge to eliminate; this upsets the natural function of the body.)

6. Practicing regular habits of oral hygiene. Never neglect your teeth. See your dentist at least yearly.

7. Balancing hours of activity with recreation. Spend some time out of doors in fresh air. Give your body proper exercise.

8. Taking care of hands. Apply lotion to keep them soft. Cut off hangnails that may tear and produce a gateway for infection. Protect breaks in the skin which may allow for entry of microorganisms.

9. Protecting eyes when you are in an isolation unit. Do not touch the eyes with your fingers while caring for a patient. (Remember—the most common causes of eye infections are the fingers.) If irrigation fluid happens to get into the eye, rinse the eye immediately with normal saline.

10. Keeping hands away from mouth when caring for a patient who is in an isolation unit. Always wash hands before handling food that enters your mouth.

11. Protecting hair from contamination. Wear a cap when you are in a highly contagious situation.

12. Removing jewelry when you are caring for a patient in an isolation unit. Rings can harbor microorganisms that may not be removed with regular handwashing. Your watch may also harbor microorganisms and interfere with proper handwashing.

Human beings are fortunate in natural body defenses. The unbroken skin serves to protect the body from microorganisms. However, microorganisms do enter the body through the respiratory tract, digestive, and genitourinary openings. The defenses which serve to protect these entry sites are body secretions and cilia which act as barriers to bacteria. These barriers include the acid reaction of the urine, digestive juices which kill bacteria, and threadlike projections and mucus which remove dust and bacteria from the respiratory tract.

The skin is called the first line of body defense, and secretions form the second line of defense. If microorganisms break through these two barriers and reach the blood stream, antibodies are formed which fight harmful bacteria.

Fever is another defense. (Fever is the heat that heals.) Moderate fever, from 102° to 104°F., is a desirable response since few bacteria can survive this temperature. Fever higher than this may be destructive to the body tissues.

Leukocytes (phagocytes or white blood corpuscles) are wandering cells in the blood which ingest and destroy bacteria. When the body is injured, they increase in number and surround and engulf invading bacteria. Other phagocytes are fixed in the body, as in the liver, spleen, bone marrow and lymph nodes which are strategic spots of body function. Destruction of bacteria is also carried out here.

The ability to resist contracting disease is called *immunity.* There are two different general classifications of immunity—natural and acquired. *Natural immunity* is the resistance with which one is born. It is inherited and considered permanent. Human beings are subject to many diseases that animals have, but are immune to certain other diseases of animals. Immunity is characteristic of certain races, i.e., yellow fever attacks Caucasians, but native Indians and Negroes are immune to it. Eskimos and Negroes are more susceptible to tuberculosis than the white man.

Acquired immunity is developed during life. This is classified further as *active acquired immunity* and *passive acquired immunity.* To develop active acquired immunity, the person must have:

(1) contracted the disease and recovered from it. Example: One who has had measles does not ordinarily have them a second time.

(2) had a mild (sometimes unnoticed) infection of the disease.

(3) been given, a suitable vaccine or antigen (a substance which stimulates antibodies within the person's body). Example: One who is vaccinated with smallpox vaccine will not have the disease.

The process of increasing the resistance of an individual to a particular infection by artificial means is called immunization.

Passive acquired immunity is made possible by injecting into one person the antibodies from the blood of other persons or animals. This type of immunity is immediate in effect, but is of short duration because the human body is not stimulated to produce its own antibodies.

Most microorganisms that invade the body have a substance called antigen. An *antigen* is a substance that causes the body to manufacture antibodies to fight against allergens. An *allergen* is a substance to which the body reacts. Let us say a microorganism invades a human being: the body reacts to the antigen by producing a protein substance called *antibodies.* These antibodies are formed in the liver, spleen, bone marrow, and other organs. They are carried by the blood and lymph throughout the body and destroy toxins of the micro-organisms, or render them incapable of harming the body.

Gamma globulin injections are another method of providing a defense. This substance consists of a fraction of plasma of human blood which contains antibodies against certain diseases. Gamma globulin is often used to modify the effects of hepatitis or measles, although we now have a specific vaccine against measles.

There are ways of *testing immunity.* This is done through skin tests. *Skin tests* determine the presence of certain antibodies in an individual. When immunity is present, a minute (small) amount of the antibody injected under the skin will produce in a given time a localized skin reaction. Skin tests are done for diphtheria (Schick test), scarlet fever (Dick test), tuberculosis (Pirquet's reaction), and histoplasmosis with histoplasmin. Skin tests are also available to investigate an individual's sensitivity to foods, pollens, and various other substances.

The extent of damage from an infection is the result of two factors: the individual's resistance to injury and the microorganism's power to injure.

The person's resistance is influenced by his age, state of nutrition, presence of disease (especially of metabolic origin), hormones such as glucocorticoids, adequacy of blood supply, location of the infection, and natural or acquired antibodies.

The microorganism's power to inflict damage to the individual is dependent on its ability to produce certain enzymes. The enzymes may destroy tissues, damage blood vessels and cause hemorrhage, block lymphatic drainage in the body by clot formation, or dissolve blood clots, allowing the infection to spread. In addition, some bacteria are ingested by phagocytes in the body as mentioned earlier. Other bacteria not readily destroyed by the phagocyte's enzymes may be transported to new locations and produce new or additional areas of infection. Rinsing your hands with an antiseptic solution removes harmful bacteria. Common germicidal solutions in use today are phenol, iodine, and hydrogen peroxide. The germicidal solutions can be very injurious to the skin if used in highly concentrated solutions.

To sum up the body's defenses against infection, we have:

1. Healthy unbroken skin and mucous membranes. It is up to the person to keep the first line of defense strong.

2. Removal of bacteria by secretions of mucous membranes and by cilia (hair-like projections) in the nose and bronchial tree. The bacteria are removed by coughing and sneezing.

3. Bacteria may be destroyed by the gastric juice and acid reaction of urine and vaginal discharges.

4. Lymph nodes act as filters to remove bacteria from the body system.

5. Increased number of white blood cells upon invasion of bacteria.

6. Antibody formation, which keeps numbers of microorganisms from multiplying.

U
N
I
T
36

7. The body reacts to an invasion of microorganisms by inflammation. Inflammation represents warfare between the offending organism and the white cells as well as the body reaction to the invasion.

Some thought should be given to the patient and how he may react to being placed in an isolation unit. He may feel that he is not only contaminated, but will not be acceptable to other members of society. When one considers the high value placed on a person's capacity to be useful in society and to accomplish what he wishes, when and where he chooses, it becomes clear how the image he has of himself and his body at this time may influence his behavior. Can you imagine a more devastating situation than being required to lie totally immobile, completely dependent on someone else to feed you and provide for body elimination—as though you were an infant?

Loss of control of one's activities and functions may produce depression and shame. There is nothing shameful about needing such care, but the human being may view the inability to control his own body as shameful. Society expects the adult to be in control of himself, and being placed in a situation of isolation intensifies his awareness of being without command of himself. You must therefore understand the patient's right to feel depressed. Make every effort to help him work through this temporary state. Frustration and anger turned inward are sometimes reflected in negative behavior by the patient and the use of abusive words and actions. Accept this as a part of his illness. Visit him often so he does not continue to feel so isolated. Some patients may accept isolation willingly. In any event, make every effort to understand your patient's needs.

COMMON COMMUNICABLE DISEASES AND COMMON ISOLATION TECHNIQUES

Codes were taken from the 1970 Isolation for Infectious Diseases as recommended by the National Communicable Disease Center. However, these may vary depending on State Public Health laws and your agency policy (check your agency's isolation procedure). Each agency usually has its own Isolation Manual; you should follow that procedure. This chart is presented as an example of an Isolation Chart.

R	=	Recommended
X	=	With Direct Contact
+	=	For Susceptibles
D	=	Desirable, but Optional

Route of Transmission	Private Room	Mask	Gown	Gloves	Excreta & Excreta-Soiled Articles	Blood	Secreta & Secreta-Soiled Articles
Mouth and Nose (Respiratory)							
Chickenpox	R	+					R
Coccidioidomycosis							R
Diphtheria	R	R	X				R
Measles	R	+					R
Meningococcal Meningitis	R	R					
Mumps	R	+					R
Plague (Bubonic, Pneumonia)	R	R	R	R			R
Pneumonias (Bacterial)							R
Poliomyelitis					R		
Q Fever					R		
Rubella	R	R					R
Smallpox	R	R	R	R			R
Tuberculosis	R	+					R
Whooping Cough	R	+					R
Skin and Mucous Membranes							
Anthrax	R	R	R	R			R
Conjunctivitis (Bacterial)							R
Gonorrhea							R
Granuloma inguinale							R
Rabies	R			X			R
Staphylococcal (skin or wound)	D	X	X	X			R
Streptococcal infections	R	R	X	X			R
Syphilis							R
Gastrointestinal							
Cholera	D	X	X	R			
Hepatitis, Infectious	D				R	R	
Salmonellosis	D		X	X	R		
Typhoid Fever	D		X	X	R		

POST-TEST

Circle the "T" if the statement is true. Circle "F" if the statement is false.

T F   1. A communicable disease may be transferred from one person to another.

T F   2. All articles of use in an isolation unit are considered contaminated.

T F   3. It is necessary to wear a gown when giving a bedpan.

T F   4. Unused articles and linen in an isolation unit may not be removed and placed with other articles and linen for use by other patients.

T F   5. Microorganisms inflict damage to the patient by their ability to produce certain enzymes.

T F   6. After discharge of an "isolation patient," it is sufficient terminal disinfection practice to air the room for one hour.

T F   7. Linen removed from an isolation unit must be placed in an additional bag, as well as the original bag in which it is placed.

T F   8. If your mask slips down from your nose on your neck, it is safe to replace it and wear it.

T F   9. Patients in an isolation unit should not have a backrub with the bare hands.

T F   10. The faucet in the isolation bathroom is considered clean and suitable to turn on and off without protection.

T F   11. In an isolation ward, a safe distance between beds is 3 feet.

T F   12. In an isolation ward, all patients have communicable diseases and respiratory tract infections; g.i. tract infections and skin infections may be placed every other bed for care convenience.

T F   13. Isolation technique dictates that a mask must always be worn.

T F   14. Food trays may be served to the patient in isolation in regular fashion since all dishes are sterilized in the dishwasher.

T F   15. It is all right to give a bedpan in an isolation unit without a gown as long as you do not touch your uniform against anything.

T F   16. TPR may be taken without a gown as long as the uniform does not touch anything.

T F   17. Discarded tissues from an isolation unit may be placed in the regular trash can since all trash is burned anyway.

T F   18. One must wear a mask when doing terminal disinfection.

T F   19. Diseases which can be communicated from one person to another are called isolated.

T F   20. One disease that cannot be contracted through respiration is syphilis.

POST-TEST ANNOTATED ANSWER SHEET

1. T   (p. 744)

2. T   (pp. 744 and 757)

3. F   (p. 752)

4. T   (p. 757)

5. T   (p. 760)

6. F   (p. 756)

7. T   (p. 756)

8. F   (p. 746)

9. F   (p. 759)

10. F   (p. 759)

11. F   (p. 744)

12. F   (p. 759)

13. F   (p. 746)

14. F   (p. 751)

15. T   (p. 752) (Note: This does not include patients on reverse isolation.)

16. T   (p. 755)

17. F   (p. 754)

18. F   (p. 756)

19. F   (p. 743)

20. T   (p. 763)

PERFORMANCE TEST

You will discuss with your instructor the differences between isolation technique and reverse isolation technique, as well as the procedure for terminal cleaning following an isolation case.

In the skills laboratory with a student partner, you will correctly demonstrate the isolation technique used in caring for a patient having a staphylococcal wound infection. You will demonstrate the procedure for gowning, masking, gloving, removal of soiled items from the patient's room, serving, and removing a meal tray.

PERFORMANCE CHECKLIST

ISOLATION TECHNIQUE

Gowning

1. Remove rings and wristwatch.

2. Wash hands.

3. Select gown (from cabinet or clothes hook).

4. Put arms into sleeves, work on arms, and adjust shoulders without contaminating hands.

5. Tie neck tapes, close gown at back, and tie waist belt without contaminating hands.

Removing Gown

1. Untie waist belt, push up sleeves, and wash hands.

2. Untie neck ties without contaminating hands.

3. Remove sleeves of gown.

 A. Place forefinger under one cuff of sleeve.

 B. Pull sleeve over hand without touching outside of gown.

 C. For other sleeve, work sleeve off using the gown-covered second hand.

4. Slip out of gown—either:

 A. Fold gown so that interior is together and hang it over hook so that open edge is easily accessible for next person using it, or

 B. Dispose of gown in laundry hamper taking care not to touch uniform or shake gown.

5. Wash hands as you leave the unit, and turn off faucet with paper towels.

Masking

1. Obtain mask from container.

2. Unfold mask, and place over nose and mouth.

3. Tie top strings at back of head. (Strings *over* ears and top edge of mask under glasses.)

4. Remove mask by untying lower strings, then top strings, and discard into designated receptacle.

5. Change mask when it becomes moist (or be able to explain when and why).

6. Rewash hands and apply clean mask.

Gloving

1. Obtain and unfold glove wrapper, and powder hands if powder pack is available.

2. Remove first glove from wrapper, at folded edge of cuff, and pull up on hand.

3. With first gloved hand grasp second glove under loose edge of cuff (sterile surface to sterile surface) and pull glove up on hand.

4. Adjust glove cuffs over gown cuffs, without contaminating gloves or gown, and adjust fingers of gloves.

5. Remove gloves before gown is removed.

   A. Pull glove off first hand without contaminating skin.

   B. Dispose of glove in receptacle.

6. Pull second glove off by placing fingers inside cuff of remaining glove, pull down over hand, and discard into receptable.

7. Wash hands before removing mask.

Removal of Waste Materials

1. Empty waste materials into designated bag (brown paper or plastic) in room.

2. Seal bag securely with string, tape, etc.

3. Place sealed bag carefully inside clean bag being held by "clean person" outside room.

   A. Take care to touch only inside of bag. (The clean person then closes, secures, and labels the double-bagged package for disposal.)

Removal of Meal Tray

1. Remove dishes from tray (one at a time).

2. Dispose of liquids down toilet, and flush toilet.

3. Dispose of solid foods in brown paper bag(s).

4. Place disposable dishes in designated receptacle.

5. Place reusable dishes (after foods have been removed) in brown bag, and seal the bag.

6. Hand sealed bag to "clean person" for double-bagging.

7. Close and secure bag, label, transport for sterilization.

NOTES

INDEX

Note: Page numbers in *italics* indicate illustrations.

INDEX